T0198200

Data Science in Critical Care

Editors

ANDRE L. HOLDER
RISHIKESAN KAMALESWARAN

CRITICAL CARE CLINICS

www.criticalcare.theclinics.com

Consulting Editor
GREGORY S. MARTIN

October 2023 • Volume 39 • Number 4

ELSEVIER

1600 John F. Kennedy Boulevard ● Suite 1800 ● Philadelphia, Pennsylvania, 19103-2899

http://www.theclinics.com

CRITICAL CARE CLINICS Volume 39, Number 4
October 2023 ISSN 0749-0704, ISBN-13: 978-0-443-18193-1

Editor: Joanna Gascoine
Developmental Editor: Saswoti Nath

Critical Care Clinics (ISSN: 0749-0704) is published quarterly by Elsevier Inc., 360 Park Avenue South, New York, NY 10010-1710. Months of issue are January, April, July, and October. Business and Editorial Offices: 1600 John F. Kennedy Blvd., Suite 1800, Philadelphia, PA 19103-2899. Customer Service Office: 6277 Sea Harbor Drive, Orlando, FL 32887-4800. Periodicals postage paid at New York, NY and additional mailing offices. Subscription prices are $274.00 per year for US individuals, $779 per year for US institutions, $100.00 per year for US students and residents, $305.00 per year for Canadian individuals, $976.00 per year for Canadian institutions, $348.00 per year for international individuals, $976.00 per year for international institutions, $100.00 per year for Canadian students/residents, and $150.00 per year for foreign students/residents. To receive student/resident rate, orders must be accompanied by name of affiliated institution, date of term, and the signature of program/residency coordinator on institution letterhead. Orders will be billed at individual rate until proof of status is received. Foreign air speed delivery is included in all *Clinics* subscription prices. All prices are subject to change without notice. POSTMASTER: Send address changes to *Critical Care Clinics*, Elsevier Periodicals Customer Service, 11830 Westline Industrial Drive, St. Louis, MO 63146. **Customer Service: 1-800-654-2452 (US). From outside of the US, call 1-314-447-8871. Fax: 1-314-447-8029. E-mail: journalscustomerservice-usa@elsevier.com (for print support) or journalsonlinesupport-usa@elsevier.com (for online support).**

Reprints. For copies of 100 or more of articles in this publication, please contact the Commercial Reprints Department, Elsevier Inc., 360 Park Avenue South, New York, NY 10010-1710. Tel.: 212-633-3874; Fax: 212-633-3820; E-mail: reprints@elsevier.com.

Critical Care Clinics is also published in Spanish by Editorial Inter-Medica, Junin 917, 1er A, 1113, Buenos Aires, Argentina.

Critical Care Clinics is covered in *MEDLINE/PubMed (Index Medicus), EMBASE/Excerpta Medica, Current Concepts/ Clinical Medicine, ISI/BIOMED,* and *Chemical Abstracts.*

Contributors

CONSULTING EDITOR

GREGORY S. MARTIN, MD, MSC
Professor, Division of Pulmonary, Allergy, Critical Care and Sleep Medicine, Research Director, Emory Critical Care Center, Director, Emory/Georgia Tech Predictive Health Institute, Co-Director, Atlanta Center for Microsystems Engineered Point-of-Care Technologies (ACME POCT), President, Society of Critical Care Medicine, Atlanta, Georgia, USA

EDITORS

ANDRE L. HOLDER, MD, MS
Assistant Professor, Division of Pulmonary, Allergy, Critical Care and Sleep Medicine, Emory University School of Medicine, Atlanta, Georgia, USA

RISHIKESAN KAMALESWARAN, PhD
Associate Professor, Departments of Biomedical Informatics and Emergency Medicine, Emory University School of Medicine, Atlanta, Georgia, USA

AUTHORS

ANKITA AGARWAL, MD, MSc
Assistant Professor of Medicine, Division of Pulmonary, Allergy, Critical Care and Sleep Medicine, Emory University School of Medicine, Emory Critical Care Center, Emory Healthcare, Atlanta, Georgia, USA

GIOVANNI ANGELOTTI, MSc
Artificial Intelligence Center, IRCCS Humanitas Research Hospital, Milan, Italy

MIHIR R. ATREYA, MD, MPH
Division of Critical Care Medicine, Department of Pediatrics, Cincinnati Children's Hospital Medical Center, University of Cincinnati College of Medicine, Cincinnati, Ohio, USA

SIVASUBRAMANIUM V. BHAVANI, MD
Department of Medicine, Emory University, Atlanta, Georgia, USA

ALAN C. BOVIK, PhD
Department of Electrical and Computer Engineering, The University of Texas at Austin, Austin, Texas, USA

JOSEPH BYERS
Respiratory Therapy, Beth Israel Deaconess Medical Center, Boston, Massachusetts, USA

STEPHANIE CABRAL, MD
Department of Medicine, Beth Israel Deaconess Medical Center, Boston, Massachusetts, USA

MAXIME CANNESSON, MD, PhD
Department of Anesthesiology and Perioperative Medicine, University of California, Los Angeles, Los Angeles, California, USA

PIER FRANCESCO CARUSO, MD
Department of Biomedical Sciences, Humanitas University, Department of Anesthesiology and Intensive Care, IRCCS Humanitas Research Hospital, Milan, Italy

MAURIZIO CECCONI, MD
Department of Biomedical Sciences, Humanitas University, Department of Anesthesiology and Intensive Care, IRCCS Humanitas Research Hospital, Milan, Italy

LEO ANTHONY CELI, MD, MSc, MPH
Laboratory for Computational Physiology, Massachusetts Institute of Technology, Cambridge, Massachusetts, USA; Division of Pulmonary, Critical Care and Sleep Medicine, Beth Israel Deaconess Medical Center, Department of Biostatistics, Harvard T.H. Chan School of Public Health, Boston, Massachusetts, USA

MARIE-LAURE CHARPIGNON, MSc
Institute for Data, Systems and Society, Massachusetts Institute of Technology, Cambridge, Massachusetts, USA

GILLES CLERMONT, MD, CM, MSc
Professor, Critical Care Medicine, University of Pittsburgh, VA Pittsburgh Heath System, Pittsburgh, Pennsylvania, USA

CLAUDIA EBM, MD
Department of Biomedical Sciences, Humanitas University, Milan, Italy

CHRYSTINNE FERNANDES, PhD
Laboratory for Computational Physiology, Massachusetts Institute of Technology, Cambridge, Massachusetts, USA

JACK GALLIFANT
Imperial College London NHS Trust, London, United Kingdom

MASSIMILIANO GRECO, MD
Department of Biomedical Sciences, Humanitas University, Department of Anesthesiology and Intensive Care, IRCCS Humanitas Research Hospital, Milan, Italy

CHRISTOPHER M. HORVAT, MD, MHA
UPMC Children's Hospital of Pittsburgh, Department of Critical Care Medicine, University of Pittsburgh School of Medicine, Pittsburgh, Pennsylvania, USA

DAVID T. HUANG, MD, MPH
Department of Critical Care Medicine, University of Pittsburgh School of Medicine, Pittsburgh, Pennsylvania, USA

JEREMY M. KAHN, MD, MSc
Professor, Department of Critical Care Medicine, University of Pittsburgh School of Medicine, Department of Health Policy and Management, University of Pittsburgh School of Public Health, Pittsburgh, Pennsylvania, USA

SUNGSOO KIM, MD, MS
Department of Anesthesiology and Perioperative Medicine, University of California, Los Angeles, Los Angeles, California, USA; Department of Electrical and Computer Engineering, The University of Texas at Austin, Austin, Texas, USA

ANDREW J. KING, PhD
Assistant Professor, Department of Critical Care Medicine, University of Pittsburgh School of Medicine, Pittsburgh, Pennsylvania, USA

SOHEE KWON, MD, MPH
Department of Anesthesiology and Perioperative Medicine, University of California, Los Angeles, Los Angeles, California, USA

JOSHUA PEI LE, BS
School of Medicine, University of Limerick, Castletroy, Co, Limerick, Ireland

VINCENT X. LIU, MD, MS
Kaiser Permanente Division of Research, Oakland, California, USA

MARY E. LOUGH, PhD, RN, CCNS, FCCM, FAHA, FCNS, FAAN
Stanford Health Care, Stanford University, Stanford, California, USA

ATUL MALHOTRA, MD
Division of Pulmonary, Critical Care and Sleep Medicine, University of California, San Diego, San Diego, California, USA

JOSEPH MARION, PhD
Statistical Scientist, Berry Consultants

MIA K. MARKEY, PhD
Department of Biomedical Engineering, The University of Texas at Austin, Austin, Texas, USA

DONALD MLOMBWA
Zomba Central Hospital, Zomba, Malawi; Kamuzu College of Health Sciences, Blantyre, Malawi; St. Luke's College of Health Sciences, Chilema-Zomba, Malawi

LAMA MOUKHEIBER, MSc
Institute for Medical Engineering and Science, Massachusetts Institute of Technology, Cambridge, Massachusetts, USA

PAUL NAGY, PhD
Associate Professor of Radiology and Radiological Science, Departments of Medicine, and Biomedical Engineering, Johns Hopkins School of Medicine, Baltimore, Maryland, USA

LAMA NAZER, PharmD, BCPS, FCCM
King Hussein Cancer Center, Amman, Jordan

SHAMIM NEMATI, PhD
Division of Biomedical Informatics, University of California, San Diego, San Diego, California, USA

BRADLEY ASHLEY ONG, MD
College of Medicine, University of the Philippines Manila, Manila, Philippines

RAVI PAL, PhD
Department of Anesthesiology and Perioperative Medicine, University of California, Los Angeles, Los Angeles, California, USA

ANUPOL PANITCHOTE, MD
Faculty of Medicine, Khon Kaen University, Thailand

MICHAEL J. PATTON, BA
Medical Scientist Training Program, Heersink School of Medicine, Hugh Kaul Precision Medicine Institute, The University of Alabama at Birmingham, Birmingham, Alabama, USA

MATTHEW ROBINSON, MD
Assistant Professor of Medicine, Division of Infectious Diseases, Johns Hopkins School of Medicine, Baltimore, Maryland, USA

JUAN C. ROJAS, MD, MS
Assistant Professor, Department of Internal Medicine, Rush University, Chicago, Illinois, USA

AKOS RUDAS, PhD
Department of Computational Medicine, University of California, Los Angeles, Los Angeles, California, USA

LAZARO N. SANCHEZ-PINTO, MD
Departments of Pediatrics and Preventive Medicine, Northwestern University Feinberg School of Medicine, Ann & Robert H. Lurie Children's Hospital of Chicago, Chicago, Illinois, USA

JONATHAN SEVRANSKY, MD, MHS
Professor of Medicine, Division of Pulmonary, Allergy, Critical Care and Sleep Medicine, Emory University School of Medicine, Emory Critical Care Center, Emory Healthcare, Atlanta, Georgia, USA

SUPREETH PRAJWAL SHASHIKUMAR, PhD
Division of Biomedical Informatics, University of California, San Diego, San Diego, California, USA

PRATIK SINHA, MD, PhD
Divisions of Clinical and Translational Research, and Critical Care, Department of Anesthesia, Washington University School of Medicine, St Louis, Missouri, USA

MARIO TERAN, MD
Clinical Informaticist for the Division of Digital Healthcare Research (DDHR), Agency for Healthcare Research and Quality, Rockville, Maryland, USA

CRAIG A. UMSCHEID, MD, MS
Director of the Evidence-Based Practice Center Division and Senior Science Advisor, Agency for Healthcare Research and Quality, Rockville, Maryland, USA

ALLAN WALKEY, MD, MSc
Professor, Department of Medicine, Section of Pulmonary, Allergy, Critical Care and Sleep Medicine, Boston University School of Medicine, Boston, Maryland, USA

GABRIEL WARDI, MD, MPH
Division of Pulmonary, Critical Care, and Sleep Medicine, Department of Emergency Medicine, University of California, San Diego, San Diego, California, USA

WASSWA WILLIAM
Mbarara University of Science and Technology, Mbarara, Uganda

AN-KWOK IAN WONG, MD, PhD
Duke Medical Center, Durham, North Carolina, USA

Contents

> Precision medicine aims to identify treatments that are most likely to result in favorable outcomes for subgroups of patients with similar clinical and biological characteristics. The gaps for the development and implementation of precision medicine strategies in the critical care setting are many, but the advent of data science and multi-omics approaches, combined with the rich data ecosystem in the intensive care unit, offer unprecedented opportunities to realize the promise of precision critical care. In this article, the authors review the data-driven and technology-based approaches being leveraged to discover and implement precision medicine strategies in the critical care setting.

> The rapid adoption of electronic health record (EHR) systems in US hospitals from 2008 to 2014 produced novel data elements for analysis. Concurrent innovations in computing architecture and machine learning (ML) algorithms have made rapid consumption of health data feasible and a powerful engine for clinical innovation. In critical care research, the net convergence of these trends has resulted in an exponential increase in outcome prediction research. In the following article, we explore the history of outcome prediction in the intensive care unit (ICU), the growing use of EHR data, and the rise of artificial intelligence and ML (AI) in critical care.

> Perioperative morbidity and mortality are significantly associated with both static and dynamic perioperative factors. The studies investigating static perioperative factors have been reported; however, there are a limited number of previous studies and data sets analyzing dynamic perioperative factors, including physiologic waveforms, despite its clinical importance. To fill the gap, the authors introduce a novel large size perioperative

Large volumes of data are collected on critically ill patients, and using data
science to extract information from the electronic medical record (EMR)
and to inform the design of clinical trials represents a new opportunity in
critical care research. Using improved methods of phenotyping critical illnesses, subject identification and enrollment, and targeted treatment
group assignment alongside newer trial designs such as adaptive platform
trials can increase efficiency while lowering costs. Some tools such as the
EMR to automate data collection are already in use. Refinement of data
science approaches in critical illness research will allow for better clinical
trials and, ultimately, improved patient outcomes.

Syndromic conditions, such as sepsis, are commonly encountered in the
intensive care unit. Although these conditions are easy for clinicians to
grasp, these conditions may limit the performance of machine-learning algorithms. Individual hospital practice patterns may limit external generalizability. Data missingness is another barrier to optimal algorithm
performance and various strategies exist to mitigate this. Recent advances
in data science, such as transfer learning, conformal prediction, and continual learning, may improve generalizability of machine-learning algorithms in critically ill patients. Randomized trials with these approaches
are indicated to demonstrate improvements in patient-centered outcomes
at this point.

Predictive analytics based on artificial intelligence (AI) offer clinicians the
opportunity to leverage big data available in electronic health records
(EHR) to improve clinical decision-making, and thus patient outcomes. Despite this, many barriers exist to facilitating trust between clinicians and AI-
based tools, limiting its current impact. Potential solutions are available at
both the local and national level. It will take a broad and diverse coalition of
stakeholders, from health-care systems, EHR vendors, and clinical educators to regulators, researchers and the patient community, to help facilitate
this trust so that the promise of AI in health care can be realized.

This article provides an overview of the most useful artificial intelligence algorithms developed in critical care, followed by a comprehensive outline of the benefits and limitations. We begin by describing how nurses and physicians might be aided by these new technologies. We then move to the possible changes in clinical guidelines with personalized medicine that will allow tailored therapies and probably will increase the quality of the care provided to patients. Finally, we describe how artificial intelligence models can unleash researchers' minds by proposing new strategies, by increasing the quality of clinical practice, and by questioning current knowledge and understanding.

Critical care data contain information about the most physiologically fragile patients in the hospital, who require a significant level of monitoring. However, medical devices used for patient monitoring suffer from measurement biases that have been largely underreported. This article explores sources of bias in commonly used clinical devices, including pulse oximeters, thermometers, and sphygmomanometers. Further, it provides a framework for mitigating these biases and key principles to achieve more equitable health care delivery.

CRITICAL CARE CLINICS

SERIES OF RELATED INTEREST

Emergency Medicine Clinics
https://www.emed.theclinics.com/
Clinics in Chest Medicine
https://www.chestmed.theclinics.com/

THE CLINICS ARE AVAILABLE ONLINE!
Access your subscription at:
www.theclinics.com

Preface

Facilitating the Next Paradigm Shift in Critical Care Through Artificial Intelligence

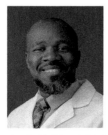 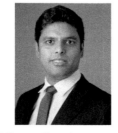

Andre L. Holder, MD, MS   Rishikesan Kamaleswaran, PhD
Editors

From the mechanical ventilator to extracorporeal circulatory support, every few years those who facilitate, practice, or study critical care are introduced to new technologies that redefine the status quo and introduce new challenges and possibilities. Machines that can exhibit artificial intelligence (AI), defined as the ability of computer systems to mirror behaviors once thought unique to humans (such as pattern recognition and decision making), may be the next major change seen in the study and practice of critical care. The field of Machine Learning (ML), how machines utilize AI using statistical and mathematical constructs, is evolving as quickly as the capacity of modern computing. While statistics is foundational to these new approaches, especially in the context of supervised learning (training a system to recognize or predict an outcome defined within the data), other areas of ML, such as unsupervised learning (training a system to recognize new, previously unseen patterns in data), deep learning (through the use of "neural nets," modeled after the human brain), and computer vision, have made this field uniquely suited to tackle many challenges of contemporary critical care. The rapid pace of advancements in this area has made it difficult to predict even how the near term may present itself, yet what is clear is the transformational change that will be felt across all facets of human knowledge, including the critical care field in general.

This collection is designed to provide an overview of the promise and potential challenges of AI in the practice, oversight, and study of critical care medicine. The first few articles discuss how AI might directly impact bedside clinicians of the future. Dr Sanchez-Pinto and colleagues introduce the potent methods that exist in reducing heterogeneity across critical care and improving treatment effectiveness through precision medicine approaches. Dr Liu and colleagues present the broad area of AI/ML

Crit Care Clin 39 (2023) xiii–xiv
https://doi.org/10.1016/j.ccc.2023.03.001
0749-0704/23/© 2023 Published by Elsevier Inc.

applied to the electronic health record (EHR) and highlight the key advantages and challenges in the domain. Dr Kim and colleagues introduce novel data sets and modalities that may provide incredible insights into physiologic dynamics of critical illness. Dr Clermont introduces how the EHR may be used within the context of an interactive learning framework through advanced interoperable tools and standards. The next article reviews how AI can improve deployment of critical care. Dr King and colleagues discuss how data science may be a powerful tool to advance implementation science, moving from population-based methods to incorporating individualized approaches. Next, we have two articles that discuss the implications of AI on the execution of critical care research. Dr Horvat reviews how Bayesian analysis can increase the efficiency and effectiveness of clinical trials, with lessons learned from the Randomized, Embedded, Multifactorial Adaptive Platform for Community-Acquired Pneumonia platform. Dr Agarwal and colleagues shed light on how the EHR can streamline clinical trial recruitment. The collection then talks about the challenges faced by the use of AI systems in the critical care landscape. Dr Wardi and colleagues give a very comprehensive overview of the different techniques applied to predictive models that make them more generalizable, especially for heterogenous syndromes like sepsis and acute respiratory distress syndrome. Dr Rojas and colleagues provide an excellent synopsis of why the right amount of clinician trust in AI is needed for appropriate use in the critically ill, and the systemic changes necessary to reach that goal. Finally, the collection closes with two bioethical dilemmas of using AI in critical care medicine. Dr Caruso and colleagues provide a balanced discussion of the possible benefits and costs of AI in critical care, indicating that the potential benefits of continuous surveillance of patients and decreased use of hospital resources may outweigh the upfront costs to infrastructure and workflow changes. Dr Charpignon and colleagues highlight the potential of AI to perpetuate inequitable care through biases in measurement, calibration, and patient selection that adversely affect segments of the population and provide possible solutions to mitigate these problems in future algorithms.

Our goal is to provide a roadmap for effective integration of AI into critical care systems, practice, and research. We hope that this collection will help revolutionize critical care to improve outcomes of those who need it.

Andre L. Holder, MD, MS
Division of Pulmonary, Allergy, Critical Care
and Sleep Medicine
Emory University School of Medicine
Woodruff Education Building
46 Armstrong Street, Room 215
Atlanta, GA 30303, USA

Rishikesan Kamaleswaran, PhD
Departments of Biomedical Informatics and
Emergency Medicine
Emory University School of Medicine
101 Woodruff Circle, Suite 4127
Atlanta, GA 30322, USA

E-mail addresses:
Andre.holder@emory.edu (A.L. Holder)
rkamaleswaran@emory.edu (R. Kamaleswaran)

Promise 1: Targeted, Personalized Bedside Care

Leveraging Data Science and Novel Technologies to Develop and Implement Precision Medicine Strategies in Critical Care

Lazaro N. Sanchez-Pinto, MD[a,b,]*,
Sivasubramanium V. Bhavani, MD[c], Mihir R. Atreya, MD, MPH[d],
Pratik Sinha, MD, PhD[e,f]

KEYWORDS

- Critical care • Precision medicine • Acute respiratory distress syndrome • Sepsis
- Machine learning • Electronic health records • Biomarkers

KEY POINTS

- Precision medicine in critical care aims to identify treatments that are most likely to result in favorable outcomes for subgroups of critically ill patients who share similar clinical and biological characteristics.
- Data science and multiomics approaches are increasingly being used to discover and implement precision medicine strategies in the critical care setting.
- Building collaborative data networks is imperative to advance the science of precision medicine and further refine the knowledge and technology that will transform the way we provide critical care.

Author contributions: all authors: concept, design, drafting of article, and final approval of the version to be published.
Funding: none for this article. Dr L.N. Sanchez-Pinto, S.V. Bhavani, and P. Sinha received funding from the NIH.
[a] Department of Pediatrics, Northwestern University Feinberg School of Medicine, Ann & Robert H. Lurie Children's Hospital of Chicago, Chicago, IL, USA; [b] Department of Preventive Medicine, Northwestern University Feinberg School of Medicine, Ann & Robert H. Lurie Children's Hospital of Chicago, Chicago, IL, USA; [c] Department of Medicine, Emory University, 100 Woodruff Circle, Atlanta, GA 30322, USA; [d] Division of Critical Care Medicine, Department of Pediatrics, Cincinnati Children's Hospital Medical Center, University of Cincinnati College of Medicine, 3333 Burnet Avenue, Cincinnati, OH 45229, USA; [e] Division of Clinical and Translational Research, Department of Anesthesia, Washington University School of Medicine, 1 Barnes Jewish Hospital Plaza, St. Louis, MO 63110, USA; [f] Division of Critical Care, Department of Anesthesia, Washington University School of Medicine, 1 Barnes Jewish Hospital Plaza, St. Louis, MO 63110, USA
* Corresponding author. Division of Critical Care Medicine, Ann & Robert H. Lurie Children's Hospital of Chicago, 225 East Chicago Avenue, Bx73, Chicago, IL 60611.
E-mail address: lsanchezpinto@luriechildrens.org

Crit Care Clin 39 (2023) 627–646
https://doi.org/10.1016/j.ccc.2023.03.002
0749-0704/23/© 2023 Elsevier Inc. All rights reserved.

INTRODUCTION

Heterogeneity is a pervasive feature of critical illness syndromes. Patients in the intensive care unit (ICU) are injured or develop critical illness for a plethora of reasons. On any given day, an intensivist may be taking care of a patient with a severe traumatic brain injury (TBI) and a few minutes later be at the bedside of a liver transplant patient with new-onset gram-negative sepsis. Critical illness, even when defined under common syndromes such as TBI, sepsis, or acute respiratory distress syndrome (ARDS), is inherently complex. The biological pathways involved in the various responses to stress and injury (such as immune, autonomic, neuroendocrine, or metabolic); the nonlinear interactions of these pathways; and the compounding effects of comorbidities, secondary injuries, and ongoing treatments make the unraveling of each form of critical illness an extremely challenging task.[1,2] Finally, critical illness is often dynamic and rapidly evolving, with clinical deterioration or response to treatment sometimes evident within minutes to hours.

This heterogeneity, complexity, and dynamicity of critical illness stands as a major hurdle in the path toward achieving higher precision in critical care medicine. Precision medicine aims to identify the treatments and interventions that are most likely to result in favorable outcomes for a group of patients based on similar unifying characteristics[3] and has been met with great clinical success in diseases such as leukemia, asthma, and heart failure.[1,4,5] In critical care, the gaps for the development and implementation of precision medicine strategies are many, but growth in this field has been identified as a major research priority.[3] Fortunately, the ICU is also a data-intense environment, with detailed data (including physiologic, laboratory, interventional, imaging, and so forth) being collected in electronic health records (EHRs) and other clinical information systems often at a very high time resolution.[6] When coupled with novel data science techniques, including unsupervised and supervised machine learning algorithms, these data have been used to identify and characterize various phenotypes of sepsis, ARDS, and other forms of critical illness.[7–10] Furthermore, when used to reanalyze randomized controlled trial (RCT) data or when studied in causal inference analyses, these phenotypes (also called subphenotypes, subtypes, subclasses, or subgroups) have been associated with heterogeneity of treatment effect (HTE), which is a key feature of precision medicine in critical care.[11] In parallel, thanks to advances in "omic" technologies and large biorepository studies, there have been substantial advances in the characterization of disease endotypes (ie, subtypes largely based on genomic, transcriptomic, or other biological information alone or in combination with clinical data).[3,12–17] Accordingly, there is a strong impetus for integrative approaches to achieve real-time prediction of patient phenotypes for identification of driving biological mechanisms and to test their significance in the context of future clinical trials (**Fig. 1**).

Despite these foundational developments, there remain several gaps and challenges between the current state and the prospective implementation, evaluation, and use of precision medicine strategies in the ICU. In this paper the authors (1) review the state-of-the-art and future directions of the discovery and characterization of disease phenotypes in critical care using data science approaches, with a focus on sepsis and ARDS; (2) describe the data-driven and technology-based approaches being developed to facilitate the implementation of precision medicine strategies in the ICU; and (3) discuss the opportunities and challenges for building critical care research data networks to advance the science of precision medicine.

A
Phenotypes of critical illness can be studied at different clinical and biological levels.

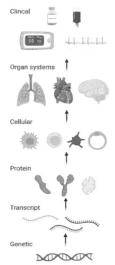

Clincal

Organ systems ↑

Cellular ↑

Protein ↑

Transcript ↑

Genetic ↑

B
Clinical and biological data combined with data-driven approaches can be used to classify patients into relevant phenotypes in real time.

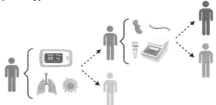

C **Phenotype identification can enable the implementation of precision therapies and care pathways in the ICU and test these in next generation clinical trials.**

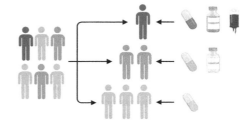

Fig. 1. Leveraging clinical and biological data to discover and implement precision medicine strategies in the intensive care unit (ICU). (*A*) Phenotypes studied at different biological levels; (*B*) Use of clinical and biological data to classify patients in real time; (*C*) Phenotype identification to enable precision medicine.

UNCOVERING RELEVANT DISEASE PHENOTYPES FROM OBSERVATIONAL DATA
Secondary Use of Clinical Data

State-of-the-art
Studies using machine learning for identifying clusters in critical illness are numerous and growing. When interpreting results from such studies, be it in secondary analyses of RCTs or large observational data, it is important to consider that most clustering algorithms are incredibly powerful and remarkably adept at delivering results that seem compelling. Irrespective of data quality or structure, clusters will emerge. The risks for overfitting, however, are high, and the generalizability of such studies can be limited. It is, therefore, incumbent on investigators to design studies that lend credibility to their findings, usually delivered through showing reproducibility and/or potential utility.[2] Although numerous studies have sought to enhance our understanding of critical illness through application of machine learning approaches, few, if any, are currently in use in clinical practice. Given the scope of their review, in this subsection the authors only present studies that have been validated in multiple datasets.

In ARDS, several investigators have sought to characterize phenotypes using machine learning approaches applied to a combination of clinical and biological data. Among these, the work by Calfee and colleagues is the most developed in terms of reproducibility and therapeutic potential. In their landmark study, they applied latent class analysis (LCA), a probabilistic modeling algorithm,[18] in 2 completed ARDS RCTs.[16] They used baseline clinical data such as demographics, vital signs, ARDS risk factors, routine laboratory values, and research protein biomarkers (eg, IL-6, IL-8, protein C, and so forth) as class-defining variables in their models. In both RCTs, they identified 2 distinct phenotypes, called the hypoinflammatory and hyperinflammatory phenotypes, with the latter defined by higher levels of proinflammatory cytokines, markers of organ failure, lower protein C, and shock. Unsurprisingly, given its characteristics, the hyperinflammatory phenotype was associated with worse clinical outcomes including fewer ventilator-free days and higher mortality. Importantly, in the ALVEOLI trial, which tested the efficacy of higher positive end-expiratory pressure (PEEP) strategy versus usual care, they observed HTE in the phenotypes.[16] Subsequently, they have applied the same LCA approach to 3 other ARDS RCTs,[19–21] identifying the same 2 phenotypes with the divergent clinical and biological characteristics and outcomes. In 2 of these trials, they observed differential treatment responses in interventions as diverse as fluid management in the FACTT trial and simvastatin in the HARP-2 trial.[19,20]

In recent advances, the same investigators have recapitulated their work, identifying the same 2 phenotypes in observational and pediatric ARDS cohorts,[17,22] as well as COVID-19–associated ARDS.[23] Notably, in the latter, they observed HTE with corticosteroid therapy. Although they adjusted for potential confounders, the analysis should be interpreted with caution given that the intervention was neither protocolized nor randomized. Outside of this research group, other investigators have also identified similar phenotypes in patients with acute hypoxic respiratory failure, with and without ARDS.[24–26] Taken together, these findings suggest that the biological pathways that describe the hyperinflammatory and hypoinflammatory phenotypes seem to be common among critically ill patients and they offer opportunity to test effective therapies in more uniform subgroups. Several key knowledge gaps remain in relation to these phenotypes: (1) it is unclear if these phenotypes are limited to ARDS or whether they are also seen in sepsis and other inflammatory critical illnesses; (2) the longitudinal stability of these phenotypes also remain uncertain and the clinical and biological implication of phenotype switching is also unknown; (3) the clinical implementation of LCA-derived molecular phenotypes remains uncertain (see further discussion later); and (4) as the field expands, it is likely that more phenotypes will be observed, particularly in the hypoinflammatory phenotype, which remains largely undifferentiated despite being the majority class in these analyses.

In sepsis, leveraging clinical data from the EHR for phenotype discovery, Seymour and colleagues used k-means clustering to describe 4 phenotypes of early sepsis (α, β, γ, and δ).[8] The α phenotype was the largest subgroup, had lowest rate of organ failure, and had the lowest mortality; the β phenotype was older with more chronic illness and more renal dysfunction; the γ phenotype had more inflammation and was more febrile; and the δ subgroup had the lowest prevalence and was associated with higher lactate, markers of liver dysfunction, and the highest mortality. They validated their findings in a larger cohort from the same health care system. Notably, the 4 phenotypes had distinct patterns of molecular biology. Further, in the PROCESS trial, which tested the efficacy of early goal-directed therapy in early sepsis, they observed significant HTE that was driven by the δ and γ subgroups.[8] Compared with the molecular phenotyping schema in ARDS, this approach has the distinct advantage of not needing plasma biomarkers to identify the phenotypes. Important limitations of this analysis include high levels of missingness in several critical phenotype defining variables such as lactate and liver enzymes (60%–80% missing) and a lack of recapitulation beyond the original investigator group.[8]

Future directions
There are various aspects related to the use of data science techniques and various data types for the discovery and characterization of relevant phenotypes that will

require further attention in future research. For example, the type of modeling approach to identify therapeutically relevant subgroups of patients and the added value of including protein biomarkers in machine learning clustering algorithms remain uncertain. Sinha and colleagues evaluated 9 machine learning clustering algorithms in 3 previously completed ARDS RCTs using baseline clinical and biological data, as described in LCA studies discussed earlier.[7] "Success" for the identified clusters was determined if there was significant HTE with the randomized intervention. They observed that supervised approaches, such as causal forest or x-learners, were better at identifying clusters with HTE than unsupervised approaches. Among unsupervised approaches, LCA was equivalent to the supervised algorithms and outperformed other unsupervised algorithms such as k-means and hierarchical clustering. Except LCA, which is based on modeling for maximum likelihood, all other approaches were subject to substantial instability with changing the initiation seed of the clustering and imputation runs.[7] Finally, excluding protein biomarkers from the clustering algorithms led to a marked decrease in the ability to detect HTE irrespective of the algorithm and RCT, suggesting that in these RCTs, inclusion of protein biomarkers was critical to identifying clusters with HTE.[7]

Clinical Trajectories

State-of-the-art

Critical illness syndromes are dynamic processes representing biological and physiologic responses evolving over minutes to hours.[27,28] Sepsis, ARDS, and vasopressor-dependent shock, all exemplify this paradigm of dynamic syndromes. Studies have shown that dynamic measures of clinical severity are more accurate predictors of mortality.[29–31] Similarly, time series analyses have demonstrated rapidly shifting transcription patterns and immune responses in critical illness.[28,32–34] The "temporal instability" of critical illness suggests that static snapshots of laboratory test results, vitals, or biomarkers may not identify clinically meaningful phenotypes that are consistent over time.[35,36] For instance, almost half of patients classified on admission to a sepsis endotype using gene expression switched subgroups within days.[37] To overcome the "temporal instability" of critical illness phenotypes, recent precision medicine approaches have incorporated longitudinal measures that better reflect the dynamic nature of critical illness syndromes.[38–41]

Bos and colleagues investigated whether there were latent phenotypes within COVID-19 ARDS using both cross-sectional and longitudinal ventilator data. Using cross-sectional data, the investigators found that there were no consistent phenotypes of COVID-19 ARDS. However, using dynamic data, the investigators found 2 distinct phenotypes with divergent trajectories of ventilatory ratio and mechanical power.[38]

Bhavani and colleagues used longitudinal body temperature measurements to identify 4 sepsis phenotypes.[39] The investigators found that the phenotypes had distinct clinical characteristics and outcomes, which have been subsequently replicated in patients with COVID-19, septic shock, and *Staphylococcus aureus* bacteremia.[42–44] In a study of biomarker profiles of the temperature trajectory phenotypes, the investigators found significant associations between temperature phenotypes and temporal changes in cytokine levels, suggesting that longitudinal temperature trajectories reflect the dynamic changing host response to infection.[44] In subsequent work, the addition of longitudinal heart rate, respiratory rate, and blood pressure measurements to temperature trajectories resulted in the identification of HTE to balanced crystalloids versus normal saline.[9] Specifically, a phenotype characterized by low temperatures, normal heart rate, normal respiratory rate, and hypotension demonstrated significant benefit from balanced crystalloids compared with normal saline, with a number-needed-to-treat of only 7 patients for a 30-day mortality benefit. This study highlights the potential precision medicine implications of dynamic trajectories.

In pediatric shock, Perizes and colleagues demonstrated that there were 4 trajectories of vasopressor-dependent shock, with distinct outcomes and potentially differential benefit from hydrocortisone.[40] Importantly, 2 of these distinct shock trajectories ("moderate slow resolving" and "moderate persistent" shock) could not be distinguished in the first 24 hours of ICU admission but had significantly different mortality. This finding underscores the importance of longitudinal trajectory phenotypes compared with baseline phenotypes in dynamic processes such as shock.

Future directions

The future directions for the study of patient trajectory phenotypes are (1) to determine the minimal time window required to accurately capture patient trajectories; (2) to evaluate the biological signatures of these patient trajectories; and (3) to investigate whether these patient trajectory phenotypes respond differently to therapies. The main limitation in any trajectory model is the requirement of a time window to observe the patient trajectory. Different trajectory models vary in the time window required, from 8 hours to 4 days. During the phenotyping window, treatments may be administered that affect the phenotype, and these treatments would have to be considered when classifying patients in real time. It is essential to identify the minimal time window required to phenotype patients in order to minimize the confounding effect of interventions on the trajectory and to expedite delivery of early targeted interventions. Future work should focus on incorporating static and dynamic clinical data to predict the patient's future trajectory group membership with an abbreviated time window of observation. Similarly, elucidating the biological profiles of these phenotypes is essential.[45] The biological profile could directly inform treatments that may benefit specific phenotypes. Future work should investigate the biological profiles of dynamic phenotypes through multiomic approaches, including cytokine, protein, messenger RNA (mRNA), and metabolite data. Finally, the most important clinical question is whether trajectory phenotypes benefit from specific therapies. The biological insights gained from the multiomic studies could provide hypotheses to test in clinical trials.

Physiologic Data

State-of-the-art

Monitoring of bedside monitor waveforms and other physiologic data is a mainstay of critical care medicine.[6,46] Physiologic data are near ubiquitous, widely available around the world, continuously collected, and subject to low selection bias (ie, compared with treatments or laboratory test results, it does not depend on an intensivist's decision for the data to be collected).[46] Data scientists using physiologic data have traditionally focused on prediction modeling (eg, the prediction of sepsis[47–49]), but its use for identifying disease phenotypes and implementing precision medicine strategies seems promising.[50] For example, Bhavani and colleagues' phenotypes of sepsis based on vital sign trajectory described earlier were based on intermittently recorded vitals in the EHR, but it would be easy to imagine an implementation that uses continuously recorded physiologic data to rapidly classify patients before fluid administration.[9] Other examples of use of vital signs and device-based physiologic data include the use of severe hypoxemia to select patient likely to benefit from proning,[2] the use of persistent hypoxemia to identify patients who may benefit from dexamethasone,[51] and the use of lung elastance to identify responders to low tidal volume strategies.[52]

Although simple vital signs seem to be very informative in terms of precision medicine applications, complex measures such as heart rate variability (HRV), arterial waveform contour analysis, or pulse pressure variation could also provide rich information for phenotyping.[46] For example, Morris and colleagues noticed that the subgroup of adult patients with trauma who had cosyntropin-confirmed adrenal insufficiency had an associated lower HRV and, among those who were treated with hydrocortisone, only survivors had a significant recovery of their HRV within a day after initiating therapy.[53] Badke and colleagues have studied HRV in critically ill children and have demonstrated that HRV is significantly associated with the inflammatory biomarkers,[54] which are an important component of some disease phenotypes, as the hyperinflammatory ARDS that has been described in adult and children.[16,17] Badke and colleagues have also described different trajectories of recovery of HRV among survivors of pediatric septic shock and its association with hospital readmission, which could be used to screen for patients susceptible for targeted intervention postdischarge.[55] Finally, pulse contour analysis and pulse pressure variation have been used to identify fluid responders among adults patients with hemodynamic instability.[56]

Future directions

One of the main advantages of device-based physiologic data is their pervasive and ubiquitous nature, including in lower resourced settings, urgent care centers, clinics, rural and community hospitals, and, increasingly, in patients' homes thanks to the increased use of wearable sensors. In parallel to this, intensivists are starting to embrace the continuum of care that starts well before the patient arrives to the ICU.[57] Although still relatively underdeveloped, the field of remote patient monitoring is evolving rapidly, particularly as technical advances allow for less invasive and more efficient physiologic monitoring.[58] It is not hard to imagine that within a few years, high-risk patients, as those with cancer or those recovering from a major surgery, will be routinely equipped with novel sensors and monitored remotely with the aid of machine learning algorithms.[59] This technology could not only be used for predicting clinical deterioration but also be potentially leveraged to recognize physiological-based phenotypes even before the patients arrive to the hospital.[9] Today's sensors are capable of recording cardiovascular, respiratory, thermal, and motion signal with materials that are flexible and unobtrusive,[60] and the next generation of sensors may be capable of also analyzing sweat for biomarkers and harvest energy from the body to prolong its battery life.[61,62] In addition, given their relatively low cost and portability, sensor-enabled physiology-based precision medicine approaches are likely to have a more generalizable and global impact in the care of critically ill patients around the world.

Biomarkers and Multiomics

Given the inherent complexity and dynamicity of critical illness syndromes, it is often challenging for providers caring for patients to know, early in the disease course, which patients are likely to improve with timely implementation of standard-of-care therapies and which patients will continue to deteriorate and thus potentially benefit from targeted interventions. Prognostic enrichment refers to approaches that rely on identifying patients at high risk of an outcome of interest such as mortality or persistent multiple organ dysfunctions. Several clinical and biological tools, including those based on serum protein, messenger RNA, and metabolite biomarkers, have been used as prognostic enrichment tools among critically ill patients. For instance, Wong and colleagues prospectively validated the pediatric sepsis risk biomarker

(PERSEVERE) model that include IL-1, IL-8, heat shock protein 70 (HSP70), CXC motif chemokine ligand 3 and 4 (CXCL3 and CXCL4), and matrix metalloproteinase 8 to estimate risk of mortality[63] and individual organ dysfunction among children with septic shock.[64,65] More recent iterations have incorporated markers of endothelial dysfunction to provide a unified model to simultaneously predict multiple organ dysfunctions.[66] Although in an ideal world, biomarker-based models would achieve both high sensitivity and specificity, existing models typically have achieved a high negative predictive value. Thus, a patient deemed low risk would be unlikely to have a poor outcome and may benefit from standard-of-care therapies alone. Alternative approaches have coupled EHR data with machine learning models to yield prognostic enrichment tools with a high positive predictive value.[67] Although not yet prospectively validated, it is conceivable that sequential utilization of such complementary approaches may be necessary to achieve real-time prognostic enrichment in critical care.

Patients deemed high risk based on prognostic enrichment, although a relatively smaller subset in comparison with all patients meeting criteria for critical illness syndromes, are likely constituted by a heterogeneous mix of patients with differing underlying biology. Predictive enrichment approaches, which involve identification of biologically relevant subclasses that demonstrate differential responses to any given therapy based on shared biological mechanisms, offer promise to sift through the underlying heterogeneity and identify the right treatment of the right patient.[68]

Paralleling efforts that have leveraged observational clinical data to identify relevant disease phenotypes detailed in the previous sections, several studies over the previous decade have used gene-expression profiling early in the course of disease to identify clinically relevant endotypes. Striking shifts in the host transcriptome occur within hours of critical illness syndromes. For instance, nearly 7000 genes are differentially expressed among patients with septic shock relative to healthy controls.[69] Leveraging these transcriptomic shifts, Wong and colleagues first identified pediatric septic shock subclasses based on 100 subclass-defining genes, which were enriched for differential adaptive system and glucocorticoid receptor responses.[69] Subsequently, receipt of adjuvant steroids was associated with an increased risk of mortality among endotype A patients in prospective observational studies, relative to patients with endotype B.[70,71] Response of these patient endotypes to corticosteroids will be tested in the Stress Hydrocortisone in Pediatric Septic Shock trial (NCT03401398) and may demonstrate efficacy of predictive enrichment. Comparable efforts among children with ARDS[72,73] and adults with sepsis have similarly identified biologically distinct endotypes, the latter including Sepsis Response Signatures (SRS), Molecular Diagnosis and Risk Stratification of Sepsis, and Inflammopathic, Adaptive, and Coagulopathic subclasses.[14,74,75] However, few approaches have been replicated in external validation cohorts.[76]

Despite the increase in gene-expression profiling, several critical challenges remain, including the following: (1) *temporality*: selection of an appropriate time point for sampling is challenging, as often this is based on meeting criteria for clinically defined syndromes based on meeting arbitrarily defined manifestations of underlying biology.[28] (2) *Stability*: transcriptomic shifts and endotype switching are well described, with nearly 50% of sepsis endotypes switching between day 1 and 3.[36] (3) *Reproducibility*: there is a lack of standardization of patient endotypes in critical illness syndromes, with studies showing only weak congruency between assignments based on methodological approach used.[13] (4) *Generalizability*: signatures correlated with systemic inflammation and organ dysfunction are shared by numerous critical illness syndromes. Thus an emphasis has been placed on determining generalizable endotypes that speak to potentially "treatable traits," rather than those derived for individual syndromes. (5) *Real-time endotype assignment*: all current approaches are based on time-consuming platforms that are limited to the research realm and retrospective designation of endotypes. A critical challenge remains parsimonious selection of gene markers, development of rapid molecular or gene-expression assays for diagnosis at the bedside, and development of classifier models that consistently assign clinically relevant patient endotypes.

Future directions
Scientific advances from other conditions such as cancer can inform future studies in critical illness syndromes. High-throughput multiomics that rely on information gathered from more than a single molecular dimension have been increasingly used to strengthen the biological basis for disease phenotypes by reducing noise associated with any single dimension. Multiomics approaches hold tremendous potential to detail the hierarchical flow of information from DNA to RNA to protein. Although studies among critical illness syndromes have interrogated biological layers beyond the host transcriptome, including host epigenome through DNA methylation profiles,[77,78] proteome,[79,80] lipidome,[81–83] and metabolome[84,85] individually, few have simultaneously profiled and integrated multiomic datasets to gain a comprehensive understanding of disease mechanisms. Davenport and colleagues identified changes in expression quantitative trait loci associated with patient SRS endotypes among adults.[14] More recent studies among those with COVID-19–related critical illness have integrated the proteome, metabolome, and lipidome to characterize biological pathways among patients.[86] It is conceivable that concerted efforts to leverage linked biospecimens from observational cohort studies or randomized trials, with integration of datasets, may serve to more comprehensively characterize patient subclasses and strengthen the biological basis of patient endotypes. Moreover, such information may not only allow for determination of HTE but may inform de novo drug development through computational models.[87,88] For instance, identification of gene regulatory elements and hub genes may enable identification of novel mechanistic targets for therapeutic drug development that are subclass specific. Lastly, cell-specific variation is increasingly recognized as a major contributor to sepsis heterogeneity.[89] Thus, future targeted studies that use single-cell multiomics may inform bioinformatic approaches to deconvolute existing large-scale bulk sequencing datasets to identify cell-specific molecular perturbations that ultimately drive patient endotypes and may be potentially amenable to targeted intervention.[90]

IMPLEMENTING PRECISION MEDICINE STRATEGIES IN THE CRITICAL CARE SETTING
Designing Next-Generation Clinical Trials Leveraging the Electronic Health Record

Over the past 3 decades, more than 30 pharmacologic therapies have been tested in more than 100 clinical trials of sepsis and ARDS. Unfortunately, these trials have failed to show consistent benefit from any novel treatment in the overall population of patients with sepsis.[91,92] The one-size-fits-all approach has not worked. Treating all patients with sepsis and ARDS with the same therapy has likely resulted in benefit to some, harm to others, and, in most clinical trials, a null effect in the overall group. The next generation of clinical trials will leverage the EHR and perform precision enrollment of phenotypes based on the models that are currently being developed and validated.[3] The challenge remains as to how these phenotypes will be identified in real time in the EHR to facilitate precision enrollment. First, many phenotyping models incorporate complicated imputation methods such as multiple imputation with chained equations that may be difficult to implement with real-time EHR data or are based on unsupervised machine learning algorithms that may not be amenable to prospective implementation.[8] Second, some of the approaches that use supervised machine learning approaches more amenable to prospective implementation require complex implementation pipelines that may not be computationally feasible in current EHR systems.[93] Third, both static and trajectory phenotypes require a period of observation to collect patient data before classification of the patient, and the challenge will be to determine how long to wait and how to expedite real-time classification.[39] Finally, some of the phenotyping strategies require integration of biomarker data and for these to be clinically useful they must be generated in near real time using novel point-of-care technology.[16,94] With implementation, simplicity and parsimony is key: simpler functional structure for the model, fewer required data elements, simpler imputation processes and variable transformations, shorter time windows of observations, lower computational resources, and more readily available data sources.

The road to precision enrollment in clinical trials begins by testing the feasibility of applying these phenotyping algorithms prospectively. The proof-of-concept must demonstrate that prospective classification with the phenotyping algorithm has comparable accuracy in classification to the retrospective derivation and validation studies.[74] Next, the algorithm will need to be integrated into a clinical trial aimed at targeting specific phenotypes for specific therapies. If a treatment benefit is shown in a clinical trial, the next step could be to conduct a trial of a recommendation system based on the phenotypes, in which physicians are either shown or not shown the recommended treatment of a particular phenotype. This type of recommendation trial would evaluate (1) whether recommendations are being incorporated into physician workflows and (2) whether the recommendation system improves outcomes. The road to precision medicine in sepsis will require collaboration between data scientists, implementation scientists, clinical trialists, and clinicians to move these algorithms from research laboratories to clinical practice.

Using Machine Learning to Predict Patient Phenotypes

The hyperinflammatory and hypoinflammatory phenotypes of ARDS described in previous sections present a good example of the promise and challenges of data-driven approaches to implement phenotyping strategies in real time. These ARDS phenotypes have been reproduced in multiple studies and populations and have shown differential treatment responses; however, the LCA models used to identify the phenotypes are complex, comprising 20 to 30 variables that are standardized (z-scaled) to the population mean, rendering them impractical for prospective use in clinical trials. It is here, in the domain of clinical implementation, that innovative applications of machine learning approaches have facilitated important breakthroughs. Sinha and colleagues first used multiple machine learning algorithms for feature selection, identifying the top 6 class-defining variables.[95] They used permutations of these variables to develop and validate 3 or variable parsimonious logistic regression models that can classify the molecular phenotypes accurately. In a follow-up proof-of-concept study (n = 39), using a novel point-of-care assay for IL-6 and soluble tumor necrosis factor receptor 1, they classified patients into the molecular phenotypes in real time using the parsimonious models.[94]

In parallel, the same investigators next used XGBoost, a form of gradient boosted machine, to develop and validate models that can accurately classify patients into molecular phenotypes using only readily available clinical data.[96] In a follow-up study, they used this XGBoost classifier model in LUNG SAFE, one of the largest observational cohorts of ARDS, and found the same clinical characteristics and significant adjusted HTE with PEEP strategy (high vs low), in line with what was observed in the LCA-derived phenotypes in the ALVEOLI trial.[16,97] Further, they also showed that these models accurately classified the phenotypes with data extracted from the EHR (as opposed to hand curated), which suggests these XGBoost models could be embedded in the EHR for future trials. Importantly, in the phenotypes identified by either the parsimonious or clinical classifier models, the same HTE observed in the original LCA studies were also observed here, suggesting that machine learning–derived models can capture the complexity of LCA-derived phenotypes. These studies underpin the importance of machine learning in both the identification and clinical implementation of the phenotypes.

Integrated Approaches for the Use of Real-Time Multiomics and Endotyping

Both phenotype-first and endotype-first approaches, detailed in this review, have relative strengths and weaknesses. Given the potential advantage of leveraging extant EHR data such as vital sign or organ dysfunction trajectories, phenotype-based approaches may in the future be widely available and more readily accessible across health care infrastructures. However, biological depth may be lacking when using such approaches in isolation. Conversely, endotype-based approaches, including those that incorporate high-throughput multiomic modalities, may not be pragmatic for real-time application in the near future. For instance, it is conceivable that point-of-care assays for gene-expression profiling that identify patient endotypes may become available in the near future.[70] However, such tools may be cost prohibitive and serve to stress existing health care infrastructures and further exacerbate disparities in access. Thus, there is an urgent need for development of an actionable framework for development of real-time multiomics technology that can be deployed in an equitable manner.

Several potential advances are needed for successful application of multiomics technology for precision medicine in critical illness. First, there is a need for studies using high-throughput multiomics technology to identify reproducible endotypes and correlated biological pathways using existing or new biorepositories. Second, there is a need to prospectively validate clinically relevant endotypes approaches in observational and RCT settings. Third, there is a need to develop point-of-care rapid molecular assays for protein biomarkers, polymerase chain reaction, mRNA, microRNA products that correlate with patient endotypes and may serve as biomarkers for patient classification and predictive enrichment. Finally, there is a need to test integrative approaches to predict patient phenotypes based on clinical models and a limited set of predictive biomarkers.

CHALLENGES AND OPPORTUNITIES OF DATA SCIENCE APPROACHES TO ADVANCE PRECISION MEDICINE IN CRITICAL CARE
Leveraging Real-World Data

The success of the approaches described here largely depend on the ability of researchers to leverage real-world observational data to advance precision medicine in critical care. Real-world data in health care are the data generated through the normal processes of clinical care and are oftentimes used as a synonym for EHR data, although other sources (such as device-generated data, patient-generated data, imaging, claims and billing data, registries, and so forth) are also considered forms of real-world data. Because real-world data are generated for purposes other than research, its use in research can provide as many challenges as opportunities. On the one hand, real-world data are prone to contain errors, suffer missingness and sparsity, and be recorded in nonstandardized formats that can make analysis and use challenging.[98] On the other hand, real-world data are being generated, recorded, digitalized, and stored at a much higher rate than data collected for research purposes. By some estimates, health care data now represent greater than 30% of all the data being generated in the world.[99] Furthermore, one of the major goals of leveraging real-world data in critical care is to implement data-driven systems in real time, and thus, being able to understand and engineer solution that take advantage of real-world data while dealing with its inherent limitations becomes an important goal.[6]

One of the common limitations of real-world data is data quality issues. Data quality assessment frameworks, as the one proposed by Kahn and colleagues, can be extremely helpful at answering key questions about data quality and addressing the issues that are found[100]; this includes attention to aspects such as conformance (eg, *are the data in the right format?*), completeness (eg, *are all the expected data available?*), and plausibility (eg, *is the value believable from a biological and contextual standpoint?*). Attention to the data quality across the entire real-world data life cycle, such as understanding the provenance and trustability of the data source, is also important.[101] Assessing completeness of the data usually focuses on comparing the amount of data found against the data expected, but does not fully address another important aspect of real-world data, which is data sparsity. Only a select number of data points at various time points are collected on a given patient, often dictated by the idiosyncrasies of health care and subject to the variation of care, which is pervasive in critical care. Approaches to deal with data missingness include techniques such as multiple imputation methods, which can be very handy but may introduce some bias.[102] Furthermore, when considering the generalizability and transportability of a model developed using data from one setting to a different setting, it is important to understand that issues with data quality and variability in measurements in the different settings can significantly affect the performance of the model, even if the model itself is scientifically good and mathematically accurate.[103] Ultimately, many of the inherent issues with real-world data can limit the reproducibility of research findings.[104] Using open science approaches, such as applying the Findable, Accessible, Interoperable, Reusable (FAIR) principles to share resources, analytical code, and scientific data generated by research, is advocated by the National Institute of Health and can serve as a way to ensure the quality, reproducibility, and usefulness of research findings from real-world data studies.[105]

Building Collaborative Networks

Establishing large-scale data collaboration networks is a critical step to enable the development, dissemination, and evaluation of algorithms and data-driven tools designed to implement precision medicine strategies in the ICU. In their official research statement for American Thoracic Society, Shah and colleagues proposed the creation of *knowledge networks*, with deeply phenotyped and harmonized data representing clinical, imaging, and multiomics data from EHRs, RCTs, and observational studies.[3] Attention to core tenets of data collaborations and sharing, such as data privacy and security, data harmonization, and data quality assurance, is paramount in such an endeavor and has previously represented major hurdles for large-scale collaborations.[98] Nowadays, however, standard data exchange languages such as the Fast Healthcare Interoperability Resources (FHIR)[106] and common data models such as the Observational Medical outcomes Partnership[107] allow for data collaborations to thrive and for researchers to overcome the technical bottlenecks that thwarted similar efforts in the past. Standards such as FHIR allow health care research networks to build shared data infrastructures, combine clinical data, and build algorithms using the same format and terminology, which can facilitate the implementation and reduce costs.[106] The 21st Century Act in the United States established FHIR as the standardized method for obtaining copies of EHR data through application programming interfaces, which has greatly accelerated the development and adoption of FHIR-based tools.[108] Initiatives such as the *Sepsis on FHIR* collaborative program, which leverages FHIR to develop an infrastructure for sepsis data and model sharing across multiple institutions, show the promise of this type of approach in the critical care setting.[109] Along with these technical developments, the regulatory environment in the United States has considerably increased the flexibility of the policies governing research data sharing through the new Common Rule,[110,111] further enabling these data collaborations.[109,112] However, the development of technology and standards for the collection, formatting, and representation of other data sources important in critical care precision medicine, such as device data (eg, bedside monitors, ventilators, and so forth) and multiomics assays, still remains a major area in need of attention from researchers, vendors, funders, and other stakeholders.[3,46] Ultimately, generalizability and reproducibility will be critical components of any precision medicine strategy in the ICU, and algorithms and tools that follow the FAIR principles and are designed for interoperability will facilitate dissemination, implementation, and validation and increase their chances of success.[113]

SUMMARY

In the critical care setting, the heterogeneity, complexity, and dynamicity of critical illness stands as a major hurdle in the path toward precision medicine. The gaps for the development and implementation of precision medicine strategies are many, but the advent of data science and multiomics approaches—combined with the rich data ecosystem in the ICU—offer unprecedented opportunities. These approaches have facilitated the discovery and characterization of sepsis and ARDS phenotypes using clinical and multiomics data and are now being leveraged to design real-time implementations that will enable next-generation clinical trials. Building and expanding collaborative data networks is imperative to advance the science of precision medicine in critical care and further refine the knowledge and technology that will transform the way we provide care to the most vulnerable patients.

CLINICS CARE POINTS

- Precision medicine strategies are promising in the critical care setting.
- Data science and novel technologies can enable the implementation of precision medicine strategies in critcal care.
- Further research and data collaboration is needed to make this a reality.

CONFLICTS OF INTEREST

Dr P. Sinha receives consultancy fees from Astra Zeneca. The other authors declare no conflict of interest.

REFERENCES

1. Buchman TG, Billiar TR, Elster E, et al. Precision medicine for critical illness and injury. Crit Care Med 2016;44(9):1635–8.

2. DeMerle KM, Angus DC, Baillie JK, et al. Sepsis subclasses: a framework for development and interpretation. Crit Care Med 2021;49(5):748–59.
3. Shah FA, Meyer NJ, Angus DC, et al. A research agenda for precision medicine in sepsis and acute respiratory distress syndrome: an official american thoracic society research statement. Am J Respir Crit Care Med 2021;204(8):891–901.
4. Seymour CW, Gomez H, Chang C-CH, et al. Precision medicine for all? Challenges and opportunities for a precision medicine approach to critical illness. Crit Care 2017;21(1):257.
5. Cutler DM. Early returns from the era of precision medicine. JAMA 2020;323(2): 109–10.
6. Sanchez-Pinto LN, Luo Y, Churpek MM. Big data and data science in critical care. Chest 2018;154(5):1239–48.
7. Sinha P, Spicer A, Delucchi KL, et al. Comparison of machine learning clustering algorithms for detecting heterogeneity of treatment effect in acute respiratory distress syndrome: a secondary analysis of three randomised controlled trials. EBioMedicine 2021;74:103697.
8. Seymour CW, Kennedy JN, Wang S, et al. Derivation, validation, and potential treatment implications of novel clinical phenotypes for sepsis. JAMA 2019; 321(20):2003–17.
9. Bhavani SV, Semler M, Qian ET, et al. Development and validation of novel sepsis subphenotypes using trajectories of vital signs. Intensive Care Med 2022. https://doi.org/10.1007/s00134-022-06890-z.
10. Sanchez-Pinto LN, Stroup EK, Pendergrast T, et al. Derivation and validation of novel phenotypes of multiple organ dysfunction syndrome in critically ill children. JAMA Netw Open 2020;3(8):e209271.
11. Khan YA, Fan E, Ferguson ND. Precision medicine and heterogeneity of treatment effect in therapies for ARDS. Chest 2021;1729–38.
12. Wong HR, Atkinson SJ, Cvijanovich NZ, et al. Combining prognostic and predictive enrichment strategies to identify children with septic shock responsive to corticosteroids. Crit Care Med 2016;44(10):e1000–3.
13. Wong HR, Sweeney TE, Hart KW, et al. Pediatric sepsis endotypes among adults with sepsis. Crit Care Med 2017;45(12):e1289–91.
14. Davenport EE, Burnham KL, Radhakrishnan J, et al. Genomic landscape of the individual host response and outcomes in sepsis: a prospective cohort study. Lancet Respir Med 2016;4(4):259–71.
15. Sweeney TE, Perumal TM, Henao R, et al. A community approach to mortality prediction in sepsis via gene expression analysis. Nat Commun 2018;9(1):694.
16. Calfee CS, Delucchi K, Parsons PE, et al. Subphenotypes in acute respiratory distress syndrome: latent class analysis of data from two randomised controlled trials. Lancet Respir Med 2014;2(8):611–20.
17. Dahmer MK, Yang G, Zhang M, et al. Identification of phenotypes in paediatric patients with acute respiratory distress syndrome: a latent class analysis. Lancet Respir Med 2022;10(3):289–97.
18. Sinha P, Calfee CS, Delucchi KL. Practitioner's guide to latent class analysis: methodological considerations and common pitfalls. Crit Care Med 2021;e63–79. https://doi.org/10.1097/ccm.0000000000004710.
19. Famous KR, Delucchi K, Ware LB, et al. Acute respiratory distress syndrome subphenotypes respond differently to randomized fluid management strategy. Am J Respir Crit Care Med 2017;195(3):331–8.

20. Calfee CS, Delucchi KL, Sinha P, et al. Acute respiratory distress syndrome sub-phenotypes and differential response to simvastatin: secondary analysis of a randomised controlled trial. Lancet Respir Med 2018;6(9):691–8.

21. Sinha P, Delucchi KL, Thompson BT, et al. Latent class analysis of ARDS sub-phenotypes: a secondary analysis of the statins for acutely injured lungs from sepsis (SAILS) study. Intensive Care Med 2018;44(11):1859–69.

22. Sinha P, Delucchi KL, Chen Y, et al. Latent class analysis-derived subpheno-types are generalisable to observational cohorts of acute respiratory distress syndrome: a prospective study. Thorax 2022;77(1):13–21.

23. Sinha P, Furfaro D, Cummings MJ, et al. Latent class analysis reveals COVID-19-related acute respiratory distress syndrome subgroups with differential re-sponses to corticosteroids. Am J Respir Crit Care Med 2021;204(11):1274–85.

24. Bos LD, Schouten LR, van Vught LA, et al. Identification and validation of distinct biological phenotypes in patients with acute respiratory distress syndrome by cluster analysis. Thorax 2017;72(10):876–83.

25. Heijnen NFL, Hagens LA, Smit MR, et al. Biological subphenotypes of acute res-piratory distress syndrome show prognostic enrichment in mechanically venti-lated patients without acute respiratory distress syndrome. Am J Respir Crit Care Med 2021;203(12):1503–11.

26. Kitsios GD, Yang L, Manatakis DV, et al. Host-response subphenotypes offer prognostic enrichment in patients with or at risk for acute respiratory distress syndrome. Crit Care Med 2019;1724–34. https://doi.org/10.1097/ccm. 0000000000004018.

27. Cazalis M-A, Lepape A, Venet F, et al. Early and dynamic changes in gene expression in septic shock patients: a genome-wide approach. Intensive Care Med Exp 2014;2(1):20.

28. Maslove DM, Wong HR. Gene expression profiling in sepsis: timing, tissue, and translational considerations. Trends Mol Med 2014;20(4):204–13.

29. Peelen L, de Keizer NF, Jonge E de, et al. Using hierarchical dynamic Bayesian networks to investigate dynamics of organ failure in patients in the intensive care unit. J Biomed Inform 2010;43(2):273–86.

30. Klein Klouwenberg PMC, Spitoni C, van der Poll T, et al. Predicting the clinical trajectory in critically ill patients with sepsis: a cohort study. Crit Care 2019; 23(1):1–9.

31. Thorsen-Meyer H-C, Nielsen AB, Nielsen AP, et al. Dynamic and explainable machine learning prediction of mortality in patients in the intensive care unit: a retrospective study of high-frequency data in electronic patient records. Lancet Digital Health 2020;2(4):e179–91.

32. Hollen MK, Stortz JA, Darden D, et al. Myeloid-derived suppressor cell function and epigenetic expression evolves over time after surgical sepsis. Crit Care 2019;23(1):355.

33. Talwar S, Munson PJ, Barb J, et al. Gene expression profiles of peripheral blood leukocytes after endotoxin challenge in humans. Physiol Genomics 2006;25(2): 203–15.

34. Calvano SE, Xiao W, Richards DR, et al. A network-based analysis of systemic inflammation in humans. Nature 2005;437(7061):1032–7.

35. Kwan A, Hubank M, Rashid A, et al. Transcriptional instability during evolving sepsis may limit biomarker based risk stratification. PLoS One 2013;8(3): e60501.

36. Wong HR, Cvijanovich NZ, Anas N, et al. Endotype transitions during the acute phase of pediatric septic shock reflect changing risk and treatment response. Crit Care Med 2018;46(3):e242–9.

37. Burnham KL, Davenport EE, Radhakrishnan J, et al. Shared and distinct aspects of the sepsis transcriptomic response to fecal peritonitis and pneumonia. Am J Respir Crit Care Med 2017;196(3):328–39.

38. Bos LDJ, Sjoding M, Sinha P, et al. Longitudinal respiratory subphenotypes in patients with COVID-19-related acute respiratory distress syndrome: results from three observational cohorts. Lancet Respir Med 2021;9(12):1377–86.

39. Bhavani SV, Carey KA, Gilbert ER, et al. Identifying novel sepsis subphenotypes using temperature trajectories. Am J Respir Crit Care Med 2019;200(3):327–35.

40. Perizes EN, Chong G, Sanchez-Pinto LN. Derivation and validation of vasoactive inotrope score trajectory groups in critically ill children with shock. Pediatr Crit Care Med 2022. https://doi.org/10.1097/PCC.0000000000003070.

41. Xu Z, Mao C, Su C, et al. Sepsis subphenotyping based on organ dysfunction trajectory. Crit Care 2022;26(1):197.

42. Bhavani SV, Verhoef PA, Maier CL, et al. Coronavirus disease 2019 temperature trajectories correlate with hyperinflammatory and hypercoagulable subphenotypes. Crit Care Med 2022;50(2):212–23.

43. Bhavani SV, Huang ES, Verhoef PA, et al. Novel temperature trajectory subphenotypes in COVID-19. Chest 2020;158(6):2436–9.

44. Bhavani SV, Wolfe KS, Hrusch CL, et al. Temperature trajectory subphenotypes correlate with immune responses in patients with sepsis. Crit Care Med 2020; 48(11):1645–53.

45. Bongers KS, Chanderraj R, Woods RJ, et al. The gut microbiome modulates body temperature both in sepsis and health. Am J Respir Crit Care Med 2022. https://doi.org/10.1164/rccm.202201-0161OC.

46. Maslove DM, Elbers PWG, Clermont G. Artificial intelligence in telemetry: what clinicians should know. Intensive Care Med 2021;47(2):150–3.

47. Nemati S, Holder A, Razmi F, et al. An interpretable machine learning model for accurate prediction of sepsis in the ICU. Crit Care Med 2018;46(4):547–53.

48. Kamaleswaran R, Akbilgic O, Hallman MA, et al. Applying artificial intelligence to identify physiomarkers predicting severe sepsis in the PICU. Pediatr Crit Care Med 2018;19(10):e495–503.

49. Griffin MP, Moorman JR. Abnormal heart rate variability precedes the clinical diagnosis of late-onset neonatal sepsis. Pediatric Research 1999;200A. https://doi.org/10.1203/00006450-199904020-01187.

50. Chambers DA, Feero WG, Khoury MJ. Convergence of implementation science, precision medicine, and the learning health care system: a new model for biomedical research. JAMA 2016;315(18):1941–2.

51. Villar J, Ferrando C, Martínez D, et al. Dexamethasone treatment for the acute respiratory distress syndrome: a multicentre, randomised controlled trial. Lancet Respir Med 2020;8(3):267–76.

52. Goligher EC, Costa ELV, Yarnell CJ, et al. Effect of lowering Vt on mortality in acute respiratory distress syndrome varies with respiratory system elastance. Am J Respir Crit Care Med 2021;203(11):1378–85.

53. Morris JA Jr, Norris PR, Waitman LR, et al. Adrenal insufficiency, heart rate variability, and complex biologic systems: a study of 1,871 critically ill trauma patients. J Am Coll Surg 2007;204(5):885–92 [discussion: 892–3].

54. Badke CM, Carroll MS, Weese-Mayer DE, et al. Association Between Heart Rate Variability and Inflammatory Biomarkers in Critically Ill Children. Pediatr Crit Care Med 2022;23(6):e289–94.

55. Badke CM, Swigart L, Carroll MS, et al. Autonomic nervous system dysfunction is associated with re-hospitalization in pediatric septic shock survivors. Front Pediatr 2021;9:745844.

56. Goligher EC, Telias I, Sahetya SK, et al. Physiology is vital to precision medicine in acute respiratory distress syndrome and sepsis. Am J Respir Crit Care Med 2022;206(1):14–6.

57. Cabrini L, Landoni G, Antonelli M, et al. Critical care in the near future: patient-centered, beyond space and time boundaries. Minerva Anestesiol 2015.

58. Vegesna A, Tran M, Angelaccio M, et al. Remote patient monitoring via non-invasive digital technologies: a systematic review. Telemed J E Health 2017; 23(1):3–17.

59. Xu S, Jayaraman A, Rogers JA. Skin sensors are the future of health care. Nature 2019;571(7765):319–21.

60. Lee SP, Ha G, Wright DE, et al. Highly flexible, wearable, and disposable cardiac biosensors for remote and ambulatory monitoring. NPJ Digit Med 2018;1:2.

61. Heikenfeld J, Jajack A, Feldman B, et al. Accessing analytes in biofluids for peripheral biochemical monitoring. Nat Biotechnol 2019;37(4):407–19.

62. Wu W, Haick H. Materials and wearable devices for autonomous monitoring of physiological markers. Adv Mater 2018;30(41):e1705024.

63. Wong HR, Caldwell JT, Cvijanovich NZ, et al. Prospective clinical testing and experimental validation of the Pediatric Sepsis Biomarker Risk Model. Sci Transl Med 2019;11(518). https://doi.org/10.1126/scitranslmed.aax9000.

64. Stanski NL, Stenson EK, Cvijanovich NZ, et al. PERSEVERE biomarkers predict severe acute kidney injury and renal recovery in pediatric septic shock. Am J Respir Crit Care Med 2020;201(7):848–55.

65. Lautz AJ, Wong HR, Ryan TD, et al. Pediatric sepsis biomarker risk model biomarkers and estimation of myocardial dysfunction in pediatric septic shock. Pediatr Crit Care Med 2021. https://doi.org/10.1097/PCC.0000000000002830.

66. Atreya MR, Cvijanovich NZ, Fitzgerald JC, et al. Integrated PERSEVERE and endothelial biomarker risk model predicts death and persistent MODS in pediatric septic shock: a secondary analysis of a prospective observational study. Crit Care 2022;26(1):210.

67. Bose SN, Greenstein JL, Fackler JC, et al. Early prediction of multiple organ dysfunction in the pediatric intensive care unit. Front Pediatr 2021;9:711104.

68. Stanski NL, Wong HR. Prognostic and predictive enrichment in sepsis. Nat Rev Nephrol 2020;16(1):20–31.

69. Wong HR, Cvijanovich N, Lin R, et al. Identification of pediatric septic shock subclasses based on genome-wide expression profiling. BMC Med 2009;7:34.

70. Wong HR, Cvijanovich NZ, Anas N, et al. Developing a clinically feasible personalized medicine approach to pediatric septic shock. Am J Respir Crit Care Med 2015;191(3):309–15.

71. Wong HR, Hart KW, Lindsell CJ, et al. External corroboration that corticosteroids may be harmful to septic shock endotype A patients. Crit Care Med 2021;49(1): e98–101.

72. Yehya N, Thomas NJ, Wong HR. Evidence of endotypes in pediatric acute hypoxemic respiratory failure caused by sepsis. Pediatr Crit Care Med 2019;20(2): 110–2.

73. Yehya N, Varisco BM, Thomas NJ, et al. Peripheral blood transcriptomic sub-phenotypes of pediatric acute respiratory distress syndrome. Crit Care 2020; 24(1):681.

74. Scicluna BP, van Vught LA, Zwinderman AH, et al. Classification of patients with sepsis according to blood genomic endotype: a prospective cohort study. Lancet Respir Med 2017;5(10):816–26.

75. Sweeney TE, Azad TD, Donato M, et al. Unsupervised analysis of transcriptomics in bacterial sepsis across multiple datasets reveals three robust clusters. Crit Care Med 2018;46(6):915–25.

76. Sweeney TE, Liesenfeld O, Wacker J, et al. Validation of inflammopathic, adaptive, and coagulopathic sepsis endotypes in coronavirus disease 2019. Crit Care Med 2021;49(2):e170–8.

77. Binnie A, Walsh CJ, Hu P, et al. Epigenetic profiling in severe sepsis: a pilot study of DNA methylation profiles in critical illness. Crit Care Med 2020;48(2): 142–50.

78. Lorente-Pozo S, Navarrete P, Garzón MJ, et al. DNA methylation analysis to unravel altered genetic pathways underlying early onset and late onset neonatal sepsis. A Pilot Study. Front Immunol 2021;12.

79. Miao H, Chen S, Ding R. Evaluation of the molecular mechanisms of sepsis using proteomics. Front Immunol 2021;12:733537.

80. Shubin NJ, Navalkar K, Sampson D, et al. Serum protein changes in pediatric sepsis patients identified with an aptamer-based multiplexed proteomic approach. Crit Care Med 2020;48(1):e48–57.

81. Mecatti GC, Messias MCF, de Oliveira Carvalho P. Lipidomic profile and candidate biomarkers in septic patients. Lipids Health Dis 2020;19(1):68.

82. Maile MD, Standiford TJ, Engoren MC, et al. Associations of the plasma lipidome with mortality in the acute respiratory distress syndrome: a longitudinal cohort study. Respiratory Research 2018. https://doi.org/10.1186/s12931-018-0758-3.

83. Wu J, Cyr A, Gruen DS, et al. Lipidomic signatures align with inflammatory patterns and outcomes in critical illness. Nat Commun 2022;13(1):6789.

84. Metwaly SM, Winston BW. Systems biology ARDS research with a focus on metabolomics. Metabolites 2020;207. https://doi.org/10.3390/metabo10050207.

85. Grunwell JR, Rad MG, Stephenson ST, et al. Cluster analysis and profiling of airway fluid metabolites in pediatric acute hypoxemic respiratory failure. Sci Rep 2021;11(1):23019.

86. Ahern DJ, Ai Z, Ainsworth M, et al. A blood atlas of COVID-19 defines hallmarks of disease severity and specificity. Cell 2022;185(5). 916–38.e58.

87. Ruan X, Ye Y, Cheng W, et al. Multi-omics integrative analysis of lung adenocarcinoma: an in silico profiling for precise medicine. Frontiers in Medicine 2022. https://doi.org/10.3389/fmed.2022.894338.

88. Mao K, Zhao Y, Ding B, et al. Integrative analysis of multi-omics data-identified key genes With KLRC3 as the core in a gene regulatory network related to immune phenotypes in lung adenocarcinoma. Frontiers in Genetics 2022. https://doi.org/10.3389/fgene.2022.810193.

89. Reyes M, Filbin MR, Bhattacharyya RP, et al. An immune cell signature of bacterial sepsis. Nat Med 2020-3;26(3):333–40.

90. Newman AM, Liu CL, Green MR, et al. Robust enumeration of cell subsets from tissue expression profiles. Nat Methods 2015;12(5):453–7.

91. Santacruz CA, Pereira AJ, Celis E, et al. Which multicenter randomized controlled trials in critical care medicine have shown reduced mortality? A systematic review. Crit Care Med 2019;47(12):1680–91.
92. Wenzel RP, Edmond MB. Septic shock—evaluating another failed treatment. N Engl J Med 2012;2122–4.
93. Chaudhary K, Vaid A, Duffy Á, et al. Utilization of deep learning for subphenotype identification in sepsis-associated acute kidney injury. Clin J Am Soc Nephrol 2020;15(11):1557–65.
94. Sinha P, Calfee CS, Cherian S, et al. Prevalence of phenotypes of acute respiratory distress syndrome in critically ill patients with COVID-19: a prospective observational study. Lancet Respir Med 2020;8(12):1209–18.
95. Sinha P, Delucchi KL, McAuley DF, et al. Development and validation of parsimonious algorithms to classify acute respiratory distress syndrome phenotypes: a secondary analysis of randomised controlled trials. Lancet Respir Med 2020; 8(3):247–57.
96. Sinha P, Churpek MM, Calfee CS. Machine learning classifier models can identify acute respiratory distress syndrome phenotypes using readily available clinical data. Am J Respir Crit Care Med 2020;202(7):996–1004.
97. Maddali MV, Churpek M, Pham T, et al. Validation and utility of ARDS subphenotypes identified by machine-learning models using clinical data: an observational, multicohort, retrospective analysis. Lancet Respir Med 2022;10(4): 367–77.
98. Sanchez-Pinto LN, Dziorny AC. From bedside to bytes and back: data quality and standardization for research, quality improvement, and clinical decision support in the era of electronic health records. Pediatr Crit Care Med 2020;780–1.
99. Thomason J. Big tech, big data and the new world of digital health. Global Health Journal 2021;165–8. https://doi.org/10.1016/j.glohj.2021.11.003.
100. Kahn MG, Callahan TJ, Barnard J, et al. A harmonized data quality assessment terminology and framework for the secondary use of electronic health record data. EGEMS (Wash DC) 2016;4(1):1244.
101. Liaw S-T, Guo JGN, Ansari S, et al. Quality assessment of real-world data repositories across the data life cycle: a literature review. J Am Med Inform Assoc 2021;28(7):1591–9.
102. Beaulieu-Jones BK, Lavage DR, Snyder JW, et al. Characterizing and managing missing structured data in electronic health records: data analysis. JMIR Med Inform 2018;6(1):e11.
103. Pajouheshnia R, van Smeden M, Peelen LM, et al. How variation in predictor measurement affects the discriminative ability and transportability of a prediction model. J Clin Epidemiol 2019;105:136–41.
104. Hripcsak G, Schuemie MJ, Madigan D, et al. Drawing reproducible conclusions from observational clinical data with OHDSI. Yearb Med Inform 2021;30(1): 283–9.
105. Kush RD, Warzel D, Kush MA, et al. FAIR data sharing: the roles of common data elements and harmonization. J Biomed Inform 2020;107:103421.
106. Braunstein ML. SMART on FHIR. Health Informatics on FHIR: How HL7's New API Is Transforming Healthcare 2018:205–225. https://doi.org/10.1007/978-3-319-93414-3_10.
107. Quiroz JC, Chard T, Sa Z, et al. Extract, transform, load framework for the conversion of health databases to OMOP. PLoS One 2022;17(4):e0266911.

108. Gordon WJ, Mandl KD. The 21st century cures act: a competitive apps market and the risk of innovation blocking. J Med Internet Res 2020;22(12):e24824.
109. Brant EB, Kennedy JN, King AJ, et al. Developing a shared sepsis data infrastructure: a systematic review and concept map to FHIR. NPJ Digit Med 2022;5(1):44.
110. Menikoff J, Kaneshiro J, Pritchard I. The common rule, updated. N Engl J Med 2017;613–5. https://doi.org/10.1056/nejmp1700736.
111. Mandl KD, Kohane IS. Data citizenship under the 21st century cures act. N Engl J Med 2020;382(19):1781–3.
112. Angus DC, Berry S, Lewis RJ, et al. The REMAP-CAP (Randomized embedded multifactorial adaptive platform for community-acquired pneumonia) study. rationale and design. Ann Am Thorac Soc 2020;17(7):879–91.
113. Bates DW, Gawande AA. Improving safety with information technology. N Engl J Med 2003;348(25):2526–34.

Predictive Modeling Using Artificial Intelligence and Machine Learning Algorithms on Electronic Health Record Data
Advantages and Challenges

Michael J. Patton, BA[a,b,*], Vincent X. Liu, MD, MS[c,*]

KEYWORDS

- Critical care outcome prediction • Machine learning • Sepsis prediction
- Mortality prediction • Data science • Clinical informatics
- Model performance evaluation • Electronic medical record analysis

KEY POINTS

- Rapid adoption of electronic health record systems and concurrent innovations in artificial intelligence and machine learning (AI/ML) produced an exponential increase in critical care outcome prediction research.
- ML algorithms using novel data elements like medical free text and temporal laboratory/vital trend data have superior performance.
- Despite recent innovations in ML, 20-year-old outcome prediction scoring systems are only modestly outperformed by novel ML methods.
- Clinical implementation of AI/ML systems for prospective outcome prediction remains a challenge.

OVERVIEW

Starting in 2008, the adoption of electronic health records (EHR) in US hospitals has grown exponentially from 9% to 96% of hospitals, while also exhibiting substantial uptake in ambulatory settings (**Fig. 1**, lines).[1] As structured and unstructured clinical data, laboratory measurements, medical images, sensor readings, and multi-omic test results have gradually become digitized, vast quantities of data are now available

[a] Medical Scientist Training Program, Heersink School of Medicine, University of Alabama at Birmingham, Birmingham, AL, USA; [b] Hugh Kaul Precision Medicine Institute at the University of Alabama at Birmingham, 720 20th Street South, Suite 202, Birmingham, Alabama, 35233, USA; [c] Kaiser Permanente Division of Research, Oakland, CA, USA
* Corresponding author.
E-mail addresses: mjpatton@uab.edu (M.J.P.); vincent.x.liu@kp.org (V.X.L.)

Crit Care Clin 39 (2023) 647–673
https://doi.org/10.1016/j.ccc.2023.02.001
0749-0704/23/© 2023 Elsevier Inc. All rights reserved.

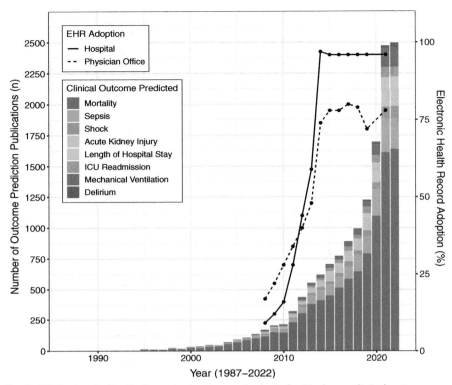

Fig. 1. US Electronic Health Record adoption and selected critical care clinical outcome prediction publications from 1987 to 2022. (*Data from* 1. National Trends in Hospital and Physician Adoption of Electronic Health Records from the American Hospital Association (AHA) Annual Survey Information Technology Supplement, 2008-present |HealthIT.gov. Available at: https://www.healthit.gov/data/quickstats/national-trends-hospital-and-physician-adoption-electronic-health-records.Accessed October 30, 2022.)

for analysis. Concurrent innovations in computing architecture and algorithms have made rapid consumption of health data feasible and a powerful engine for clinical innovation.[2,3] In critical care research, as in other fields, the net convergence of these trends has resulted in a tremendous increase in the number of publications related to outcomes prediction.

Although critical care research already had a rich and storied history with mortality prediction, the emerging availability of large-scale data has driven expansion into assessment of more diverse outcomes, including sepsis, acute kidney injury, and delirium, among others (see **Fig. 1**, bars). Similarly, the availability of novel artificial intelligence and machine learning algorithms (AI/ML) has pushed researchers beyond traditional regression-based approaches as they seek to improve prediction accuracy and model performance. In the following article, we explore the history of outcome prediction in the intensive care unit (ICU), the growing use of EHR data, and the rise of AI/ML in critical care in three sections: (1) a brief overview of AI/ML algorithms; (2) a review of outcome prediction scoring systems that preceded the use of AI/ML; and (3) selected case studies exhibiting the progress and challenges for AI/ML in ICU mortality and sepsis. Finally, we address the translation gap whereby promising in silico models fail to be implemented and proven effective in bedside clinical care settings.

ARTIFICIAL INTELLIGENCE AND MACHINE LEARNING ALGORITHMS

Broadly speaking, AI is focused on creating computer programs that can self-learn approaches to perform tasks, make decisions, or predict outcomes from data. ML describes a sub-discipline within AI that seeks to use algorithms to automatically derive insights from data. Much like human learning, AI/ML systems require repeated observations (data) and iteratively improving rules (algorithms) to learn. Take the example of a dropped glass shattering on the floor. Through repeated observations, a young child formulates an implicit "notion" of gravity; however, codifying the rules that govern these observations would only become an explicit "algorithm" when Newton's equation for gravitational force was described.[4] In the same way, the use of AI/ML in critical care and health care asks whether algorithms can identify and predict the underlying patterns present by examining repeated observations of patient encounters and treatments. In nearly all cases, these patterns have already begun to be identified through clinical experience and codified through some criteria. However, advances in AI/ML approaches seek to realize the promise of more timely, precise, and useful insights.

The most common AI/ML approaches used with EHR data include supervised and unsupervised ML. Supervised ML uses a labeled outcome for training an algorithm. For example, starting with a set of labeled outcomes (eg, hospital mortality, sepsis onset, delirium), supervised ML algorithms identify patterns based on inputs or features (eg, variables) to make predictions. Commonly used examples of supervised ML algorithms or 'models' include regression-based approaches (logistic, regularized [ridge, lasso, elastic net], and Cox regression), support vector machines, tree-based models (decision trees, random-forest, gradient-boosted machines), nearest neighbors, and artificial neural networks (recurrent, convolutional, or multi-layered architecture termed 'deep' learning networks). Promising approaches seek to further combine the most valuable information from each modeling approach in so-called 'ensemble modeling' that aggregates the predictions from several methods.[5–11]

In contrast to supervised ML, unsupervised ML models use data without a pre-defined outcome label and seek to categorize observations into similar groups by quantifying statistical relationships and patterns within the data features/variables. Because these approaches lack a pre-defined outcome, unsupervised ML is most often used to postulate novel subgroups, clusters, or phenotypes within a patient population or based on a clinical outcome (eg, subtypes of patients with septic shock).[12,13] Commonly used examples of unsupervised ML techniques include dimensionality reduction methods (eg, principal component analysis [PCA]) and clustering (consensus, k-means, and hierarchical clustering).[12,14–18]

Recent applications in critical care have further begun to explore a promising new methodology in AI/ML: reinforcement learning (RL). RL describes an algorithmic approach to generating optimal decisions through trial and error, so that desirable choices are 'rewarded', and undesirable choices are 'punished' within an overall reward function.[19] The application of RL to games (eg, Go, chess, video games) has allowed computers to rapidly acquire capabilities that rival, and even greatly exceed, human players, in part by gaining an incredible wealth of experience playing games repeatedly.[19] In many cases, entirely new strategies of game-play have emerged from these RL methodologies which have surprised human experts trained through traditional means. As a result, there is broad excitement about the potential for RL approaches to identify optimal treatment patterns for clinical decisions in critical care (eg, whether to use vasopressors or intravenous fluids for hypotension).[20]

OUTCOME PREDICTION BEFORE THE RISE OF MACHINE LEARNING

Before the swift adoption of EHRs and rise of ML in outcome prediction, four decades of research had already been dedicated to severity-of-illness scoring systems. These well-known scores have produced highly robust precursors with more recent updated models which seek to improve risk stratification and prediction in critical care. Historically, three major purposes of severity-of-illness have been identified. First, scoring systems have been used to adjust for cohort severity of illness.[21–24] In practice, randomized control trial managers can evaluate the balance of the control and treatment group severity-of-illness with a validated score.[25–28] In observational clinical research, these scores can be used with inferential statistical techniques (eg, matching, causal inference methods, or propensity scoring) to identify potentially causal effects of treatments on outcomes.[29,30]

A second use of severity-of-illness scoring systems has been to inform the operation, structure, and organization of ICU.[31] For example, scores can quantify the severity of illness within individual patients and across ICUs for health care system administrative planning, including resource allocation.[32,33] Severity scores are also used to assess ICU performance and compare the quality of care between different institutions through benchmarking evaluations.[34–37] These scores have also been used to estimate the impact of planned changes to an ICU, such as changes in staffing composition, shift duration, unit size, and clinical specialist coverage on patient outcomes.[38–41]

The third purpose of scoring systems has been to inform decisions about clinical care. In a small number of use cases, scores have been used to evaluate patient prognosis so that they could potentially assist patients, families, and medical providers in making decisions about ICU care.[31,42] In limited circumstances, scoring systems have also been used to assess the suitability of patients for interventions. For example, the Acute Physiology and Chronic Health Evaluation II (APACHE -II) score was used to assess sepsis patient candidacy for recombinant human–activated protein C (Drotrecogin Alfa) use.[43,44] Scores have also been used to characterize patient disease states. For example, an increase of two or more points in the Sequential (or Sepsis-related) Organ Failure Assessment (SOFA) score was incorporated as a key criterion in the revised consensus clinical definition of sepsis (Sepsis 3).[45,46]

In addition to these traditional uses of severity-of-illness scoring systems, the rise of ML in clinical outcomes research has found these traditional severity scores useful as performance benchmarks. For example, a 2016 study conducted by Churpek and colleagues trained a set of ML mortality prediction models (logistic regressions and a random forest [RF]) and bench-marked them against the Modified Early Warning score (MEWS), a well-described points-based severity-of-illness score.[47] Beyond benchmarking, severity scores are also now routinely treated as ML model features and are even directly integrated into models.[48–51]

The underlying design of many severity-of-illness scoring systems is quite similar because they tend to incorporate variables that are familiar to clinicians as key clinical and physiologic phenomena that are major predictors and, in some cases, causal determinants of mortality (**Table 1** for details selected system scoring criteria).[43,52,53] Associations have been reproduced repeatedly between features such as age, type of ICU admission, vital signs, neurologic function, respiratory dysfunction, renal

Table 1
Derivation of Select Severity-of-Illness Scores

Scoring System	Total Score	Variables Required for Score (Total Points)	
APACHE-II *Acute Physiology and Chronic Health Evaluation* (Knaus et al. 1985) Study Size: 5030 patients	71 total points	Demographic (0–6) • Age (0–6)	Chronic Health (0–7) • Nonoperative or emergency postoperative (0–5) • Elective postoperative (0–2)
		Physiologic (0–58) • Temperature (0–4) • Mean Arterial Pressure (0, 2–4) • Heart Rate (0, 2–4) • Respiratory Rate (0–1, 3–4) • Pao$_2$[a] (0, 2–4) • Arterial pH (0–1, 3–4)	• Serum Sodium (0–4) • Serum Potassium (0–1, 3–4) • Serum Creatinine (0, 2–4) • Hematocrit (0–2, 4) • White Blood Cell Count (0–2, 4) • Glasgow Coma Scale (1–15)
SAPS-II *Simplified Acute Physiology Score* (le Gall et al. 1993) Study Size: 12,997 patients	161 total points	Demographics, Chronic Health, and Admission Type (0–43) • Age (0–18) • Metastatic Cancer (9) or Hematologic Malignancy (10) or HIV Diagnosis (17)	• Scheduled surgical (0) or Medical admission (6) or Unscheduled surgical (8)
		Physiologic (0–118) • Heart Rate (0–11) • Systolic Blood Pressure (0–13) • Temperature (0–3) • Pao$_2$/Fio$_2$ Ratio (0–11) • Urine Output (0–11) • Serum Urea Nitrogen (0–10)	• White Blood Cell Count (0–12) • Serum Potassium (0–3) • Serum Sodium (0–3) • Serum Bicarbonate (0–6) • Bilirubin (0–9) • Glasgow Coma Scale (0–26)
SOFA *Sepsis-Related Organ Failure Assessment* (Vincent et al. 1996) Study Size 1643 patients	24 total points	Physiologic (0–24) • Pao$_2$/Fio$_2$ (0–2); with respiratory support (2–4) • Platelet Count (0–4) • Bilirubin (0–4) • Mean Arterial Pressure (0–1); with increasing vasopressor (2–4) • Glasgow Coma Scale (0–4) • Creatinine (0–2); decreased urine output (3–4)	

[a] Serum Bicarbonate if blood-gas data unavailable (0–1, 3–4).

dysfunction, and the presence of specific comorbid conditions and clinically meaningful ICU outcomes. Several other variables which describe additional aspects of physiologic derangement, organ dysfunction, and/or the context of ICU admission (eg, surgery vs medical admission, pre-ICU length of stay, planned or emergent need for critical care, diagnosis, cardiopulmonary resuscitation) have also become incorporated within scoring systems through iterative updates.[54]

The most well-known scoring system, APACHE-II score from 1985, uses age, type of admission, chronic health evaluation, and 12 physiologic features within the first 24 hours after ICU admission to predict hospital mortality (see **Table 1**).[43] The initial score was based on data from 5030 ICU admission across 13 hospitals and, despite its age, it remains an industry standard for its quantification of the severity of illness. APACHE-III followed a similar approach to model development and was based on 17,440 admissions in 40 US hospitals published in 1991 with 18 variables and a total score ranging from 0 to 300.[55] Several aspects of the APACHE-III were made proprietary which may have curtailed its uptake and use outside of proprietary systems while generating some controversy in the ICU research community. The APACHE-IV, published in 2006, was developed based on 129 variables derived from the worst values within the first 24 hours of ICU admission on a sample of greater than 100,000 patients from 104 ICUs in the United States and exhibited an AUROC of 0.88. Supplemental Figure 1[16,56]

The Simplified Acute Physiology Score II (SAPS-II) was developed using a sample of 13,152 admissions from 12 European and North American countries in 1993 (see **Table 1**).[52] In contrast to APACHE, the SAPS-II is not disease-specific and has an explicit goal of quick calculation early after a patient's ICU admission.[52] SAPS-II uses 17 variables selected by logistic regression including 12 physiologic variables, age, type of admission (medical, scheduled vs unscheduled surgical), and three co-morbid conditions (metastatic cancer, Acquired immunodeficiency syndrome [AIDS], and hematologic malignancy). Because the APACHE scoring systems were developed in US cohorts, the SAPS is often used more commonly in Europe and includes customized models for different geographies.

The Sequential (or Sepsis-related) Organ Failure Assessment (SOFA) score is the most well-known of the organ dysfunction scores and was originally developed in 1994 to quantify a continuum of morbidity in 1643 critically ill patients in 16 countries (see **Table 1**).[53] The SOFA score is composed of six organ sub-scores (respiratory, cardiovascular, hepatic, coagulation, neurologic, renal), each graded from 0 to 4 according to the degree of dysfunction. Although the score was primarily designed to describe organ dysfunction, subsequent studies have validated its association with mortality, with studies confirming a strong correlation between the mean or worst SOFA score over the course of an ICU admission with adverse outcomes.[57] Importantly, in the acute surge periods of the SARS-CoV-2 severe acute respiratory syndrome coronavirus 2 (SARS-CoV-2), the causative pathogen of Coronavirus disease 2019 (COVID-19) pandemic, SOFA scores were proposed, and also questioned, as a severity-of-illness metric that could help guide resource allocation (eg, mechanical ventilators, renal replacement therapy) under crisis conditions.[58]

PROGRESS AND CHALLENGES IN ARTIFICIAL INTELLIGENCE AND MACHINE LEARNING ALGORITHMS MODELING: MORTALITY OUTCOME PREDICTION

Between 1980 and 2000, successive iterations in severity scores have produced mortality prediction models that have exhibited improved model discrimination. For example, the APACHE-II exhibited an AUROC of 0.83 which improved to an AUROC of 0.90 in APACHE-III (**Fig. 2**).[43,59] From 2000 onward, pre-existing and newly altered scoring systems such as the National and Modified Early Warning Score (NEWS, AUROC = 0.89; MEWS = 0.73) and the quick SOFA score (qSOFA; a simplified version of the SOFA score, AUROC = 0.69) have been developed, proposed, and assessed for mortality prediction.[46,47,60,88-90] The Systemic Inflammatory Response Syndrome (SIRS) score, originally developed in 1992 for ICU infection detection and

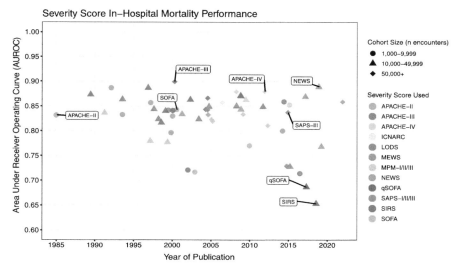

Fig. 2. In-Hospital Mortality Prediction With Severity Score Models. Severity score model performance for predicting in-hospital mortality for adult inpatient encounters from 1985 to 2022. Sequential Organ Failure Score (SOFA), quick SOFA (qSOFA), Systemic Inflammatory Response Syndrome (SIRS), Logistic Organ Dysfunction Score (LODS), Simplified Acute Physiology Score (SAPS), Modified Early Warning Score (MEWS), National Early Warning Score (NEWS), Mortality Prediction Model (MPM), Intensive Care National Audit and Research Center (ICNARC), Acute physiologic assessment and chronic health evaluation (APACHE). Data visualized was collected from references cited. (*Data from* Refs[7,43,47,52,55,56,59–87])

derived from less than 1000 ICU patients, has also been evaluated for mortality prediction, albeit with relatively poor performance (AUROC = 0.65).[47,91] Despite the large number of severity score mortality models and outcomes comparisons, the 1999 study conducted by Siro and colleagues exhibited the highest AUROC = 0.90 with the APACHE-III score.[59] Similar performance was observed in the Veteran's Affairs model developed by Render and colleagues in 2003 (AUROC = 0.88, **Fig. 3**) described more than two decades ago.[92]

Historically, ML methods for mortality prediction have predominantly used regression-based techniques. However, the widespread adoption of EHRs in the United States has spurred an increase in the volume and diversity of ML techniques used. From 2015 forward, numerous ML techniques have been applied to the mortality outcome including gradient-boosted decision trees, Bayesian networks, RF, artificial neural networks (ANNs), along with logistic regressions and have been reported as showing AUROCs $\geq$0.90.[6,51,82,93] In the following section, we evaluate select examples that highlight some of the challenges that face ML outcome models and suggest areas of novel improvement in the field.

An exciting development has been the use of novel features beyond structured EHR data elements, such as clinical documentation. For example, Marafino and colleagues assessed the impact of multiple clinical measurements along with medical free text from clinician notes on in-hospital mortality prediction using a large ICU cohort from the University of California at San Francisco (UCSF; n = 15,666) and two separate external validation cohorts (Mills-Peninsula Medical Center, n = 38,624; Beth Israel Deaconess Medical Center, n = 46,906).[6] In the study, three different logistic regression models were trained, including (1) a baseline model (using minimum and

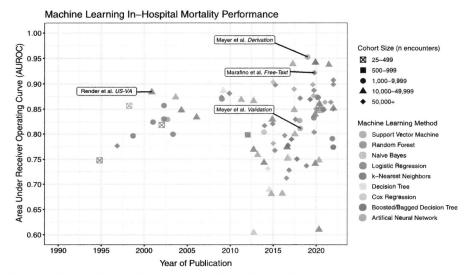

Fig. 3. In-Hospital Mortality Prediction with ML Models. ML model performance for predicting in-hospital mortality for adult inpatient encounters (ICU and general admission) from 1990 to 2022. Specific studies are highlighted, with "Derivation" and "Validation" labels referring to study-specific training/testing data and external validation data, respectively. "Free-Text" labels refer to newer ML studies that have incorporated these respective datatypes as model features. Abbreviations: United States Veterans Association data (US-VA). Data visualized was collected from references cited. (*Data from* Refs[6,7,45,48–51,75,82,84,92–131])

maximum laboratory and vitals measurements); (2) a trajectory model (using coefficient for linear trend of a lab or vitals measurement); and (3) a natural language processing (NLP)-augmented trajectory model (addition of unstructured text describing patient condition). Using data collected within 24 hours of ICU admission, model performance improved significantly from the baseline model (AUROC = 0.83) with the addition of trajectory features (AUROC = 0.89) and NLP-augmented features (AUROC = 0.92).[6] A particular strength of the study was the external validation of the models and approaches that allowed for an assessment of institutional differences in laboratory measurement time and clinical documentation that could have impacted model performance.

Another key aspect of the Marafino study was the use of 'trajectory' data (eg, features for linear trends and last-minus-first-values) derived from each set of laboratory measurements gathered within 24 hours of ICU admission. The use of trajectory data resulted in consistently higher performance (AUROC ≥ 0.10) than the baseline model. The use of summary statistics and derivative features of individual features has also been tested in many other studies that have similarly revealed that trends of data elements can significantly enhance overall model performance. This strategy quantifies early trajectories among ICU patients, including those who exhibit: (1) an initially poor prognosis with steady recovery; (2) an initially good prognosis that steadily declines; (3) a persistently poor prognosis; and (4) patients with drastic variation in the laboratory or vital measurements that regain stability and recover. These trajectory features, when coupled with clinical documentation features, produced the highest performance. Interestingly, an exploration of clinical documentation found that terms indicative of acute organ failure ("sepsis", "shock", "coagulopathy"), complex interventions ("ECMO" [extra-corporal membrane oxygenation]), and poor clinical exam signs ("fixed pupils", "gag reflex", and "ascites") had the greatest impact on model performance. The overall implications of this study are two-fold. First, the prognostic signs used by clinicians in documentation can be reliably identified and used as informative features for outcomes assessment. Second, even with a standard regression-based approach, improvements through feature engineering of temporal or longitudinal variables can still substantially improve performance.

Generalizable model performance in external settings remains a challenge in AI/ML broadly with fewer studies that routinely validate models in independent external, compared with internal, datasets. In a 2018 study by Meyer and colleagues, a recurrent neural network (RNN; a type of ANN model) and a SAPS-II-adapted model were applied to predict mortality in a large cohort of cardiac surgery encounters with ICU admissions in which 11,492 (25%) encounters met inclusion criteria.[82] However, to normalize the dataset to maintain a mortality rate of 50% in each group, a substantial number of potential training observations were excluded. After evaluation of the internal test dataset, the authors reported higher performance for the RNN (accuracy = 0.88, PPV = 0.90, NPV = 0.86, sensitivity = 0.85, specificity = 0.91, F1 = 0.88, and AUROC = 0.95) compared with the SAPS-II model (accuracy = 0.71, PPV = 0.68, NPV = 0.74, sensitivity = 0.78, specificity = 0.68, F1 = 0.73, and AUROC = 0.71) on all metrics.

In external validation, 5898 encounters from the Medical Information Mart for Intensive Care-III (MIMIC-III) dataset were used.[132] Despite the particular care taken to find similar encounters in the MIMIC-III dataset to those in their original sample, the authors documented a significant decline in RNN (0.81) and SAPS-II (0.63) AUROC values (see **Fig. 3**, Meyer and colleagues Validation). Importantly, when the authors performed a supplemental evaluation of the RNN and SAPS-II models with the native mortality rates in both the training (6.2% mortality rate) and MIMIC-III validation data (1.3% mortality rate), they found that the performance of the RNN on the unadjusted test data and MIMIC-III validation set was significantly lower (AUROC 0.78 and 0.81, respectively). This highlights a theme demonstrating the challenges of maintaining generalizable performance in external datasets in different settings, as well as the limitations of even advanced AI/ML modeling approaches to overcome brittle performance across datasets.

PROGRESS AND CHALLENGES IN ARTIFICIAL INTELLIGENCE AND MACHINE LEARNING ALGORITHMSMODELING: SEPSIS OUTCOME PREDICTION

Historical accounts of sepsis (from the Greek word "sepo," meaning "to rot") have been documented in ancient cultures dating as far back as 4000 BCE.[133] Despite centuries of documented cases and the rise of microbial research in the 1800s, the first multi-national effort to clinically define sepsis and related terminology was conducted in 1991 and published the following year.[91,134] Although there is a rich history of research in sepsis outcomes, unlike mortality prediction, comparing the performance of sepsis risk assessment models research is significantly more complex because of substantial changes in the clinical criteria used in definitions of sepsis that have occurred over the past 30 years. For example, because the cohort characteristics and outcomes of patients identified by the 1991 Sepsis-1 SIRS criteria, compared with the expanded criteria enumerated in Sepsis-2[135] or the Sepsis-3 definition (including a ≥2 point SOFA score increase) differs, comparisons are of variable utility.[46] Additional definitions, including those in use by the US Center for Disease Control or Center for Medicare and Medicaid Services (CMS) have also produced thematically similar, but operationally distinct, sepsis criterion for surveillance studies.[136,137] To reflect this evolution, we examine sepsis models predicting several outcomes including sepsis, bacteremia, and septic shock.[46,91,135]

Another distinction, compared with mortality prediction, is that many serum biomarkers have been evaluated for sepsis outcomes prediction (**Fig. 4**). The predictive performance of these biomarkers has been described as ranging widely from a nearly perfect AUROC ($\geq$0.95) to no better than random chance (AUROC $\geq$0.50).[153,168,178] Broadly speaking, since 2000, the highest-performing blood-based biomarkers include procalcitonin and C-reactive protein (CRP). However, neither has been assessed with the sample size and patient diversity present in the SIRS, SOFA, and qSOFA severity scores studies, in part, because these biomarkers are assessed during clinical care in only a relatively minority of all infected or septic patients (outside of more recent clinical experience with COVID-19, in which CRP values are used to assess patient candidacy for certain treatments).

Over the past two decades, along with the treatment guidelines published by the Surviving Sepsis Campaign, there has been a profound emphasis on earlier identification and treatment of sepsis. This has been driven by accumulated observational studies assessing that even a single hour's delay in antimicrobial treatment in sepsis conferred a significant increase in the likelihood of hospital mortality.[181,182] Starting in 2003, and continuing on into 2021, each campaign meeting has produced and published best practice recommendations for the management of sepsis and septic shock.[181,183–186] These observations have had a profound impact on the sepsis prediction field, pushing researchers to develop and test ML models that could identify sepsis hours before the onset of severe sepsis or septic shock.

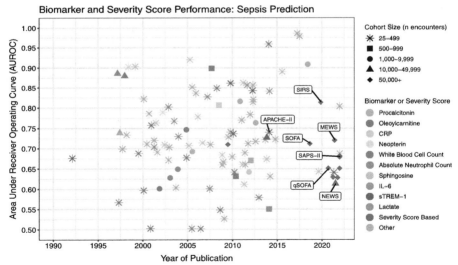

Fig. 4. Sepsis Prediction with Blood-Based Biomarker and Severity-of-Illness Scoring Systems Models. Blood-based biomarker (top-10 AUROCs color labeled with remainder denoted as "Other") and severity score model performance for predicting sepsis, septic shock, and bacteremia in pediatric and adult hospital encounters from 1990 to 2022. Abbreviations: C-reactive protein (CRP), Interleukin-6 (IL-6), Soluble Triggering Receptor Expressed on Myeloid Cells-1 (sTREM-1), Sequential Organ Failure Score (SOFA), quick SOFA (qSOFA), Systemic Inflammatory Response Syndrome (SIRS), Simplified Acute Physiology Score (SAPS), Modified Early Warning Score (MEWS), National Early Warning Score (NEWS), Acute physiologic assessment and chronic health evaluation (APACHE). Data visualized were collected from references cited. (*Data from* Refs[11,138–180])

In 2016, Desautels and colleagues trained a regularized elastic net regression model (InSight) to predict sepsis onset using 20,276 encounters (11% septic, n = 2257) selected from the publicly available MIMIC-III dataset.[187] Based on a relatively simple set of eight model features derived solely from vitals obtained at the bedside (systolic blood pressure, pulse pressure, respiration rate, heart rate, SpO_2, body temperature, and a Glasgow Coma Score), the authors reported that their model produced an AUROC of 0.88 and an area under the precision recall curve (AUPRC) of 0.60 for sepsis occurring at any time during a hospitalization (**Fig. 5**). However, when the performance was evaluated for a more clinically actionable time frame (within the next 4 hours), the model performance fell sharply (AUROC = 0.75, AUPRC = 0.28; see **Fig. 5**) and was not substantially different from the simpler points-based MEWS score (AUROC = 0.73, AUPRC = 0.25) developed in the late 1990s.

Over the past 5 years, a large number of models have been reported for predicting the onset of sepsis. For example, the Artificial Intelligence Sepsis Expert (AISE) model by Nemati and colleagues utilized a custom regularized Weilbull-Cox regression to predict sepsis at 4-, 6-, 8-, and 12-hour time-points before onset (with time-zero defined as the time patients met the sepsis criteria). The time-to-event approach can enhance model performance for a time-sensitive outcome through censoring which allows for the removal of patients who were transferred out of the ICU or died before a septic outcome, rather than labeling them as negative sepsis events. Beyond the modeling approach, AISE also expanded its feature set to include 57 other high-resolution dynamic features (time-series calculations of vitals), 10 clinical (all of which are in the AISE model), 30 laboratory measurements, and 19 demographic, medical history, and treatment features. The AISE model exhibited AUROC values of 0.87 (training) and 0.82 (independent test).

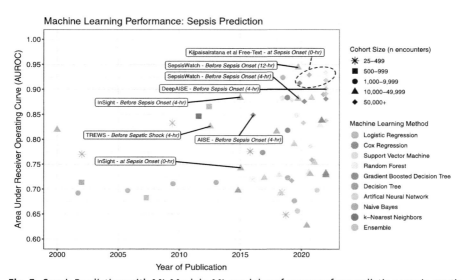

Fig. 5. Sepsis Prediction with ML Models. ML model performance for predicting sepsis, septic shock, and bacteremia in pediatric and adult hospital encounters from 1990 to 2022. Specific studies are highlighted with the author describing the name of the ML model. "Free-Text" label refers to newer ML studies that have incorporated this datatype as a model feature. Abbreviations: Artificial Intelligence Sepsis Expert (AISE), Targeted Real-time Early Warning Score (TREWS). (*Data from* Refs[11,117,138,152,154,155,187–210])

DeepAISE, the 2021 artificial neural network successor to AISE, expanded the scope of training and testing data to three ICU cohorts from Emory University (n = 25,820 encounters, 1445 septic 6%), the University of California San Diego University (UCSD; n = 18,752 encounters, 1073 septic 5.7%), and the publicly available MIMIC-III dataset (n = 40,473, 2276 septic 5.6%).[206] DeepAISE reported consistently high performance across all three datasets (Emory AUROC = 0.90, UCSD AUROC = 0.88, MIMIC-III AUROC = 0.87). The study also confirmed the importance of features comprising the SOFA and SIRS scores (heart rate, temperature, Glasgow Coma Score, and white blood cell count), whereby simulated missingness in these variables resulted in significant degradations in prediction performance.

The incorporation of clinical documentation has also been seen as promising for improving sepsis prediction through NLP approaches. For example, Kijpaisalratana and colleagues examined a cohort of 133,502 encounters (n = 1203 septic 1%) with RF, logistic regression, neural network, and gradient-boosted tree ML models with and without clinical documentation drawn from patient chief complaints and AUROCs ≥ 0.91 were reported for every model trained with free-text features. Although this study has not been externally validated, it confirms the broad interest in evaluating novel features, including free text, for improving early detection of sepsis within EHR data.

A critical future step for any ML-based predictive outcome model is implementation into live hospital EHRs and prospective validation on patients in real time. Already, several sepsis alerting and prediction systems have been embedded within EHR systems, with a growing number of subsequent reports that these systems are being deprecated or decommissioned due to clinician burden or frustration with the tools. The Targeted Real-time Early Warning Score (TREWS) was developed using an ensemble modeling approach with regularized logistic regression and a time-to-event Cox regression algorithm to evaluate the risk of septic shock at a given time post-admission.[138] A TREWS model modified for sepsis detection was subsequently implemented and evaluated at five hospital sites in the Maryland and Washington DC area. Physician interaction with the TREWS alert system resulted in a 1.85-hour reduction in median time to first antibiotic order and a 3.34% reduction in mortality for patients with suspected sepsis, although the cohort described in the study represented only a small fraction of the overall cohort in which the tool was deployed.[211]

In 2020, a Gaussian RNN model from Duke University called SepsisWatch reported an AUROC of 0.94 for 12-hour sepsis detection in a retrospective evaluation. These exciting results have laid the foundation for a prospective sepsis detection study (NCT:036556260), the results of which are not available at this time.[11] Although both of these tools using advanced AI/ML approaches are promising, lead investigators from TREWS and SepsisWatch studies have commented on the limited geographic implementation of their models. Recent attempts to tackle this limitation have been undertaken with the Epic Sepsis Model (ESM), which saw implementation in many US health systems, including several hospital sites in Michigan.[203] Overall, the performance of the ESM was heavily affected by the time horizon of data given to the model with an AUROC = 0.73 for 12-hour pre-sepsis detection and an AUROC = 0.80 with data from 3-hour post-sepsis detection.[203] However, concerns about the performance of ESM have been raised with suggestions that in one setting its performance was found to be 'wanting'.[212] At the same, when deployed prospectively, a randomized evaluation suggested it resulted in faster time to treatment as well as favorable improvements in mortality.[213] Epic is currently deploying a second version of ESM which customizes the model to each health system setting in which it is deployed, so that performance can be tuned to the local setting in which it will be used.

OVERCOMING THE 'TRANSLATION GAP' IN ARTIFICIAL INTELLIGENCE AND MACHINE LEARNING ALGORITHMS-DRIVEN EHR TOOLS

Although there is incredible enthusiasm about the role that AI/ML will play in improving health care delivery and patient outcomes, the clinical integration of these tools remains in a nascent stage today. Applying the 'technology hype cycle' framework to AI/ML in health care, it remains unclear if we are yet past the 'peak of inflated expectations', caught in the 'trough of disillusionment', or if we are now on the 'slope of enlightenment' and moving toward the 'plateau of productivity'.[214] Although the number of peer-reviewed studies applying AI/ML to EHR data in in silico experiments appears to be rising exponentially, there is a tremendous 'translation gap' in terms of evidence that such tools robustly improve outcomes in patients. If such models were drug products, it would give the appearance that the drug pipeline is very rich, although there would be a paucity of proven drug therapies available for treatment. Similarly, if these models were laboratory or diagnostic tests, despite their promise, there would be very few that were available to reliably improve diagnostic excellence.

Many factors have contributed to this 'translation gap' that still needs to be overcome. The incredible scale of data, computing power, and innovative algorithms available today with relatively easy access have made the process of producing AI/ML models nearly trivial, compared with the painstaking efforts of prior decades. For example, highly impactful open-source ICU data resources like the MIMIC program, as well as other emerging data collaboratives, have unlocked tremendous opportunities for model development. These efforts should be celebrated and replicated, however, model developers tapping into these data are often siloed and lack critical insight into the clinical context of model deployment.

Understanding the context into which a model is placed within a clinical or operational workflow is incredibly important. For example, one of the reasons that sepsis alerting systems and risk scores have been decommissioned is because they often alert after a clinician has already identified a patient that is at risk for sepsis. Thus, the alerting system only serves to burden the clinician with an unnecessary distraction while also often requiring a 'hard stop' (ie, a mandatory action in the EHR that stops the clinician from moving forward in their work) in response. If that same alert were to come at a different time point in the clinical workflow—in sepsis, even minutes earlier in clinical care perhaps—the sustainability and effectiveness of the tool might be dramatically different.

Grasping the concept that a predictive model needs to be seamlessly integrated into a clinical workflow may also change a modeler's approach to assessing model performance. Although the literature is rife with examples of an 'arms race' for improved AUROC values, a focus on reducing clinical burden while achieving acceptable performance would likely accelerate actual model instantiation into clinical settings. For example, at the specific risk threshold in which clinicians are making decisions (ie, 'we will keep patients for observation if their risk of myocardial infarction is anything >1%'), the incremental loss of discrimination by moving from an advanced modeling approach like neural networks to simpler models like regression may not impact the models' effect on outcomes in a significant manner. Thus, performance measures should be reported at the specific risk thresholds relevant to clinical decision-making in context, rather than across the entire range of operating characteristics, with quantification of incremental gains or losses in performance between modeling approaches. In many cases, starting clinical implementation at a very high-risk threshold (which nearly always favors specificity over sensitivity) will improve the clinical acceptability of a tool at the implementation outset, with the opportunity to gradually dial back the threshold as the model's impact on care and clinical burden are familiarized and accepted.

These considerations highlight two other limitations in today's environment. First, the data infrastructure and computing platforms for moving from modeling to instantiation to deployment to maintenance are insufficient for long-term model sustainability. Few groups have effectively crossed from modeling to clinical deployment, which is critical for examining the impact of the model, much less onto issues related to model maintenance. How is data drift tracked and mitigated? What impact does an alert-driven intervention have on the appropriate risk thresholds after model deployment? How does a model's performance remain stable or degrade over time? Each of these questions has important implications for designing the infrastructure and architecture of truly sustainable AI/ML platforms in health care. They also highlight the need for strong collaboration between clinicians, data scientists, computing architects, and EHR builders to ensure that economies of scale and sustainability can be achieved well into the future. Translators, for example, those who are clinicians but are also deeply familiar with the advantages and limitations presented by data science, are needed to ensure that these opportunities are not squandered.

Finally, emerging research has shown us how biased data and algorithms can result in unintended consequences that can propagate inequities and disparities in patient care. Notably, this potential for bias can arise from a diversity of areas within the AI/ML implementation including non-representative datasets, differential missingness and informativeness, algorithmic and label bias, and the potential for discriminatory care resulting from the clinical or operational use of models. These phenomena represent a critical risk to the safe and equitable deployment of algorithms and there is growing scrutiny over this area. However, potentially discriminatory algorithms are not exclusive to AI/ML, as highly familiar data elements (eg, glomerular filtration rate calculations, pulse oximeters, SOFA scores) have also been found to potentially result in disparate or inequitable practice.[215] Regulatory agencies including the Food and Drug Administration (FDA), Center for Medicare and Medicaid Services (CMS), and the White House, among many others, are increasing the scrutiny of models to justifiably protect the interests and safety of patients. However, the process of quantifying, measuring, and judging trade-offs in model bias and performance remains poorly understood and impending regulations will exert an uncertain impact on progress in the field.

SUMMARY

Critical care has a long and rich history of using detailed clinical data for predicting a diversity of outcomes, most importantly ICU mortality. The rapid expansion of data availability through the EHR as well as innovations in computing platforms and algorithms have produced substantial new advances in outcomes predictions marked by a growing breadth of outcomes of interest as well as novel methods for improving performance. Although some of these innovations are now entering into routine clinical care, through EHR-embedded real-time platforms, robust studies demonstrating their value at the bedside remain limited. Nonetheless, the future is bright for AI/ML applications in intensive care.

AUTHOR CONTRIBUTIONS

Michael J. Patton (MJP) and Vincent X. Liu (VXL) prepared and wrote the main text. Michael J. Patton produced all figures and tables from data extracted from the references cited.

CLINICS CARE POINTS

- Critical care has a rich history of data-driven risk scoring for prognostication and risk adjustment with novel approaches yielding only moderate incremental improvements
- Although there is tremendous enthusiasm about ML and AI in risk prediction, few studies have robustly demonstrated their value in improving patient-specific outcomes
- Novel risk stratification tools need to be carefully integrated and contextualized within a well-defined workflow to produce benefits and minimize drawbacks

DISCLOSURE

The authors have nothing to disclose.

SUPPLEMENTARY DATA

Supplementary data related to this article can be found online at https://doi.org/10.1016/j.ccc.2023.02.001.

REFERENCES

1. National trends in hospital and physician adoption of electronic health records from the American hospital association (AHA) annual survey information technology supplement, 2008-present |HealthIT.gov. Available at: https://www.healthit.gov/data/quickstats/national-trends-hospital-and-physician-adoption-electronic-health-records.
2. Murdoch TB, Detsky AS. The inevitable application of big data to health care. JAMA, J Am Med Assoc 2013;309:1351–2.
3. Kuo AMH. Opportunities and challenges of cloud computing to improve health care services. J Med Internet Res 2011;13:e67.
4. Newton I. The mathematical Principles of natural philosophy, 1728, Vol 1. In B. Motte.
5. Liu Y, Chen PHC, Krause J, et al. How to read articles that use machine learning: users' guides to the medical literature. JAMA, J Am Med Assoc 2019;322:1806–16.
6. Marafino BJ, Park M, Davies JM, et al. Validation of prediction models for critical care outcomes using natural language processing of electronic health record data. JAMA Netw Open 2018;1:e185097.
7. Churpek MM, Yuen TC, Winslow C, et al. Multicenter comparison of machine learning methods and conventional regression for predicting clinical deterioration on the wards. Crit Care Med 2016;44:368–74.
8. Gulshan V, Peng L, Coram M, et al. Development and validation of a deep learning algorithm for detection of diabetic retinopathy in retinal fundus photographs. JAMA, J Am Med Assoc 2016;316:2402–10.
9. Ting DSW, Cheung CYL, Lim G, et al. Development and validation of a deep learning system for diabetic retinopathy and related eye diseases using retinal images from multiethnic populations with diabetes. JAMA, J Am Med Assoc 2017;318:2211–23.
10. Ehteshami Bejnordi B, Veta M, Johannes van Diest P, et al. Diagnostic assessment of deep learning algorithms for detection of lymph node metastases in women with breast cancer. JAMA, J Am Med Assoc 2017;318:2199–210.

11. Bedoya AD, Futoma J, Clement ME, et al. Machine learning for early detection of sepsis: an internal and temporal validation study. JAMIA open 2020;3:252–60.

12. Geri G, Vignon P, Aubry A, et al. Cardiovascular clusters in septic shock combining clinical and echocardiographic parameters: a post hoc analysis. Intensive Care Med 2019;45:657–67.

13. Castela Forte J, Yeshmagambetova G, Grinten MLV, et al. Identifying and characterizing highrisk clusters in a heterogeneous ICU population with deep embedded clustering. Sci Rep 2021;11:12109.

14. Vranas KC, Jopling JK, Sweeney TE, et al. Identifying distinct subgroups of ICU patients: a machine learning approach. Crit Care Med 2017;45:1607–15.

15. Castela Forte J, Perner A, Horst van der ICC. The use of clustering algorithms in critical care research to unravel patient heterogeneity. Intensive Care Med 2019; 45(7):1025–8.

16. Hanley JA, McNeil BJ. The meaning and use of the area under a receiver operating characteristic (ROC) curve. Radiology 1982;143:29–36.

17. Pearson K. On the theory of contingency and its relation to association and normal correlation. London: Drapers Company Research Memoirs; 1904.

18. Rijsbergen C van. Information retrieval. London: Butterworths; 1979.

19. Schrittwieser J, Antonoglou I, Hubert T, et al. Mastering Atari, Go, chess and shogi by planning with a learned model. Nature 2020;588(7839):604–9.

20. Komorowski M, Celi LA, Badawi O, et al. The Artificial Intelligence Clinician learns optimal treatment strategies for sepsis in intensive care. Nat Med 2018; 24(11):1716–20.

21. Zimmerman JE, Kramer AA. A history of outcome prediction in the ICU. Curr Opin Crit Care 2014;20:550–6.

22. Breslow MJ, Badawi O. Severity scoring in the critically ill: part 2: maximizing value from outcome prediction scoring systems. Chest 2012;141:518–27.

23. Vincent JL, Moreno R. Clinical review: scoring systems in the critically ill. Crit Care 2010;14:207.

24. Keegan MT, Gajic O, Afessa B. Severity of illness scoring systems in the intensive care unit. Crit Care Med 2011;39:163–9.

25. Sevransky JE, Rothman RE, Hager DN, et al. Effect of vitamin C, thiamine, and hydrocortisone on Ventilator- and vasopressor-free days in patients with sepsis: the VICTAS randomized clinical trial. JAMA 2021;325:742–50.

26. Investigators NSS, Finfer S, Chittock DR, et al. Intensive versus conventional glucose control in critically ill patients. N Engl J Med 2009;360:1283–97.

27. Bouadma L, Luyt CE, Tubach F, et al. Use of procalcitonin to reduce patients' exposure to antibiotics in intensive care units (PRORATA trial): a multicentre randomised controlled trial. Lancet (London, England) 9713 2010;375:463–74.

28. Sprung CL, Annane D, Keh D, et al. Hydrocortisone therapy for patients with septic shock. N Engl J Med 2008;358:111–24.

29. Knaus WA, Wagner DP, Zimmerman JE, et al. Variations in mortality and length of stay in intensive care units. Ann Intern Med 1993;118:753–61.

30. Seymour CW, Kennedy JN, Wang S, et al. Derivation, validation, and potential treatment implications of novel clinical phenotypes for sepsis. JAMA 2019; 321:2003–17.

31. Breslow MJ, Badawi O. Severity scoring in the critically ill: part 1–interpretation and accuracy of outcome prediction scoring systems. Chest 2012;141:245–52.

32. Christian MD, Joynt GM, Hick JL, et al. Chapter 7. Critical care triage. Recommendations and standard operating procedures for intensive care unit and

hospital preparations for an influenza epidemic or mass disaster. Intensive Care Med 2010;36(Suppl 1):S55–64.

33. Pronovost PJ, Angus DC, Dorman T, et al. Physician staffing patterns and clinical outcomes in critically ill patients: a systematic review. JAMA 2002;288: 2151–62.

34. Afessa B, Keegan MT, Hubmayr RD, et al. Evaluating the performance of an institution using an intensive care unit benchmark. Mayo Clin Proc 2005;80: 174–80.

35. Cook SF, Visscher WA, Hobbs CL, et al. Project IMPACT: results from a pilot validity study of a new observational database. Crit Care Med 2002;30:2765–70.

36. Teres D, Lemeshow S. Using severity measures to describe high performance intensive care units. Crit Care Clin 1993;9:543–54.

37. Becker RB, Zimmerman JE. ICU scoring systems allow prediction of patient outcomes and comparison of ICU performance. Crit Care Clin 1996;12:503–14.

38. Carson SS, Stocking C, Podsadecki T, et al. Effects of organizational change in the medical intensive care unit of a teaching hospital: a comparison of 'open' and 'closed' formats. JAMA, J Am Med Assoc 1996;276:322–8.

39. Li TC, Phillips MC, Shaw L, et al. On-site physician staffing in a community hospital intensive care unit. Impact on test and procedure use and on patient outcome. JAMA 1984;252:2023–7.

40. Nathanson BH, Higgins TL, Teres D, et al. A revised method to assess intensive care unit clinical performance and resource utilization. Crit Care Med 2007;35: 1853–62.

41. Multz AS, Chalfin DB, Samson IM, et al. A "closed" medical intensive care unit (MICU) improves resource utilization when compared with an "open" MICU. Am J Respir Crit Care Med 1998;157:1468–73.

42. Knaus WA. Apache 1978-2001: the development of a quality assurance system based on prognosis: milestones and personal reflections. Arch Surg 2002;137: 37–41.

43. Knaus WA, Draper EA, Wagner DP, et al. Apache II: a severity of disease classification system. Crit Care Med 1985;13:818–29.

44. Bernard GR, Vincent JL, Laterre PF, et al. Efficacy and safety of recombinant human activated protein C for severe sepsis. N Engl J Med 2001;344:699–709.

45. Seymour CW, Liu VX, Iwashyna TJ, et al. Assessment of clinical criteria for sepsis: for the third international consensus definitions for sepsis and septic shock (Sepsis-3). JAMA, J Am Med Assoc 2016;315:762–74.

46. Singer M, Deutschman CS, Seymour CW, et al. The third international consensus definitions for sepsis and septic shock (Sepsis-3). JAMA, J Am Med Assoc 2016;315:801–10.

47. Churpek MM, Snyder A, Han X, et al. Quick sepsis-related organ failure assessment, systemic inflammatory response syndrome, and early warning scores for detecting clinical deterioration in infected patients outside the intensive care unit. Am J Respir Crit Care Med 2017;195:906–11.

48. Hunziker S, Celi LA, Lee J, et al. Red cell distribution width improves the simplified acute physiology score for risk prediction in unselected critically ill patients. Crit Care 2012;16:R89.

49. Raffa JD, Johnson AEW, O'Brien Z, et al. The global open source severity of illness score (GO). Crit Care Med 2022;50:1040–50.

50. Keller MB, Wang J, Nason M, et al. Preintubation sequential organ failure assessment score for predicting COVID-19 mortality: external validation using

electronic health record from 86 U.S. Healthcare systems to appraise current ventilator triage algorithms. Crit Care Med 2022;50:1051–62.

51. Iwase S, Nakada TA, Shimada T, et al. Prediction algorithm for ICU mortality and length of stay using machine learning. Sci Rep 2022;12:12912.

52. Le Gall JR, Lemeshow S, Saulnier F. A new Simplified Acute Physiology Score (SAPS II) based on a European/North American multicenter study. JAMA, J Am Med Assoc 1993;270:2957–63.

53. Vincent JL, Moreno R, Takala J, et al. The SOFA (Sepsis-related organ failure assessment) score to describe organ dysfunction/failure. On behalf of the working group on sepsis-related problems of the European society of intensive care medicine. Intensive Care Med 1996;22:707–10.

54. Marik PE, Varon J. Severity scoring and outcome assessment. Computerized predictive models and scoring systems. Crit Care Clin 1999;15:633–46, viii.

55. Knaus WA, Wagner DP, Draper EA, et al. The Apache III prognostic system. Risk prediction of hospital mortality for critically ill hospitalized adults. Chest 1991; 100:1619–36.

56. Zimmerman JE, Kramer AA, McNair DS, et al. Acute Physiology and Chronic Health Evaluation (Apache) IV: hospital mortality assessment for today's critically ill patients. Crit Care Med 2006;34:1297–310.

57. Ferreira FL, Bota DP, Bross A, et al. Serial evaluation of the SOFA score to predict outcome in critically ill patients. JAMA 2001;286:1754–8.

58. Schmidt H, Roberts DE, Eneanya ND. Sequential organ failure assessment, ventilator rationing and evolving triage guidance: new evidence underlines the need to recognise and revise, unjust allocation frameworks. Journal of medical ethics 2 2022;48:136–8.

59. Sirio CA, Shepardson LB, Rotondi AJ, et al. Community-wide assessment of intensive care outcomes using a physiologically based prognostic measure: implications for critical care delivery from Cleveland Health Quality Choice. Chest 1999;115:793–801.

60. Redfern OC, Pimentel MAF, Prytherch D, et al. Predicting in-hospital mortality and unanticipated admissions to the intensive care unit using routinely collected blood tests and vital signs: development and validation of a multivariable model. Resuscitation 2018;133:75–81.

61. Harrison DA, Brady AR, Parry GJ, et al. Recalibration of risk prediction models in a large multicenter cohort of admissions to adult, general critical care units in the United Kingdom. Crit Care Med 2006;34:1378–88.

62. Moreno R, Vincent JL, Matos R, et al. The use of maximum SOFA score to quantify organ dysfunction/failure in intensive care. Results of a prospective, multicentre study. Working Group on Sepsis related Problems of the ESICM. Intensive Care Medicine 1999;25:686–96.

63. Brinkman S, Bakhshi-Raiez F, Abu-Hanna A, et al. External validation of acute physiology and chronic health evaluation IV in Dutch intensive care units and comparison with acute physiology and chronic health evaluation II and simplified acute physiology score II. J Crit Care 2011;26:105, e11–8.

64. Harrison DA, Rowan KM. Outcome prediction in critical care: the ICNARC model. Curr Opin Crit Care 2008;14:506–12.

65. Rivera-Fernández R, Vázquez-Mata G, Bravo M, et al. The Apache III prognostic system: customized mortality predictions for Spanish ICU patients. Intensive Care Med 1998;24:574–81.

66. Beck DH, Smith GB, Pappachan JV, et al. External validation of the SAPS II, Apache II and Apache III prognostic models in South England: a multicentre study. Intensive Care Med 2003;29:249–56.

67. Poole D, Rossi C, Anghileri A, et al. External validation of the Simplified Acute Physiology Score (SAPS) 3 in a cohort of 28,357 patients from 147 Italian intensive care units. Intensive Care Med 2009;35:1916–24.

68. Kramer AA, Higgins TL, Zimmerman JE. Comparison of the mortality probability admission model III, national quality forum, and acute physiology and chronic health evaluation IV hospital mortality models: implications for national benchmarking. Crit Care Med 2014;42:544–53.

69. Oh TE, Hutchinson R, Short S, et al. Verification of the acute physiology and chronic health evaluation scoring system in a Hong Kong intensive care unit. Crit Care Med 1993;21:698–705.

70. Higgins TL, Kramer AA, Nathanson BH, et al. Prospective validation of the intensive care unit admission Mortality Probability Model (MPM0-III). Crit Care Med 2009;37:1619–23.

71. Rowan KM, Kerr JH, Major E, et al. Intensive Care Society's Apache II study in Britain and Ireland–II: outcome comparisons of intensive care units after adjustment for case mix by the American Apache II method. Br Med J 1993;307: 977–81.

72. Moreno R, Miranda DR, Fidler V, et al. Evaluation of two outcome prediction models on an independent database. Crit Care Med 1998;26:50–61.

73. Engerström L, Nolin TMC, et al. Impact of missing physiologic data on performance of the simplified acute physiology score 3 risk-prediction model. Crit Care Med 2017;45:2006–13.

74. Lee H, Shon YJ, Kim H, et al. Validation of the Apache IV model and its comparison with the Apache II, SAPS 3, and Korean SAPS 3 models for the prediction of hospital mortality in a Korean surgical intensive care unit. Korean Journal of Anesthesiology 2014;67:115–22.

75. Duke GJ, Santamaria J, Shann F, et al. Critical care outcome prediction equation (COPE) for adult intensive care. Critical Care and Resuscitation 2008;10:41.

76. Timsit JF, Fosse JP, Troché G, et al. Calibration and discrimination by daily Logistic Organ Dysfunction scoring comparatively with daily Sequential Organ Failure Assessment scoring for predicting hospital mortality in critically ill patients. Crit Care Med 2002;30:2003–13.

77. Zimmerman JE, Wagner DP, Draper EA, et al. Evaluation of acute physiology and chronic health evaluation III predictions of hospital mortality in an independent database. Crit Care Med 1998;26:1317–26.

78. Moreno RP, Metnitz PGH, Almeida E, et al. SAPS 3–From evaluation of the patient to evaluation of the intensive care unit. Part 2: development of a prognostic model for hospital mortality at ICU admission. Intensive Care Med 2005;31: 1345–55.

79. Wong DT, Crofts SL, Gomez M, et al. Evaluation of predictive ability of Apache II system and hospital outcome in Canadian intensive care unit patients. Crit Care Med 1995;23:1177–83.

80. Markgraf R, Deutschinoff G, Pientka L, et al. Comparison of acute physiology and chronic health evaluations II and III and simplified acute physiology score II: a prospective cohort study evaluating these methods to predict outcome in a German interdisciplinary intensive care unit. Crit Care Med 2000;28:26–33.

81. Livingston BM, MacKirdy FN, Howie JC, et al. Assessment of the performance of five intensive care scoring models within a large Scottish database. Crit Care Med 2000;28:1820–7.

82. Meyer A, Zverinski D, Pfahringer B, et al. Machine learning for real-time prediction of complications in critical care: a retrospective study. Lancet Respir Med 2018;6:905–14.

83. Liu VX, Lu Y, Carey KA, et al. Comparison of early warning scoring systems for hospitalized patients with and without infection at risk for in-hospital mortality and transfer to the intensive care unit. JAMA Netw Open 2020;3:e205191.

84. Kim S, Kim W, Park RW. A comparison of intensive care unit mortality prediction models through the use of data mining techniques. Healthcare Informatics Research 2011;17:232–43.

85. Cárdenas-Turanzas M, Ensor J, Wakefield C, et al. Cross-validation of a Sequential Organ Failure Assessment score-based model to predict mortality in patients with cancer admitted to the intensive care unit. J Crit Care 2012;27: 673–80.

86. Higgins TL, Teres D, Copes WS, et al. Assessing contemporary intensive care unit outcome: an updated Mortality Probability Admission Model (MPM0-III). Crit Care Med 2007;35:827–35.

87. Lemeshow S, Teres D, Klar J, et al. Mortality Probability Models (MPM II) based on an international cohort of intensive care unit patients. JAMA, J Am Med Assoc 1993;270:2478–86.

88. Subbe CP, Kruger M, Rutherford P, et al. Validation of a modified early warning score in medical admissions. QJM : monthly journal of the Association of Physicians 10 2001;94:521–6.

89. Prytherch DR, Smith GB, Schmidt PE, et al. ViEWS–Towards a national early warning score for detecting adult inpatient deterioration. Resuscitation 2010; 81:932–7.

90. Smith GB, Prytherch DR, Meredith P, et al. The ability of the National Early Warning Score (NEWS) to discriminate patients at risk of early cardiac arrest, unanticipated intensive care unit admission, and death. Resuscitation 4 2013;84: 465–70.

91. Bone RC, Balk RA, Cerra FB, et al. Definitions for sepsis and organ failure and guidelines for the use of innovative therapies in sepsis. Chest 1992;101: 1644–55.

92. Render ML, Kim HM, Welsh DE, et al. Automated intensive care unit risk adjustment: results from a National Veterans Affairs study. Crit Care Med 2003;31: 1638–46.

93. Tang F, Xiao C, Wang F, et al. Predictive modeling in urgent care: a comparative study of machine learning approaches. JAMIA open 2018;1:87–98.

94. Adrie C, Francais A, Alvarez-Gonzalez A, et al. Model for predicting short-term mortality of severe sepsis. Crit Care 2009;13:R72.

95. Render ML, Welsh DE, Kollef M, et al. Automated computerized intensive care unit severity of illness measure in the department of Veterans Affairs: preliminary results. SISVistA investigators. Scrutiny of ICU severity Veterans health sysyems technology architecture. Crit Care Med 2000;28:3540–6.

96. Moran JL, Solomon PJ. Outcome AC for, Australian RE(of, and (ANZICS) NZICS. Fixed effects modelling for provider mortality outcomes: analysis of the Australia and New Zealand intensive care society (ANZICS) adult patient data-base. PLoS One 2014;9:e102297.

97. Dybowski R, Weller P, Chang R, et al. Prediction of outcome in critically ill patients using artificial neural network synthesised by genetic algorithm. Lancet 1996;347:1146–50.

98. Wang Y, Chen W, Heard K, et al. Mortality prediction in ICUs using A novel time-slicing Cox regression method. AMIA Annual Symposium Proceedings 2015; 2015:1289–95.

99. Moran JL, Bristow P, Solomon PJ, et al. Mortality and length-of-stay outcomes, 1993-2003, in the binational Australian and New Zealand intensive care adult patient database. Crit Care Med 2008;36:46–61.

100. Angus DC, Linde-Zwirble WT, Sirio CA, et al. The effect of managed care on ICU length of stay: implications for medicare. JAMA, J Am Med Assoc 1996;276: 1075–82.

101. Clermont G, Angus DC, DiRusso SM, et al. Predicting hospital mortality for patients in the intensive care unit: a comparison of artificial neural networks with logistic regression models. Crit Care Med 2001;29:291–6.

102. Minne L, Toma T, Jonge E de, et al. Assessing and combining repeated prognosis of physicians and temporal models in the intensive care. Artif Intell Med 2013;57:111–7.

103. Churpek MM, Yuen TC, Edelson DP. Predicting clinical deterioration in the hospital: the impact of outcome selection. Resuscitation 2013;84:564–8.

104. Keizer NF de, Bonsel GJ, Goldfad C, et al. The added value that increasing levels of diagnostic information provide in prognostic models to estimate hospital mortality for adult intensive care patients. Intensive Care Med 2000;26: 577–84.

105. Duke GJ, Barker A, Rasekaba T, et al. Development and validation of the critical care outcome prediction equation, version 4. Critical Care and Resuscitation 2013;15:191–7.

106. Render ML, Deddens J, Freyberg R, et al. Veterans Affairs intensive care unit risk adjustment model: validation, updating, recalibration. Crit Care Med 2008;36:1031–42.

107. Timsit JF, Fosse JP, Troché G, et al. Accuracy of a composite score using daily SAPS II and LOD scores for predicting hospital mortality in ICU patients hospitalized for more than 72 h. Intensive Care Med 2001;27:1012–21.

108. Markgraf R, Deutschinoff G, Pientka L, et al. Performance of the score systems Acute Physiology and Chronic Health Evaluation II and III at an interdisciplinary intensive care unit, after customization. Crit Care 2001;5:31–6.

109. Raith EP, Udy AA, Bailey M, et al. Prognostic accuracy of the SOFA score, SIRS criteria, and qSOFA score for in-hospital mortality among adults with suspected infection admitted to the intensive care unit. JAMA, J Am Med Assoc 2017;317: 290–300.

110. Awad A, Bader-El-Den M, McNicholas J, et al. Early hospital mortality prediction of intensive care unit patients using an ensemble learning approach. Int J Med Inf 2017;108:185–95.

111. Silva A, Cortez P, Santos MF, et al. Mortality assessment in intensive care units via adverse events using artificial neural networks. Artif Intell Med 2006;36: 223–34.

112. Shickel B, Loftus TJ, Adhikari L, et al. A continuous acuity score for critically ill patients using clinically interpretable deep learning. Sci Rep 2019;9:1879.

113. Kim SY, Kim S, Cho J, et al. A deep learning model for real-time mortality prediction in critically ill children. Crit Care 2019;23:279.

114. Raita Y, Goto T, Faridi MK, et al. Emergency department triage prediction of clinical outcomes using machine learning models. Crit Care 2019;23:64.
115. Brajer N, Cozzi B, Gao M, et al. Prospective and external evaluation of a machine learning model to predict in-hospital mortality of adults at time of admission. JAMA Netw Open 2020;3:e1920733.
116. Holmgren G, Andersson P, Jakobsson A, et al. Artificial neural networks improve and simplify intensive care mortality prognostication: a national cohort study of 217,289 first-time intensive care unit admissions. Journal of intensive care 2019; 7:44.
117. Parreco JP, Hidalgo AE, Badilla AD, et al. Predicting central line-associated bloodstream infections and mortality using supervised machine learning. J Crit Care 2018;45:156–62.
118. Wong RSY, Ismail NA. An application of bayesian approach in modeling risk of death in an intensive care unit. PLoS One 2016;11:e0151949.
119. He F, Page JH, Weinberg KR, et al. The development and validation of simplified machine learning algorithms to predict prognosis of hospitalized patients with COVID-19: multicenter, retrospective study. J Med Internet Res 2022;24: e31549.
120. Hug CW, Szolovits P. ICU acuity: real-time models versus daily models. AMIA Annual Symposium Proceedings 2009;2009:260–4.
121. Ren Y, Loftus TJ, Datta S, et al. Performance of a machine learning algorithm using electronic health record data to predict postoperative complications and report on a mobile platform. JAMA Netw Open 2022;5:e2211973.
122. Hsu YT, He YT, Ting CK, et al. Administrative and claims data help predict patient mortality in intensive care units by logistic regression: a nationwide database study. BioMed Res Int 2020;2020:9076739.
123. Elhazmi A, Al-Omari A, Sallam H, et al. Machine learning decision tree algorithm role for predicting mortality in critically ill adult COVID-19 patients admitted to the ICU. Journal of infection and public health 2022;15:826–34.
124. Higgins TL, Freeseman-Freeman L, Stark MM, et al. Benchmarking inpatient mortality using electronic medical record data: a retrospective, multicenter analytical observational study. Crit Care Med 2022;50:543–53.
125. Zhang Z, Hong Y. Development of a novel score for the prediction of hospital mortality in patients with severe sepsis: the use of electronic healthcare records with LA regression. Oncotarget 2017;8:49637–45.
126. Xu Y, Trivedi A, Becker N, et al. Machine learning-based derivation and external validation of a tool to predict death and development of organ failure in hospitalized patients with COVID-19. Sci Rep 2022;12:16913.
127. Reina Reina A, Barrera JM, Valdivieso B, et al. Machine learning model from a Spanish cohort for prediction of SARS-COV-2 mortality risk and critical patients. Sci Rep 2022;12:5723.
128. Daly K, Beale R, Chang RW. Reduction in mortality after inappropriate early discharge from intensive care unit: logistic regression triage model. Br Med J 2001;322:1274–6.
129. Edelson M, Kuo TT. Generalizable prediction of COVID-19 mortality on worldwide patient data. JAMIA open 2022;5:ooac036.
130. Houthooft R, Ruyssinck J, Herten van der J, et al. Predictive modelling of survival and length of stay in critically ill patients using sequential organ failure scores. Artif Intell Med 2015;63:191–207.
131. Sigakis MJG, Bittner EA, Wanderer JP. Validation of a risk stratification index and risk quantification index for predicting patient outcomes: in-hospital mortality,

30-day mortality, 1-year mortality, and length-of-stay. Anesthesiology 2013;119: 525–40.

132. Johnson AEW, Pollard TJ, Shen L, et al. MIMIC-III, a freely accessible critical care database. Sci Data 2016;3:160035.

133. Majno G. The ancient riddle of sigma eta psi iota sigma (sepsis). J Infect Dis 1991;163:937–45.

134. Funk DJ, Parrillo JE, Kumar A. Sepsis and septic shock: a history. Crit Care Clin 2009;25:83–101, viii.

135. Levy MM, Fink MP, Marshall JC, et al. 2001 SCCM/ESICM/ACCP/ATS/SIS international sepsis definitions conference. Crit Care Med 2003;31:1250–6.

136. Hospital inpatient specifications manuals version 5.13 – discharges 01/01/2023 through 06/30/2023. Available at: https://qualitynet.cms.gov/inpatient/specifications-manuals.

137. Centers for Disease Control and Prevention. Available at: https://www.cdc.gov/sepsis/pdfs/Sepsis-Surveillance-Toolkit-Aug-2018_508.pdf.

138. Henry KE, Hager DN, Pronovost PJ, et al. A targeted real-time early warning score (TREWScore) for septic shock. Sci Transl Med 2015;7. 299ra122.

139. Lee GM, Harper MB. Risk of bacteremia for febrile young children in the post-Haemophilus influenzae type b era. Arch Pediatr Adolesc Med 1998;152:624–8.

140. Kallio R, Surcel HM, Bloigu A, et al. Admission neopterin and interleukin 12 concentrations in identifying infections in adult cancer patients. Cytokine 2001;13: 371–4.

141. Groeneveld AB, Bossink AW, Mierlo GJ van, et al. Circulating inflammatory mediators in patients with fever: predicting bloodstream infection. Clin Diagn Lab Immunol 2001;8:1189–95.

142. Isaacman DJ, Burke BL. Utility of the serum C-reactive protein for detection of occult bacterial infection in children. Arch Pediatr Adolesc Med 2002;156: 905–9.

143. Groeneveld ABJ, Tacx AN, Bossink AWJ, et al. Circulating inflammatory mediators predict shock and mortality in febrile patients with microbial infection. Clin Immunol 2003;106:106–15.

144. Bonsu BK, Harper MB. A low peripheral blood white blood cell count in infants younger than 90 days increases the odds of acute bacterial meningitis relative to bacteremia. Acad Emerg Med 2004;11:1297–301.

145. Cuello García CA, Tamez Gómez L, Valdez Ceballos J. [Total white blood cell count, erythrosedimentation rate and C-reactive protein for the detection of serious bacterial infections in 0to 90-day-old infants with fever without a source]. Anales de Pediatria 2008;68:103–9.

146. Kruif MD de, Limper M, Sierhuis K, et al. PTX3 predicts severe disease in febrile patients at the emergency department. J Infect 2010;60:122–7.

147. Matono T, Yoshida M, Koga H, et al. Diagnostic accuracy of quick SOFA score and inflammatory biomarkers for predicting community-onset bacteremia. Sci Rep 2022;12:11121.

148. Huttunen R, Hurme M, Aittoniemi J, et al. High plasma level of long pentraxin 3 (PTX3) is associated with fatal disease in bacteremic patients: a prospective cohort study. PLoS One 2011;6:e17653.

149. Aikawa N, Fujishima S, Endo S, et al. Multicenter prospective study of procalcitonin as an indicator of sepsis. J Infect Chemother 2005;11:152–9.

150. Guinard-Barbier S, Grabar S, Chenevier-Gobeaux C, et al. Is mid-regional pro-atrial natriuretic peptide (MRproANP) an accurate marker of bacteremia in

pyelonephritis? Biomarkers: biochemical Indicators of Exposure, Response. and Susceptibility To Chemicals 2011;16:355–63.

151. Hoenigl M, Raggam RB, Wagner J, et al. Diagnostic accuracy of soluble urokinase plasminogen activator receptor (suPAR) for prediction of bacteremia in patients with systemic inflammatory response syndrome. Clin Biochem 2013;46: 225–9.

152. Kijpaisalratana N, Sanglertsinlapachai D, Techaratsami S, et al. Machine learning algorithms for early sepsis detection in the emergency department: a retrospective study. Int J Med Inf 2022;160:104689.

153. Julián-Jiménez A, Gutiérrez-Martín P, Lizcano-Lizcano A, et al. Usefulness of procalcitonin and C-reactive protein for predicting bacteremia in urinary tract infections in the emergency department. Actas Urol Esp 2015;39:502–10.

154. Kim JK, Ahn W, Park S, et al. Early prediction of sepsis onset using neural architecture search based on genetic algorithms. Int J Environ Res Publ Health 2022;19.

155. Burdick H, Pino E, Gabel-Comeau D, et al. Validation of a machine learning algorithm for early severe sepsis prediction: a retrospective study predicting severe sepsis up to 48 h in advance using a diverse dataset from 461 US hospitals. BMC Med Inf Decis Making 2020;20:276.

156. Ratzinger F, Schuardt M, Eichbichler K, et al. Utility of sepsis biomarkers and the infection probability score to discriminate sepsis and systemic inflammatory response syndrome in standard care patients. PLoS One 2013;8:e82946..

157. Milcent K, Faesch S, Gras-Le Guen C, et al. Use of procalcitonin assays to predict serious bacterial infection in young febrile infants. JAMA Pediatr 2016; 170:62–9.

158. Shorr AF, Tabak YP, Johannes RS, et al. Candidemia on presentation to the hospital: development and validation of a risk score. Crit Care 2009;13:R156.

159. Poses RM, Anthony M. Availability, wishful thinking, and physicians' diagnostic judgments for patients with suspected bacteremia. Med Decis Making 1991;11: 159–68.

160. Bossink AW, Groeneveld AB, Thijs LG. Prediction of microbial infection and mortality in medical patients with fever: plasma procalcitonin, neutrophilic elastase-alpha1-antitrypsin, and lactoferrin compared with clinical variables. Clin Infect Dis 1999;29:398–407.

161. Müller B, Harbarth S, Stolz D, et al. Diagnostic and prognostic accuracy of clinical and laboratory parameters in community-acquired pneumonia. BMC Infect Dis 2007;7:10.

162. Senthilnayagam B, Kumar T, Sukumaran J, et al. Automated measurement of immature granulocytes: performance characteristics and utility in routine clinical practice. Pathol Res Int 2012;2012:483670.

163. Mencacci A, Leli C, Cardaccia A, et al. Procalcitonin predicts real-time PCR results in blood samples from patients with suspected sepsis. PLoS One 2012;7: e53279.

164. Rintala EM, Aittoniemi J, Laine S, et al. Early identification of bacteremia by biochemical markers of systemic inflammation. Scand J Clin Lab Investig 2001;61:523–30.

165. Su L, Han B, Liu C, et al. Value of soluble TREM-1, procalcitonin, and C-reactive protein serum levels as biomarkers for detecting bacteremia among sepsis patients with new fever in intensive care units: a prospective cohort study. BMC Infect Dis 2012;12:157.

166. Pavare J, Grope I, Kalnins I, et al. High-mobility group box-1 protein, lipopoly-saccharidebinding protein, interleukin-6 and C-reactive protein in children with community acquired infections and bacteraemia: a prospective study. BMC Infect Dis 2010;10:28.
167. Pulliam PN, Attia MW, Cronan KM. C-reactive protein in febrile children 1 to 36 months of age with clinically undetectable serious bacterial infection. Pediatrics 2001;108:1275–9.
168. Zafar Iqbal-Mirza S, Serrano Romero de Ávila V, Estévez-González R, et al. Ability of procalcitonin to differentiate true bacteraemia from contaminated blood cultures in an emergency department. Enfermedades infecciosas y microbiologia clinica (English ed. 2019;37:560–8.
169. To KKW, Lee KC, Wong SSY, et al. Lipid mediators of inflammation as novel plasma biomarkers to identify patients with bacteremia. J Infect 2015;70: 433–44.
170. Pratt A, Attia MW. Duration of fever and markers of serious bacterial infection in young febrile children. Pediatr Int 2007;49:31–5.
171. Tudela P, Lacoma A, Prat C, et al. [Prediction of bacteremia in patients with suspicion of infection in emergency room]. Med Clínica 2010;135:685–90.
172. Ruiz-González A, Esquerda A, Falguera M, et al. Triggering receptor (TREM-1) expressed on myeloid cells predicts bacteremia better than clinical variables in community-acquired pneumonia. Respirology 2011;16:321–5.
173. Vijarnsorn C, Winijkul G, Laohaprasitiporn D, et al. Postoperative fever and major infections after pediatric cardiac surgery. J Med Assoc Thail 2012;95: 761–70.
174. Shi Y, Du B, Xu YC, et al. Early changes of procalcitonin predict bacteremia in patients with intensive care unit-acquired new fever. Chinese Med J 2013;126: 1832–7.
175. Wyllie DH, Bowler ICJW, Peto TEA. Relation between lymphopenia and bacteraemia in UK adults with medical emergencies. J Clin Pathol 2004;57:950–5.
176. Jager CPC de, Wijk van PTL, Mathoera RB, et al. Lymphocytopenia and neutrophil-lymphocyte count ratio predict bacteremia better than conventional infection markers in an emergency care unit. Crit Care 2010;14:R192.
177. Bilavsky E, Yarden-Bilavsky H, Ashkenazi S, et al. C-reactive protein as a marker of serious bacterial infections in hospitalized febrile infants. Acta Paediatr 2009; 98:1776–80.
178. Caterino JM, Scheatzle MD, Forbes ML, et al. Bacteremic elder emergency department patients: procalcitonin and white count. Acad Emerg Med 2004; 11:393–6.
179. Hoenigl M, Raggam RB, Wagner J, et al. Procalcitonin fails to predict bacteremia in SIRS patients: a cohort study. Int J Clin Pract 2014;68:1278–81.
180. Jeong S, Park Y, Cho Y, et al. Diagnostic utilities of procalcitonin and C-reactive protein for the prediction of bacteremia determined by blood culture. Clin Chim Acta 2012;413:1731–6.
181. Evans L, Rhodes A, Alhazzani W, et al. Executive summary: surviving sepsis campaign: international guidelines for the management of sepsis and septic shock 2021. Crit Care Med 2021;49:1974–82.
182. Seymour CW, Gesten F, Prescott HC, et al. Time to treatment and mortality during mandated emergency care for sepsis. N Engl J Med 2017;376:2235–44.
183. Dellinger RP, Carlet JM, Masur H, et al. Surviving Sepsis Campaign guidelines for management of severe sepsis and septic shock. Crit Care Med 2004;32: 858–73.

184. Dellinger RP, Levy MM, Carlet JM, et al. Surviving Sepsis Campaign: international guidelines for management of severe sepsis and septic shock: 2008. Crit Care Med 2008;36:296–327.

185. Dellinger RP, Levy MM, Rhodes A, et al. Surviving Sepsis Campaign: international guidelines for management of severe sepsis and septic shock, 2012. Intensive Care Med 2013;39:165–228.

186. Rhodes A, Evans LE, Alhazzani W, et al. Surviving sepsis campaign: international guidelines for management of sepsis and septic shock: 2016. Intensive Care Med 2017;43:304–77.

187. Desautels T, Calvert J, Hoffman J, et al. Prediction of sepsis in the intensive care unit with minimal electronic health record data: a machine learning approach. JMIR medical informatics 2016;4:e28.

188. Xiao Y, Griffin MP, Lake DE, et al. Nearest-neighbor and logistic regression analyses of clinical and heart rate characteristics in the early diagnosis of neonatal sepsis. Med Decis Making 2010;30:258–66.

189. Ratzinger F, Haslacher H, Perkmann T, et al. Machine learning for fast identification of bacteraemia in SIRS patients treated on standard care wards: a cohort study. Sci Rep 2018;8:12233.

190. Lee KH, Dong JJ, Jeong SJ, et al. Early detection of bacteraemia using ten clinical variables with an artificial neural network approach. J Clin Med 2019;8.

191. Roimi M, Neuberger A, Shrot A, et al. Early diagnosis of bloodstream infections in the intensive care unit using machine-learning algorithms. Intensive Care Med 2020;46:454–62.

192. Jaimes F, Arango C, Ruiz G, et al. Predicting bacteremia at the bedside. Clin Infect Dis 2004;38:357–62.

193. Pai KC, Wang MS, Chen YF, et al. An artificial intelligence approach to bloodstream infections prediction. J Clin Med 2021;10.

194. Lee KH, Dong JJ, Kim S, et al. Prediction of bacteremia based on 12-year medical data using a machine learning approach: effect of medical data by extraction time. Diagnostics 2022;12.

195. Bonsu BK, Chb M, Harper MB. Identifying febrile young infants with bacteremia: is the peripheral white blood cell count an accurate screen? Ann Emerg Med 2003;42:216–25.

196. Lizarralde Palacios E, Gutiérrez Macías A, Martínez Odriozola P, et al. Bacteriemia adquirida en la comunidad: elaboración de un modelo de predicción clínica en pacientes ingresados en un servicio de medicina interna. Med Clínica 2004;123:241–6.

197. Nagata K, Hirota T, Fujiwara H. [Analysis of blood cultures in patients presenting with community-acquired pneumonia at the emergency room]. J Jpn Respir Soc 2010;48:661–7.

198. Lien F, Lin HS, Wu YT, et al. Bacteremia detection from complete blood count and differential leukocyte count with machine learning: complementary and competitive with C-reactive protein and procalcitonin tests. BMC Infect Dis 2022;22:287.

199. Chase M, Klasco RS, Joyce NR, et al. Predictors of bacteremia in emergency department patients with suspected infection. Am J Emerg Med 2012;30:1691–7.

200. Kuo YY, Huang ST, Chiu HW. Applying artificial neural network for early detection of sepsis with intentionally preserved highly missing real-world data for simulating clinical situation. BMC Med Inf Decis Making 2021;21:290.

201. Jin SJ, Kim M, Yoon JH, et al. A new statistical approach to predict bacteremia using electronic medical records. Scand J Infect Dis 2013;45:672–80.
202. Rafiei A, Rezaee A, Hajati F, et al. Early prediction of sepsis using fully connected LSTM-CNN model. Comput Biol Med 2021;128:104110.
203. Wong A, Otles E, Donnelly JP, et al. External validation of a widely implemented proprietary sepsis prediction model in hospitalized patients. JAMA Intern Med 2021;181:1065–70.
204. Isaacman DJ, Shults J, Gross TK, et al. Predictors of bacteremia in febrile children 3 to 36 months of age. Pediatrics 2000;106:977–82.
205. Nemati S, Holder A, Razmi F, et al. An interpretable machine learning model for accurate prediction of sepsis in the ICU. Crit Care Med 2018;46:547–53.
206. Shashikumar SP, Josef CS, Sharma A, et al. DeepAISE - an interpretable and recurrent neural survival model for early prediction of sepsis. Artif Intell Med 2021;113:102036.
207. Lipsky BA, Kollef MH, Miller LG, et al. Predicting bacteremia among patients hospitalized for skin and skin-structure infections: derivation and validation of a risk score. Infect Control Hosp Epidemiol 2010;31:828–37.
208. Paul M, Andreassen S, Nielsen AD, et al. Prediction of bacteremia using TREAT, a computerized decision-support system. Clin Infect Dis 2006;42:1274–82.
209. Shashikumar SP, Li Q, Clifford GD, et al. Multiscale network representation of physiological time series for early prediction of sepsis. Physiol Meas 2017;38:2235–48.
210. Giannini HM, Ginestra JC, Chivers C, et al. A machine learning algorithm to predict severe sepsis and septic shock: development, implementation, and impact on clinical practice. Crit Care Med 2019;47:1485–92.
211. Adams R, Henry KE, Sridharan A, et al. Prospective, multi-site study of patient outcomes after implementation of the TREWS machine learning-based early warning system for sepsis. Nat Med 2022;28(7):1455–60.
212. Wong A, Otles E, Donnelly JP, et al. External validation of a widely implemented proprietary sepsis prediction model in hospitalized patients. JAMA Intern Med 2021;181(8):1065–70.
213. Tarabichi Y, Cheng A, Bar-Shain D, et al. Improving timeliness of antibiotic administration using a provider and pharmacist facing sepsis early warning system in the emergency department setting: a randomized controlled quality improvement initiative. Crit Care Med 2022;50(3):418–27.
214. Chen JH, Asch SM. Machine learning and prediction in medicine - beyond the peak of inflated expectations. N Engl J Med 2017;376(26):2507–9.
215. Vyas DA, Eisenstein LG, Jones DS. Hidden in plain sight - reconsidering the use of race correction in clinical algorithms. N Engl J Med 2020;383(9):874–82.

Machine Learning of Physiologic Waveforms and Electronic Health Record Data
A Large Perioperative Data Set of High-Fidelity Physiologic Waveforms

Sungsoo Kim, MD, MS[a,b,1], Sohee Kwon, MD, MPH[a,1],
Akos Rudas, PhD[c], Ravi Pal, PhD[a], Mia K. Markey, PhD[d],
Alan C. Bovik, PhD[b], Maxime Cannesson, MD, PhD[a,*]

KEYWORDS

- Machine learning • Physiologic waveforms • Deep neuronal networks
- Perioperative medicine • Surgery • Prediction

KEY POINTS

- A large data set that includes static clinical informatoin and dynamic real-time physiologic waveforms collected during the perioperative period
- Diverse outcomes including in-hospital morbity and mortality

INTRODUCTION

More than 313 million major surgical procedures are undertaken annually worldwide, and more than 42 million surgeries are performed annually in the United States.[1–3] According to the time of surgery, the perioperative period is categorized into 3 groups: preoperative, intraoperative, and postoperative periods.[4,5] Intraoperative mortality is now rare,[6,7] but the postoperative mortality still remains high, with about 2% of patients undertaking noncardiac surgery dying within 1 month after surgery.[8] The postoperative period accounts for approximately 4 million deaths per year worldwide.[9]

During the perioperative period, a variety of medical factors can be analyzed to predict the outcomes of surgery and the prognosis of patients.[4,5] The factors can be

[a] Department of Anesthesiology and Perioperative Medicine, University of California Los Angeles, Los Angeles, CA 90095, USA; [b] Department of Electrical & Computer Engineering, The University of Texas at Austin, Austin, TX, USA; [c] Department of Computational Medicine, University of California Los Angeles, Los Angeles, CA 90095, USA; [d] Department of Biomedical Engineering, The University of Texas at Austin, Austin, TX, USA
[1] Contributed equally as the first author.
* Corresponding author. Department of Anesthesiology and Perioperative Medicine, David Geffen School of Medicine at UCLA, 757 Westwood Plaza, Los Angeles, CA 90095.
E-mail address: mcannesson@mednet.ucla.edu

Crit Care Clin 39 (2023) 675–687
https://doi.org/10.1016/j.ccc.2023.03.003
0749-0704/23/© 2023 Elsevier Inc. All rights reserved.

categorized broadly into 2 classes: static versus dynamic as to the factor changes over time. The static factors, such as age, sex, and past medical history, are stationary over a substantial time period. In contrast, dynamic factors, such as vital signs (physiologic waveforms), including blood pressure, heart rate, and respiratory rate, are versatile over a short time period.

The postoperative morbidity and mortality are significantly associated with both static and dynamic perioperative factors.[7] Among the static factors, postoperative complications, including myocardial injury and acute kidney injury, are most strongly associated with postoperative mortality.[8,10] Those factors were closely related to a patient's baseline condition, which might not be modified during the perioperative period.[11] Among the dynamic factors, intraoperative or postoperative hypotension is strongly associated with postoperative myocardial injury, acute kidney injury, and mortality.[12–15] Recently, the importance of analyzing the dynamic factors has been revitalized given that the dynamic factor is potentially modifiable in the perioperative period to reduce adverse surgical outcomes.[7]

Despite the clinical importance of dynamic factors for predicting perioperative outcomes, few previous studies have analyzed perioperative dynamic factors.[16,17] Research on dynamic factors has been hindered by the lack of relevant data sets.[16] Large medical data sets, especially the MIMIC and eICU data sets, were published that include patients' vital signs that were measured at patients' bedside at the intensive care unit or emergency department.[18–20] However, these data sets do not include perioperative information of patients who underwent surgeries. Furthermore, it does not include real-time dynamic waveform data, which were measured continuously. Collecting and organizing diverse dynamic factors within different data formats along with different frequencies of occurrence is technically challenging.[18]

To fill the gap, the authors introduce a novel, large perioperative data set: MLORD data set. It has 3 unique features: (1) the data set was collected during preoperative, intraoperative, and postoperative periods; (2) the data set was composed of a large patient population (n = 17,327) under close continuous surgical observations (72,264 hours); (3) the data set was composed of continuous dynamic vital signs (real-time physiologic waveforms) with a high frequency (at the maximum rate of 256 data points in 1 second [256 Hz]).

METHOD
Patient Population

A total of 17,327 patients were enrolled in this large perioperative data set: MLORD to Predict, Diagnose, and Treat Hemodynamic Instability in Surgical Patients (NIH research funding: R01HL14469). All patients underwent surgeries between 2019 and 2022 at UCLA.

Data Definition and Description

Variables were categorized into 2 classes: static factors and dynamic factors. The authors define a factor as static if it is not changed within 5 minutes and as dynamic if the factor is changed within 5 minutes. The value of a 5-minute cutoff was selected based on the current guideline for Standards of Basic Anesthetic Monitoring.[21] Static factors include age, sex, body mass index, past medical history, drinking history, smoking history, and surgery type according to Current Procedural Terminology (CPT) code. Baseline laboratory values, such as complete blood counts or basic metabolic panel, collected during the preoperative period are likewise categorized as static factors because they occur only once. Dynamic factors include vital signs that are continuously observed by electrical monitors, such as blood pressure, heart rate, and respiratory rate. Similarly, intermittent interventions, such as infusions of medications, boluses of medications, measurements of blood loss, and measurement of urine output, are categorized as dynamic factors because they change frequently. In addition, follow-up laboratory values collected during the intraoperative and postoperative periods were categorized as dynamic factors because they are repeated within a relatively short time period.

Data Acquisition

Informed by the authors' previous research,[16] the MLORD data set consists of both clinical data and waveform data. The data mining process is depicted in **Fig 1**. Clinical data were retrieved from EHR including Epic (Verona, WI, USA) and Surgical Information Systems (Alpharetta, GA, USA).[22] The waveform data were collected in the operating room directly through the Bernoulli data collection system (Cardiopulmonary, New Haven, CT, USA). The waveforms encompassed in the MLORD data set are more than 72,264 hours of data time and 7.6 TB of data size. The waveform data consist of continuous physiologic waveforms generated from vital sign monitoring devices, such as ECG, photoplethysmography, and ventilation machines. The waveform data were collected at different, preestablished sampling rates from 1/3 Hz to 256 Hz. For example, systolic blood pressure was captured at 1/3 Hz, whereas ECG was captured at 256 Hz. All standards of Basic Anesthetic Monitoring waveform[21] were collected if it was collected in the perioperative setting. If there were data from additional devices, such as invasive arterial blood pressure monitor or muscle twitch

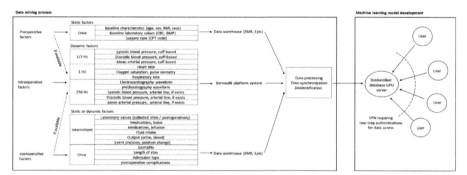

Fig. 1. Framework for data mining process and machine learning developments. During data mining process, perioperative/intraoperative/postoperative factors are collected based on patient-specific data availability. Clinical data, including baseline characteristics, laboratory values, surgery type, medications (bolus dose, infusion rate), output (urine, blood), mortality, and length of stay, are collected by data warehouse through the EMR and the Epic system. Continuous waveform data with different frequency, including blood pressure, oxygen saturation, heart rate, ECG, and photoplethysmography, are collected through the Bernoulli platform system. All collected factors are processed, synchronized by absolute time stamps, deidentified automatically, and forwarded to the deidentified database GPU server. During the machine learning model development process, each user accesses remotely into the deidentified database GPU servers and corporates to build a project-specific prediction or classification models. The users require 2 steps of independent authentications verifying the users' identification for accessing the MLORD data set through VPN. GPU, graphic processing unit; EMR, electronic medical record; Hz, hertz (one event per second); VPN, virtual private networks.

monitor, the data were also collected and stored. All alarms and warning signs that were generated by the ventilation machine during operation were also collected. All waveform data were automatically deidentified. The data were synchronized retrospectively with the clinical data from the EHR. The MLORD data set was generated securely at UCLA.

Data Accessibility

Because of institutional policies on privacy of patient and security of medical data, access to the MLORD data set is limited and cannot be made publicly available in an uncontrolled repository. Public availability is under discussion within the institution. At this point, access to the MLORD data set can be requested from the institution or individuals for research purposes. Interested parties may contact the corresponding author (mcannesson@mednet.ucla.edu) or the first author (sungsookim@mednet. ucla.edu) to request access to the MLORD data set.

RESULTS

Table 1 reports the demographics of the patients in the MLORD data set. A total of 17,327 patients were included in this study. Slightly more male patients (51.5%) than female patients were enrolled. The mean (standard deviation) age was 57.1 (17.7) years. The distribution of patients by race was white (n = 9035 [52%]), Asian (n = 790 [9.4%]), black (n = 1112 [6.4%]), and others (n = 2917 [32.6%]). A total of 65% (n = 9324) were nonsmokers, and 58% (n = 4553) were current drinkers.

 Table 2 provides a summary of participants' past medical histories. The top 30 highest conditions are presented in Supplementary Table 1. The most common past medical histories were hypertension (n = 2321 [13%]), coronary artery disease (n = 1078 [6.2%]), and hyperlipidemia (n = 1295 [7.5%]).

 Table 3 presents a list of the primary procedures represented in the data set. The top 30 primary procedures that occurred most frequently are provided in Supplementary Table 2. A total of 33,311 primary procedures with 2008 different procedure codes were included in this study. The most common primary procedures were left heart catheterization (n = 708 [4.1%]), right-left heart catheterization (n = 652 [3.8%]), and ablation of atrial fibrillation (n = 542 [3.2%]).

 As a subgroup analysis, patients who received arterial line placements were analyzed. Continuous dynamic waveform data, including invasive arterial blood pressures, were available for this subgroup. **Table 4** demonstrated the demographics of patients categorized by absence or presence of invasive arterial line placement (no vs yes). Compared with patients without invasive arterial line placements, patients with invasive arterial line placements were older and more likely to be men, a smoker, and not an alcohol user (P<.001).

 Table 5 provides a list of past medical history categorized by absence or presence of an invasive arterial line placement (no vs yes). The 30 highest incidence past medical histories in patients are presented in Supplementary Table 3. Noticeably, arterial lines were placed more frequently with patients with coronary artery disease (P<.001) or atrial fibrillation (P<.005).

 Table 6 lists primary procedures categorized by absence or presence of invasive arterial line placement (no vs yes). The 30 most frequent primary procedures in patients with invasive arterial line placement are shown in Supplementary Table 4. Noticeably, arterial lines were placed more frequently in patients who underwent right-left heart catheterization, exploratory laparotomy, coronary artery bypass graft, liver transplant, and flexible bronchoscopy (all P<.001). However, there was no

Table 1
Baseline characteristics of patients[a]

	Missing	Overall	Female	Male
n		17,327	8389	8936
Age, mean (SD)	0	57.1 (17.7)	55.8 (17.6)	58.3 (17.7)
Sex, n (%)[b]				
Female	0	8389 (48.4)	8389 (100.0)	
Male		8936 (51.6)		8936 (100.0)
Unknown		2 (0.0)		
Race, n(%)[c]				
Asian	0	1500 (8.7)	790 (9.4)	709 (7.9)
Black		1112 (6.4)	581 (6.9)	531 (5.9)
Others		5680 (32.8)	2763 (32.9)	2917 (32.6)
White		9035 (52.1)	4255 (50.7)	4779 (53.5)
Smoking status, n (%)				
Never	3077	9324 (65.4)	5049 (72.1)	4274 (59.0)
Not Asked		307 (2.2)	151 (2.2)	156 (2.2)
Passive		56 (0.4)	34 (0.5)	22 (0.3)
Quit		3684 (25.9)	1456 (20.8)	2228 (30.8)
Yes		879 (6.2)	317 (4.5)	562 (7.8)
Alcohol use, n (%)				
Never	4553	787 (6.2)	467 (7.4)	320 (4.9)
No		2943 (23.0)	1575 (25.0)	1368 (21.1)
Not asked		585 (4.6)	291 (4.6)	294 (4.5)
Not currently		1065 (8.3)	511 (8.1)	554 (8.5)
Yes		7394 (57.9)	3448 (54.8)	3946 (60.9)
Intravenous drug use, n (%)				
No	1892	15,429 (100.0)	7502 (100.0)	7926 (99.9)
Yes		6 (0.0)	2 (0.0)	4 (0.1)

Abbreviation: EMR, electric medical records.
[a] Data were obtained from all patients included in the MLORD data set (n = 17,327).
[b] Sex is categorized into female, male, and unknown based on patients' responses.
[c] For simplicity, race is recategorized into Asian, black, other, and white. In the UCLA EMR system, race is categorized into "Asian," "Black: African American," "African American," "European," "Asian: Filipino," "American Indian or Alaska Native," "Declined to Specify," "Asian: Asian Indian," "Asian: Taiwanese," "Asian: Vietnamese," "American Indian," "Asian: Pakistani," "Chinese," "Do Not Identify with Race," "Choose Not to Answer," "Asian: Japanese," "Not Listed," "Pacific Islander: Native Hawaiian," "Filipino," "Alaska Native," "Indonesian," "Asian: Indonesian," "Asian: Thai," "Iranian," "Assyrian," "Asian: Not Listed," "African," "Korean," "Indian (India)," "Taiwanese," "Pacific Islander: Other," "Native Hawaiian or Other Pacific Islander," "Caribbean/West Indian," and "Pacific Islander: Samoan."

statistically significant difference in the frequency of invasive arterial line placement in patients who underwent left heart catheterization ($P = .22$).

DISCUSSION

It is remarkable that the MLORD data set has several unique features. First, the MLORD data set contains patients' medical information obtained during preoperative,

Table 2				
The common past medical history in MLORD data set[a]				
		Overall	**Female**	**Male**
N		17,327	8389	8936
Hypertension, n (%)	False	15,006 (86.6)	7422 (88.5)	7582 (84.8)
	True	2321 (13.4)	967 (11.5)	1354 (15.2)
Coronary artery disease, n (%)	False	16,249 (93.8)	8136 (97.0)	8111 (90.8)
	True	1078 (6.2)	253 (3.0)	825 (9.2)
Hyperlipidemia, n (%)	False	16,032 (92.5)	7822 (93.2)	8208 (91.9)
	True	1295 (7.5)	567 (6.8)	728 (8.1)
GERD (gastroesophageal reflux	False	16,359 (94.4)	7876 (93.9)	8481 (94.9)
disease), n (%)	True	968 (5.6)	513 (6.1)	455 (5.1)
Hypothyroidism, n (%)	False	16,494 (95.2)	7840 (93.5)	8652 (96.8)
	True	833 (4.8)	549 (6.5)	284 (3.2)
Prediabetes, n (%)	False	16,531 (95.4)	7972 (95.0)	8557 (95.8)
	True	796 (4.6)	417 (5.0)	379 (4.2)
Anemia, n (%)	False	16,635 (96.0)	8037 (95.8)	8596 (96.2)
	True	692 (4.0)	352 (4.2)	340 (3.8)
Vitamin D deficiency, n (%)	False	16,686 (96.3)	7989 (95.2)	8695 (97.3)
	True	641 (3.7)	400 (4.8)	241 (2.7)
Dyslipidemia, n (%)	False	16,707 (96.4)	8160 (97.3)	8545 (95.6)
	True	620 (3.6)	229 (2.7)	391 (4.4)
Anxiety, n (%)	False	16,687 (96.3)	7980 (95.1)	8705 (97.4)
	True	640 (3.7)	409 (4.9)	231 (2.6)

[a]Data were obtained from all patients in MLORD data set (n = 17,327). A total of 306,976 past medical histories were reported from all patients in the MLORD data set. There are 13,021 unique disease codes (ICD codes) of past medical history. The average number of past medical history per one patient was 19.1. For simplicity, the top 10 of the most common past medical history were selected. The other past medical history was demonstrated in Supplementary Table 1.

intraoperative, and postoperative periods. Few prior data sets include patients' medical data from the operating room during surgeries.[16,23] Second, the MLORD data set contains a much larger size of the patient population (n = 17,327) than previous operating room data sets, such as Edward Lifesciences waveform database (n = 670)[23] and University of California at Irvine Medical Center waveform data set (n = 204).[16,23] The size of the MLORD data set may provide a sufficient volume of data for modern machine learning research, as the study protocol was designed[24] to enable training of prediction models. Third, the MLORD data set is composed of continuous real-time dynamic physiologic waveforms. The waveforms include all vital signs that are recommended by the American Society of Anesthesiologists[21] for monitoring patients during operations. The dynamic waveforms consist of heart signal, invasive arterial blood pressure, cuff-based blood pressure, and photoplethysmography. The waveforms provide real-time information with a high level of fidelity in diverse data structures. The physiologic waveform provides physiologic signals, which is beneficial for immediate and proactive patients' care in the operating room. Given these unique features, the MLORD data set may enable clinical informatics, epidemiology, and machine learning research to progress rapidly for advanced understanding of physiologic reactions during critical care of surgery.

The subgroup analysis of patients who received arterial line placements demonstrated findings that are consistent with prior studies and established clinical knowledge, which provides reassurance that the MLORD data set represents the patient

Table 3
The common primary procedures that are included in MLORD data set[a]

		Overall	Female	Male
n		17,327	8389	8936
Right-left heart cath, n (%)	False	16,675 (96.2)	8134 (97.0)	8539 (95.6)
	True	652 (3.8)	255 (3.0)	397 (4.4)
Left heart cath, n (%)	False	16,619 (95.9)	8185 (97.6)	8432 (94.4)
	True	708 (4.1)	204 (2.4)	504 (5.6)
Ablation A-FIB, n (%)	False	16781 (96.8)	8195 (97.7)	8584 (96.1)
	True	546 (3.2)	194 (2.3)	352 (3.9)
Magnetic Resonance angiography lower extremity without contrast, n (%)	False	16,898 (97.5)	8194 (97.7)	8702 (97.4)
	True	429 (2.5)	195 (2.3)	234 (2.6)
Exploratory laparotomy, n (%)	False	16,898 (97.5)	8194 (97.7)	8702 (97.4)
	True	429 (2.5)	195 (2.3)	234 (2.6)
Sickle cell Preparation, n (%)	False	16,949 (97.8)	8237 (98.2)	8710 (97.5)
	True	378 (2.2)	152 (1.8)	226 (2.5)
Cadaveric renal transplant, n (%)	False	16,949 (97.8)	8237 (98.2)	8710 (97.5)
	True	378 (2.2)	152 (1.8)	226 (2.5)
Coronary artery bypass graft, n (%)	False	17,021 (98.2)	8334 (99.3)	8685 (97.2)
	True	306 (1.8)	55 (0.7)	251 (2.8)
Unrestricted visitation status, n (%)	False	17,021 (98.2)	8334 (99.3)	8685 (97.2)
	True	306 (1.8)	55 (0.7)	251 (2.8)
Interleukin- 6 serum, n (%)	False	17,031 (98.3)	8093 (96.5)	8936 (100.0)
	True	296 (1.7)	296 (3.5)	

[a]Data were obtained from all patients in MLORD data set (n = 17,327). A total of 33,311 primary procedures were proceeded with all patients in MLORD data set. There are 1130 unique procedure codes (CPT codes) in MLORD data set. The average number of primary procedures per patient was 1.81. For simplicity, the top 10 of the most common primary procedures were selected. The other primary procedures were demonstrated in Supplementary Table 2.

population of interest. For example, patients with possibly worse medical conditions, including older age and smoking history, in the MLORD data set demonstrated more frequent invasive arterial line insertion placements.[4] Furthermore, MLORD patients with higher cardiac injury burdens, such as history of coronary artery disease and atrial fibrillation, also demonstrated more frequent invasive arterial line insertion placements. In addition, certain types of primary procedures, such as coronary artery bypass graft or liver transplant, were highly related with invasive arterial line placement, consistent with prior knowledge that the type of primary procedure is an important factor in the decision to place an invasive arterial line for continuous monitoring of arterial blood pressure or predicting fluid responsiveness.[4,5]

Given the large number of patients assessed and the diversity of data structures collected, the MLORD data set presents a unique opportunity to advance knowledge of perioperative morbidity and mortality.[16] Conventional statistical methods, such as a logistic regression, may be an insufficient analytical tool for the continuous physiologic waveform.[16] In the authors' previous research, quantitative methods were applied to extract physiologic characteristics of the waveforms but caused potential loss of information that waveforms may contain. Recently, machine learning/artificial intelligence approaches have been widely applied into the diverse structure of data sets.[24–27] Continuous waveforms with diverse patterns can be effectively analyzed with machine learning/artificial intelligence approaches.[24,26] In the following discussion, the authors

Table 4
Baseline characteristics of patients, categorized by categorized by a absence or an absence of invasive arterial line placement (no vs yes)[a]

	Missing	Overall	No	Yes	P Value
		17,327	12,510	4817	
Age, mean (SD)	0	57.1 (17.7)	56.2 (17.9)	59.5 (16.9)	<.001
Sex, n (%)[b]					
Female	0	8389 (48.4)	6390 (51.1)	1999 (41.5)	<.001
Male		8936 (51.6)	6119 (48.9)	2817 (58.5)	
Unknown		2 (0.0)	1 (0.0)	1 (0.0)	
Race, n (%)[c]					
Asian	0	1500 (8.7)	1091 (8.7)	409 (8.5)	.004
Black		1112 (6.4)	809 (6.5)	303 (6.3)	
Others		5680 (32.8)	4000 (32.0)	1680 (34.9)	
White		9035 (52.1)	6610 (52.8)	2425 (50.3)	
Smoking status, n (%)					
Never	3077	9324 (65.4)	7011 (67.2)	2313 (60.5)	<.001
Not asked		307 (2.2)	216 (2.1)	91 (2.4)	
Passive		56 (0.4)	40 (0.4)	16 (0.4)	
Quit		3684 (25.9)	2533 (24.3)	1151 (30.1)	
Yes		879 (6.2)	629 (6.0)	250 (6.5)	
Alcohol use, n (%)					
Never	4553	787 (6.2)	564 (6.0)	223 (6.5)	<.001
No		2943 (23.0)	2102 (22.5)	841 (24.6)	
Not asked		585 (4.6)	454 (4.9)	131 (3.8)	
Not currently		1065 (8.3)	718 (7.7)	347 (10.1)	
Yes		7394 (57.9)	5513 (59.0)	1881 (55.0)	
IV drug use, n (%)					
No	1892	15,429 (100.0)	11,293 (100.0)	4136 (100.0)	1.000
Yes		6 (0.0)	5 (0.0)	1 (0.0)	

[a] Data were obtained from patients in MLORD data set.
[b] Sex is categorized into female, male, and unknown based on patients' responses.
[c] For simplicity, race is re-categorized into Asian, black, other, and white. In UCLA EMR system, race is categorized into "Asian," "Black: African American," "African American," "European," "Asian: Filipino," "American Indian or Alaska Native," "Declined to Specify," "Asian: Asian Indian," "Asian: Taiwanese," "Asian: Vietnamese," "American Indian," "Asian: Pakistani," "Chinese," "Do Not Identify with Race," "Choose Not to Answer," "Asian: Japanese," "Not Listed," "Pacific Islander: Native Hawaiian," "Filipino," "Alaska Native," "Indonesian," "Asian: Indonesian," "Asian: Thai," "Iranian," "Assyrian," "Asian: Not Listed," "African," "Korean," "Indian (India)," "Taiwanese," "Pacific Islander: Other," "Native Hawaiian or Other Pacific Islander," "Caribbean/West Indian," and "Pacific Islander: Samoan."

provide a concise tutorial on machine learning to assist the reader in recognizing the transformative potential of the MLORD data set.

Machine learning is a subset of artificial intelligence using pattern-recognition to analyze associations within data.[24,26] The benefit of machine learning is an automated self-learning process from large data sets to extract patterns and inferences automatically. Machine learning models can be classified into the 2 following categories: linear and nonlinear approaches. Linear models include logistic regression and linear regression that demonstrate associations between risk factors and exposure. Nonlinear models include more broad categories, including decision trees, random forests, and supportive vector machines. Deep neural networks refer to a class of promising nonlinear machine learning models that learn features or representations at increasing levels of abstraction.

Table 5					
The most common past medical history, categorized by a presence or an absence of invasive arterial line placement (no vs yes)[a]					
		Overall	False	True	P Value
N		17,327	12,510	4817	
Hypertension, n (%)	False	15,006 (86.6)	10,810 (86.4)	4196 (87.1)	.237
	True	2321 (13.4)	1700 (13.6)	621 (12.9)	
Coronary artery disease, n (%)	False	16,249 (93.8)	11,869 (94.9)	4380 (90.9)	<.001
	True	1078 (6.2)	641 (5.1)	437 (9.1)	
Hypothyroidism, n (%)	False	16,494 (95.2)	11,902 (95.1)	4592 (95.3)	.630
	True	833 (4.8)	608 (4.9)	225 (4.7)	
Hyperlipidemia, n (%)	False	16,032 (92.5)	11,568 (92.5)	4464 (92.7)	.674
	True	1295 (7.5)	942 (7.5)	353 (7.3)	
GERD, n (%)	False	16,359 (94.4)	11,784 (94.2)	4575 (95.0)	.049
	True	968 (5.6)	726 (5.8)	242 (5.0)	
Prediabetes, n (%)	False	1653 1 (95.4)	11,928 (95.3)	4603 (95.6)	.582
	True	796 (4.6)	582 (4.7)	214 (4.4)	
Atrial fibrillation, n (%)	False	16,751 (96.7)	12,126 (96.9)	4625 (96.0)	.003
	True	576 (3.3)	384 (3.1)	192 (4.0)	
Anemia, n (%)	False	16,635 (96.0)	12,006 (96.0)	4629 (96.1)	.737
	True	692 (4.0)	504 (4.0)	188 (3.9)	
Dyslipidemia, n (%)	False	16,707 (96.4)	12,051 (96.3)	4656 (96.7)	.321
	True	620 (3.6)	459 (3.7)	161 (3.3)	
Vitamin D deficiency, n (%)	False	16,686 (96.3)	12,024 (96.1)	4662 (96.8)	.041
	True	641 (3.7)	486 (3.9)	155 (3.2)	

[a] Data were obtained from patients in the MLORD data set (n = 17,327). A total of 88,568 past medical histories were reported from patients with invasive arterial line placement in the MLORD data set (n = 4723). There are 8211 unique disease codes (ICD codes) of past medical history. The average number of past medical history per one patient was 19.3. For simplicity, the top 10 of the most common past medical history was selected in a subgroup of patients with invasive arterial line placement (n = 4817). Please refer to Supplementary Table 3, which demonstrates other past medical histories were frequently reported with a subgroup population who received invasive arterial line placement (n = 4817).

Compared with simpler machine learning models with only 2 layers of learning, deep learning models can be composed of millions of parameters with multiple layers of learning process. Deep learning was originally proposed in the early 1980s but only recently demonstrated dramatic progressions owing to significant progression of computing power.[25] Machine learning algorithms typically can be categorized into 2 main groups according to the presence or absence of supervised training process using a full labeling data set. Noticeably, deep learning using multilayer processing has been widely applied in both supervised and unsupervised learning and demonstrated acceptable performance.[24–27]

The MLORD data set contains diverse continuous waveforms of vital signs. A waveform is composed of sequential data with time information. Compared with conventional risk factors, such as simple numeric or categorical variables, waveforms require more sophisticated machine learning methods for analysis. Next, 3 types of deep learning algorithms are summarized that can be effective for complex data types, such as physiologic waveforms: convolutional neural networks, recurrent neural networks, and transformers.

In recent years, convolutional networks have been widely applied with tremendous success in fields such as computer vision.[24–27] It can readily scale to 2- or 3-

Table 6
Primary procedures, categorized by a presence or an absence of invasive arterial line placement (no vs yes)[a]

		Overall	False	True	P Value
n		17,327	12,510	4817	
Right-left heart cath, n (%)	False	16,675 (96.2)	12,168 (97.3)	4507 (93.6)	<.001
	True	652 (3.8)	342 (2.7)	310 (6.4)	
RIS MR Lower extremity without contrast left IP, n (%)	False	16,898 (97.5)	12,398 (99.1)	4500 (93.4)	<.001
	True	429 (2.5)	112 (0.9)	317 (6.6)	
Exploratory laparotomy, n (%)	False	16,898 (97.5)	12,398 (99.1)	4500 (93.4)	<.001
	True	429 (2.5)	112 (0.9)	317 (6.6)	
Unrestricted visitation status, n (%)	False	17,021 (98.2)	12,493 (99.9)	4528 (94.0)	<.001
	True	306 (1.8)	17 (0.1)	289 (6.0)	
Coronary artery bypass graft, n (%)	False	17,021 (98.2)	12,493 (99.9)	4528 (94.0)	<.001
	True	306 (1.8)	17 (0.1)	289 (6.0)	
Influenza A B Respiratory Syncytial Virus Infection (RSV) PCR reflex to resp virus panel, respiratory upper, n (%)	False	17,078 (98.6)	12,499 (99.9)	4579 (95.1)	<.001
	True	249 (1.4)	11 (0.1)	238 (4.9)	
Liver transplant adult, n (%)	False	17,078 (98.6)	12,499 (99.9)	4579 (95.1)	<.001
	True	249 (1.4)	11 (0.1)	238 (4.9)	
Bronchoscopy flexible, n (%)	False	17,058 (98.4)	12,433 (99.4)	4625 (96.0)	<.001
	True	269 (1.6)	77 (0.6)	192 (4.0)	
Bleeding time, n (%)	False	17,058 (98.4)	12,433 (99.4)	4625 (96.0)	<.001
	True	269 (1.6)	77 (0.6)	192 (4.0)	
Left heart cath, n (%)	False	16,619 (95.9)	11,984 (95.8)	4635 (96.2)	.220
	True	708 (4.1)	526 (4.2)	182 (3.8)	

[a] Data were obtained from patients in MLORD data set (n = 17,327). A total of 11,212 primary procedures were proceeded in patients with invasive arterial line placement in the MLORD data set (n = 4723). There are 677 unique procedure codes (CPT codes) in the MLORD data set. The average number of primary procedures per one patient was 2.01. For simplicity, the top 10 of the most common primary procedures were selected in a subgroup of patients with invasive arterial line placement (n = 4817). Please refer to Supplementary Table 4, which demonstrates other primary procedures that were frequently proceeded in a subgroup population who received invasive arterial line placement (n = 4817).

dimensional data with multiple kernels to extract spatial or temporal features of data. Convolutional neural networks can be also applied into a 1D temporal sequence. The convolution operation allows a network to share parameters across time effectively. However, the time span may be shallow if kernel sizes are insufficient. Thus, a limited number of neighboring features of the input can be analyzed simultaneously through a network. However, this drawback can be successfully addressed by appropriate kernel sizes with favorable complexity and processing time.

Recurrent neural networks provide another way to extend deep learning to sequential data. Recurrent networks can scale to longer sequences than would be practical for networks without sequence-based specialization, and most recurrent networks can also process sequences of variable length.[24–27] Each member of the network output is a function using the previous members of the output. The same update rule is applied to previous members of output as a chain. This recurrent structure results in the sharing of parameters through long computational graphs.[28] Long short-term memory refers to recurrent neural networks that use self-loops with scalable weights to generate internal paths where information can flow for long durations.[29]

Similar to recurrent neural networks, transformers are used to process sequential data. However, transformers process entire sequences at once based solely on novel attention mechanisms without any recurrent layers, in contrast to convolutional or recurrent neural networks that use the dominant sequence flow of information.[30] An advantage of transformers is that they are more parallelizable, which means that high performance can be achieved with significantly less time for network training with a sufficient amount of training data. Transformers can be effective solutions for high-performance models in data-risk tasks.

Although the performance of deep neural networks can be impressive, 3 key issues need to be considered before using the class of methods.

First, deep learning models can be overfit, especially when applied to smaller data sets.[25] Put another way, traditional machine learning or statistical models are more reliable than deep learning models for smaller sample sizes.[24] In some cases, transfer learning, a type of machine learning in which knowledge is transferred from other domains with sufficient data samples into a specific domain that suffers from a lack of data, may enable the use of a deep learning model on a smaller data set.[31]

Second, deep learning methods typically entail extensive training complexity and lengthy processing time.[30] In some cases, this concern can be mitigated by selection of representative subgroups using substantial exclusion criteria or feature reduction using feature selection algorithms. If sufficient data are available, training time can also be reduced through use of an attention-based deep learning model.

Third, lack of interpretability is a concerning challenge posed by deep learning models, particularly when they are applied in the medical field.[32,33] The nonlinear characteristic of deep learning hinders visualization of associations among factors and outcomes in contrast to traditional statistical models that can more readily support the understanding of disease and physiology. Therefore, applying deep learning algorithms to health data requires careful consideration.[32,33] With respect to the potential of the MLORD data set, notice that 2 of the 3 key concerns about deep learning models are assuaged by the availability of a large number of observations, and the MLORD data set contains data from 17,327 patients.

SUMMARY

In this research, the authors describe the MLORD data set, a large data set that includes dynamic real-time physiologic waveforms collected during the perioperative period. Because of its large size and diversity of data structures, the MLORD data set will permit the use of modern machine learning algorithms, such as deep neural networks, empowering new discoveries that will transform research on perioperative complications including myocardial infarction, kidney failure, stroke, or mortality.

AUTHOR CONTRIBUTION

Conception and design: S. Kim, S. Kwon, M. Cannesson. Administrative support: M. Cannesson Provision of study materials or patients: M. Cannesson. Collection and assembly of data: S. Kim, M. Cannesson. Data analysis and interpretation: All authors. Manuscript writing: All authors. Final approval of manuscript: All authors. Accountable for all aspects of the work: All authors.

CONFLICT OF INTEREST DISCLOSURE

None reported.

ROLE OF THE FUNDING SOURCE

This research is supported by NIH research funding (R01HL144692; Machine Learning of Physiological Waveforms and Electronic Health Record Data to Predict, Diagnose, and Treat Hemodynamic Instability in Surgical Patients) and by UCLA Anesthesiology & Perioperative Medicine Seed grant (441006-2X-75014; Application of Deep Learning for real-time noninvasive continuous monitoring for enhanced vital monitoring).

SUPPLEMENTARY DATA

Supplementary data related to this article can be found online at https://doi.org/10.1016/j.ccc.2023.03.003.

REFERENCES

1. Weiser TG, Haynes AB, Molina G, et al. Size and distribution of the global volume of surgery in 2012. Bull World Health Organ 2016;94(3):201–209F.
2. Weiser TG, Regenbogen SE, Thompson KD, et al. An estimation of the global volume of surgery: a modelling strategy based on available data. Lancet 2008; 372(9633):139–44.
3. Meara JG, Leather AJM, Hagander L, et al. Global Surgery 2030: evidence and solutions for achieving health, welfare, and economic development. Lancet 2015; 386(9993):569–624.
4. Butterworth JF, Mackey DC, Wasnick JD. Morgan and Mikhail's clinical anesthesiology. McGraw-Hill Education; 2018.
5. Barash PG. Clinical anesthesia. Lippincott Williams & Wilkins; 2009.
6. Li G, Warner M, Lang BH, et al. Epidemiology of anesthesia-related mortality in the United States, 1999–2005. Anesthesiology 2009;110(4):759–65.
7. Saugel B, Sessler DI. Perioperative blood pressure management. Anesthesiology 2021;134(2):250–61.
8. The Vascular Events in Noncardiac Surgery Patients Cohort Evaluation (VISION) Study Investigators, Spence J, LeManach Y, et al. Association between complications and death within 30 days after noncardiac surgery. Can Med Assoc J 2019; 191(30):E830–7.
9. Nepogodiev D, Martin J, Biccard B, et al. Global burden of postoperative death. Lancet 2019;393(10170):401.
10. Ahuja S, Mascha EJ, Yang D, et al. Associations of Intraoperative Radial arterial systolic, Diastolic, mean, and Pulse pressures with myocardial and acute kidney injury after noncardiac surgery. Anesthesiology 2020;132(2):291–306.
11. Mathis MR, Naik BI, Freundlich RE, et al. Preoperative risk and the association between hypotension and postoperative acute kidney injury. Anesthesiology 2020;132(3):461–75.
12. Walsh M, Devereaux PJ, Garg AX, et al. Relationship between Intraoperative mean arterial pressure and clinical outcomes after noncardiac surgery. Anesthesiology 2013;119(3):507–15.
13. Salmasi V, Maheshwari K, Yang D, et al. Relationship between Intraoperative hypotension, defined by Either reduction from baseline or absolute Thresholds, and acute kidney and myocardial injury after noncardiac surgery. Anesthesiology 2017;126(1):47–65.
14. Sessler DI, Meyhoff CS, Zimmerman NM, et al. Period-dependent associations between hypotension during and for Four Days after noncardiac surgery and a

composite of myocardial Infarction and death. Anesthesiology 2018;128(2): 317–27.

15. Mascha EJ, Yang D, Weiss S, et al. Intraoperative mean arterial pressure Variability and 30-day mortality in patients having noncardiac surgery. Anesthesiology 2015;123(1):79–91.
16. Cannesson M, Hofer I, Rinehart J, et al. Machine learning of physiological waveforms and electronic health record data to predict, diagnose and treat haemodynamic instability in surgical patients: protocol for a retrospective study. BMJ Open 2019;9(12):e031988.
17. Davies SJ, Vistisen ST, Jian Z, et al. Ability of an arterial waveform analysis–Derived hypotension prediction index to predict Future hypotensive events in surgical patients. Anesth Analg 2020;130(2):352–9.
18. Pollard TJ, Johnson AEW, Raffa JD, et al. The eICU Collaborative Research Database, a freely available multi-center database for critical care research. Sci Data 2018;5(1):180178.
19. Johnson, A., Bulgarelli, L., Pollard, T., et al., Mimic-iv. PhysioNet. 2020. Available at: https://physionet.org/content/mimiciv/1.0/. Accessed August 23, 2021.
20. Johnson A, Bulgarelli L, Pollard T, et al. MIMIC-IV-ED. PhysioNet 2021.
21. Committee on Standards and Practice Parameters (CSPP). Standards for basic Anesthetic monitoring. Available at: https://www.asahq.org/standards-and-guidelines/standards-for-basic-anesthetic-monitoring, American Society of Anesthesiologists, 2020.
22. Hofer IS, Gabel E, Pfeffer M, et al. A systematic approach to creation of a perioperative data warehouse. Anesth Analg 2016;122(6):1880–4.
23. Hatib F, Jian Z, Buddi S, et al. Machine-learning algorithm to predict hypotension based on high-fidelity arterial pressure waveform analysis. Anesthesiology 2018; 129(4):663–74.
24. Murphy KP. Machine learning: a probabilistic perspective. MIT press; 2012.
25. LeCun Y, Bengio Y, Hinton G. Deep learning. Nature 2015;521(7553):436–44.
26. Mohri M, Rostamizadeh A, Talwalkar A. Foundations of machine learning. MIT press; 2018.
27. Goodfellow I, Bengio Y, Courville A. Deep learning. MIT press; 2016.
28. Graves A, Rahman MA, Hinton G. Speech recognition with deep recurrent neural networks. In: 2013 IEEE International Conference on Acoustics, Speech and signal processing. IEEE 2013;6645–9.
29. Gers FA, Schmidhuber J, Cummins F. Learning to forget: Continual prediction with LSTM. Neural Comput 2000;12(10):2451–71.
30. Vaswani A, Shazeer N, Parmar N, et al. Attention is all you need. Adv Neural Inf Process Syst 2017;30.
31. Pan SJ, Yang Q. A survey on transfer learning. IEEE Trans Knowl Data Eng 2010; 22(10):1345–59.
32. Gianfrancesco MA, Tamang S, Yazdany J, et al. Potential biases in machine learning algorithms using electronic health record data. JAMA Intern Med 2018;178(11):1544–7.
33. Cabitza F, Rasoini R, Gensini GF. Unintended consequences of machine learning in medicine. JAMA 2017;318(6):517–8.

The Learning Electronic Health Record

Gilles Clermont, MD, CM, MSc[a,b,*]

KEYWORDS

- Electronic health records • Data science • Artificial intelligence
- Clinical decision support

KEY POINTS

- Further EHR developments targeting a balance among stakeholders are needed.
- Clinical decision support systems stand at a critical juncture in their development, and clinician involvement will likely be pivotal to their success and growing adoption.
- There exists a large disparity in access to modern EHR technology owing to financial and technological resources in underresourced environment and developing countries.

MANDATES AND THE ELECTRONIC HEALTH RECORD

The Health Information Technology for Economic and Clinical Health (HITECH) Act was signed into law in 2009 as part of the American Recovery and Reinvestment Act. HITECH was a forward-thinking piece of legislation aimed at greatly expanding the use of electronic health records (EHRs), while framing and enforcing more precisely security and privacy issues surrounding the greater availability of capability of exchanging medical data.[1] HITECH also widened the scope of security and privacy protection of patient data under the Health Insurance Portability and Accountability Act (HIPAA). As a direct result of HITECH, more than US$30 billion were invested in the modernization and digitization of health record systems. Although only 8% of hospitals had an EHR system in 2008, more than 96% including a vast majority of rural hospitals had certified EHR technology (CEHRT) in 2021. CEHRT refers to the capability of an EHR system to meet certain standards set by the Office of the National Coordinator for Health Information Technology (ONC). The list of these standards expands beyond EHRs and target health information technology more broadly.[2] This list spans 8 domains including clinical processes, care coordination, clinical quality measurement, privacy and security, public health, health IT design and performance, and

[a] VA Pittsburgh Medical Center, 1054 Aliquippa Street, Pittsburgh, PA 15104, USA; [b] Critical Care Medicine, University of Pittsburgh, 200 Lothrop Street, Pittsburgh, PA 15061, USA
* VA Pittsburgh Medical Center, 1054 Aliquippa Street, Pittsburgh, PA 15104.
E-mail address: cler@pitt.edu
Twitter: @gclermont (G.C.)

Crit Care Clin 39 (2023) 689–700
https://doi.org/10.1016/j.ccc.2023.03.004
0749-0704/23/Published by Elsevier Inc.

electronic exchange of health data. Overall, certification aims to provide a broad set of tools and standards to improving quality and efficiency of health care for patients irrespective of their entry point in the system, and the EHRs are a key component of this system.

Certification is a voluntary program, and an EHR does not have to be certified but there are certain incentives and requirements that make it beneficial for an EHR to be certified. For example, in the United States, health-care providers that use certified EHRs can qualify for federal incentives under the HITECH Act. Additionally, certain health-care providers, such as those participating in the Medicaid and Medicare programs, are required to use certified EHRs to receive reimbursement for certain services. The full list of certified providers, including EHR platform, is available at chpl. healthit.gov.[3]

THE PROMISE OF MEANINGFUL USE

A primary purpose of electronic capture of health data of medical data was to facilitate sharing of medical information. This would have tangible advantages that would meaningfully influence several aspects of health-care delivery such as quality, timeliness, and standardization. Thus, the expansion of EHR technology provided a broad roadmap of incentivization anchored around principles of meaningful use of the EHR (MU).[4] The roadmap of MU was divided in 3 stages. Stage 1 objectives (MU1) focused on data capture and sharing; stage 2 (MU2) focused on objectives relating to advanced clinical processes beyond simple collation of core components of an EHR; and stage 3 (MU3) sought to develop objectives relating to patient outcomes. The extent to which an EHR meets criteria for meaningful use (MU), as put forth by the Center for Medical Services and the ONC parallels many of the certification criteria discussed above. More specifically, MU3 sets rules around (1) protected health information; (2) electronic prescribing; (3) clinical decision support systems (CDSS) mostly focused on allergies and drug safety; (4) computerized provider order entry (CPOE) of laboratories, imaging studies, and medications; (5) patient electronic access to their records; (6) coordination of care through patient engagement and education; (7) health information exchange (HIE) through systems interoperability; and (8) public health and clinical data registry reporting including participation in an immunization registry and syndromic surveillance. Many of the objectives of the MU3 roadmap remain aspirational for clinical practices with limited resources while there are considerations beyond technical challenges preventing rapid progression toward those objectives for large corporate EHR providers including undue burden by the end-users of many of those requirements.[5] However, rapidly expanding technological advances might reprioritize some of the objectives of MU3 and, perhaps, reshape the traditional construct of the health IT ecosystem.

THE ELECTRONIC HEALTH RECORD AND THE PROVIDER

The digitization of the medical record and emergence of MU3 objectives did have tangible impacts on patient care, although early review did not substantiate impact on clinical outcomes.[6] A large number of medical errors in patients are secondary to medication and CPOE directly targeted this. In fact, up to two-thirds of medical errors in hospitalized patients relate to medication administration or omission. The impact of CPOE, and often associated rudimentary CDSS, has been studied repeatedly and found to be generally favorable, although many reports underline problems associated with some implementations.[7–10] Patients' access to their health information, another important emphasis of MU3, was found to improve self-reported levels of engagement or activation related to self-management, enhanced patient knowledge of their condition and treatment, and improved organizational efficiencies in a mental health-care facility. However, several studies did not find any statistically significant effect of patient portals on health outcomes.[11,12] However, metrics of end-user health outcomes are crude and may be required to be more fine-grained. Similarly, organization-level efficiencies may translate into improved end-user satisfaction not easily captured. HIE carries the promises of providing more informed care, better coordinated care among providers, avoiding duplication of resources, and potentially improving patient care. The impact of improved HIE seems generally positive, favorably impacting readmission rates and care.[13–15] However, there has been a documented negative impact of the increased requirements for documentation and patient–clinician interaction time. Perception of excessive stress associated with information technology is strongly correlated with physician and nurse burnout rates,[16–19] which preferentially influence late career and more experienced practitioners, possibly hastening their retirement from the active clinical workforce. Clearly, this was an unintended consequence of aggressive implementation of MU criteria on the one hand, and increasing financial accountability on the other. Complicating this already delicate balance is the need for system-level security beyond privacy concerns. A recent Ponemon Institute study, which surveyed 641 health-care IT and security practitioners, found that 89% of the organizations surveyed experienced a cyberattack in the past year. Organizations experiencing cloud compromises, ransomware, supply chain and business email compromises reported a 23% increase in patient mortality rates, although the nature of this association is unclear. Cyberattacks were associated with poor patient outcomes for 57% of those surveyed, and increased complications from medical procedures for nearly half of them.[20] This rapidly shifting environment has exposed an exquisite need for equipoise among stockholders in the design and implementation of IT-centered reforms to health-care delivery, a worldwide problem. This also offers exciting opportunities to focus future developments in health IT in general, and of the EHR more specifically, toward achieving this balance.

ELECTRONIC HEALTH RECORD AND DATA SCIENCE

EHRs have led to the creation of vast repositories of digitized data, potentially available for research but also for personalized clinical decision support. Patients have a generally positive attitude toward sharing health data for research purposes, provided very legitimate privacy concerns are addressed.[21–26] Given recent events that have threatened public trust in the health domain, and other arenas, this may well change in the near future. Leveraging data science with the ultimate goals of improving patient outcomes while ensuring the robustness and sustainability of the health-care ecosystem must therefore be anchored on strong ethical premises. It is encouraging that this social responsibility is increasingly recognized and promoted.[27,28]

In 2016, Wilkenson and colleagues published a landmark article framing the use of scientific data for research. This document proposed that scientific data should be findable, accessible, interoperable, and reusable, establishing the FAIR principles (Findable, Accessible, Interoperable, Reusable) of data use and stewardship.[29] The FAIR principles cover many important steps of the data life cycle because it pertains to health-care data and EHR data-based research.[30] Several frameworks have been suggested to implement the guiding principles outlined by FAIR to practice. In particular, data cards have a particular appeal in attempting to enhance rigor and reproducibility at several steps of the data life cycle, from choosing the data elements to collect and appropriate metadata, to minimizing bias and barriers to access, promoting democratization, and ensuring sustainability and reuse.[31] As will be discussed below, several emerging technologies in different stages of maturity are addressing existing threats to leveraging EHR data to implement MU3 and beyond.

THE ELECTRONIC HEALTH RECORD AND CLINICAL DECISION SUPPORT

The inclusion of CDSS as part of the EHR is almost as old as EHRs themselves.[32,33] Early CDSS focused on drug–drug interaction, drug dosing, allergy warnings, interpretation of laboratory values, presentation to end-users of expert-driven practice guidelines, and recommended treatment plans and clinical pathways.[34,35] The ability to extract data in real-time from the EHR ushered more efficient patient portals but also a new class of CDSS allowing just-in-time, personalized care. Indeed, more complex rules could be exerted on streaming data. Supporting technology is rapidly evolving. SMART on Fast Healthcare Interoperability Resources (FHIR) is a set of open standards and specifications for building health-care applications that can access EHRs using the FHIR standard, which includes both a growing list of data elements to be accessed and the rules to access them.[36] SMART stands for subscription, management, and authorization for resources and tasks.[37] The goal of SMART on FHIR is to make it easier for developers to create apps that can securely access patient data stored in EHR systems and to provide a consistent way for EHR systems to manage access to that data.[37,38] The ability for real-time EHR access allowing for the implementation of "sniffer" preceded the availability of FHIR. Sniffers apply simple rules to EHR data to effect syndromic surveillance. An early application pertains to the detection of acute kidney injury (AKI) and a large body of literature, including clinical trials, reported on the impact of such systems.[39–43] Although several of those reports were encouraging, suggesting improved patient-centered outcomes such as length of stay, there remains much scope for improvement, including the need for decreasing the rate of false alerting of such systems.[44,45] A major emphasis for such sniffers has been the early detection of sepsis. The ability to implement simple diagnostic rules for the existence of AKI as part of a computational phenotype[46–48] has greatly helped the development of such sniffers. Recent efforts to offer a similar computable definition for sepsis have ushered a wave of efforts toward early detection of this syndrome of great interest to critical care clinicians,[49] further fueled by evidence that early detection and intervention is likely associated with improved outcomes.[50] This interest has fueled the development of a large number of algorithms by academic groups and corporate EHR vendors. This remarkable level of activity has seen, within a decade, the emergence of a large number of such algorithms and their implementation and evaluation in clinical practice algorithms,[51–56] their usability and factors influencing adoption of sepsis detection CDSS in large hospital systems,[57–59] with varying degree of success. A recent report outlines the poor performance of a commercial system,[60] whereas other homegrown solutions have in time been rolled out for various reasons, including unacceptable rates of untimely or false-positive alarms. This particularly instructing example illustrates pitfalls and opportunities offered by such high-stake, real-time CDSS. Systems performing well in a given environment may not generalize well to other environments. Therefore, evidence of performance should include a demonstration of generalizability. Guidelines for model development, full documentation of such models, and their publications are forthcoming,[61,62] as are guidelines for trialing interventions involving artificial intelligence.[63] Individual hospital systems will inevitably carry idiosyncrasies in their case mix, and a CDSS demonstrating good generalizability may not perform well locally.[64] Methods, such as federated learning, allowing data-driven adjustments of such global models to local data while preserving local data enclaves are the topic of intense investigation.[65,66]

Yet, there will be limited tolerance for poorly performing, opaque CDSS difficult to integrate into clinical workflow. The current emphasis on human-centered design, coupled with a realization of the importance of CDSS providing clinically interpretable explanations for their predictions or recommendations, will be key to the successful adoption in clinical practice.[67] Progress may prove slower than expected and clinicians will need to be fully involved with CDSS development, with a special emphasis on nurse clinicians, typically the front-line clinicians and targets of many CDSS. Applying the familiar Dunning-Kruger effect to hype generated by technology under development,[68] the Gartner group publishes an analysis of expected progress across a large number of emerging technologies. Interestingly, the 2022 Gartner hype cycle for health-care providers suggests that the development of CDSS targeting critical care surveillance systems is just passing the peak of inflated expectations, an analysis shared by some in the academic community.[69]

EMERGING TECHNOLOGIES FOR ELECTRONIC HEALTH RECORDS

EHR can be improved in several ways. End-user interfaces could be considerably more ergonomic. Clinicians often have to navigate across several windows to extract relevant information. Recent efforts have successfully leveraged eye-tracking to understand clinicians' personal preferences in interacting with the EHR interface.[70,71] Such research could lead to personalized EHR aiming to decrease end-user frustration. Beyond technical advances in interoperability, data management systems, and security infrastructure, several other exciting developments with EHR platforms are currently under investigation targeting ease of use, ease of documentation, and verbal communication between the EHR and its end-user. A major challenge to CDSS adoption has been the relative inability of those tools to provide explanations in a form understandable to clinicians. Filling that important gap is the subject of intense research and an important component of the trustworthiness of such systems.[72,73] It is becoming increasingly apparent that clinicians will play a major role in helping machines think the way they do. In other words, explanations have to be provided in terms that are clinically relevant. Thus, contrary to intuition, a human-in-the-loop approach will likely prove essential to link data to clinical concepts and to enhance the generalizability, reproducibility, and trustworthiness of the learning process.[74,75]

Embedded clinical trials already leverage automated clinical data collection from the EHR, while activating predetermined treatment pathways.[76,77] These embedded trials designs target subjects already identified through a clinical screen of a specific laboratory test. One could imagine large-scale automated identification of more generally anomalous physiology, encounter type or frequency, medication administration, or care patterns, well beyond abnormal laboratory results. These explorations use the EHR platform outside its traditional patient-centric paradigm. Potential medical errors could be identified through some mismatch between a clinician's action, such as prescribing a certain medication, and the patient's current condition. Clearly, some of those associations are guided by a body of evidence and enshrined in practice guidelines but the vast majority of clinical actions are not the subject of existing guidelines. This evidence, however, could be hidden in the "consciousness" of the EHR and be discoverable.[78,79]

More generally, EHR anomaly detection sniffers could open the possibility of earlier detection and treatment at scale and significantly influence population well-being. This is far from being a trivial concept. The EHR being leveraged as a system to enhance the care of the individual will require an ongoing learning of existing patterns of patient features, clinical actions, and outcomes. One can imagine a system that is constantly refining such patterns, matching individuals to these patterns, and identifying best courses of actions for patients. It would be expected that best actions would be of a preventative nature as well as curative. This AI-supported EHR constantly learns from new encounters and outcomes. As new evidence is gathered outside a particular EHR system, patterns corresponding to this evidence could be positively rewarded such that patients could benefit from this external evidence. Thus, one can imagine how knowledge from different EHR systems of patients, clinical actions, and outcome patterns could be federated within a network, or ecosystem of EHRs, to benefit individual patients anywhere within this ecosystem. More standardized, yet personalized patient care could be provided at any service point within a health-care system, and patients could be proactively reached as an anomalous pattern develops within the EHR. These advances would lead to a greater democratization and hopefully more equitable care by leveling opportunity for care.

THE ELECTRONIC HEALTH RECORD IN UNDERRESOURCED ENVIRONMENTS

EHRs are becoming increasingly sophisticated and feature-rich but their implementation requires significant political leadership, as well as extensive financial and technological resources. In many low-income and middle-income countries, health-care providers may still be relying on paper-based systems, due to the lack of funding, technical expertise, and infrastructure to implement and maintain EHR systems. Although open-source or low-cost cloud-based EHR systems are potentially available, technological support remains a tenement of successful implementation. These open-source solutions offer basic functionalities, thus there exists a growing digital divide, where the benefits of EHRs are not equally distributed and underresourced environments miss out on the potential improvements in care and efficiency that EHRs can provide.[80] Improving digital literacy and technical skills in these environments is currently a high priority to build capacity and help ensure the long-term sustainability of EHR systems. Data science literacy is also of prime importance, and ongoing efforts in the form of datathons, for example, have been very effective in this respect.[81,82]

SUMMARY

The last 2 decades have witnessed an explosive adoption of EHRs in developed countries. In the United States, this was fueled by political leadership and financial incentivization, and a clear path for development embodied in the meaningful use program. A key priority of the US health-care information technology reform focused on interoperability and data sharing framed around the FAIR principles. The vast expansion in digitized health-care data has also fueled major efforts in data science and artificial intelligence, including automated processing of EHR data and bedside clinical support systems. Such systems have raised the possibility of offering personalized data-driven and evidence-driven care in a timely fashion at the bedside. Yet, hype associated with their introduction was often not matched by their performance. Ongoing and central involvement of clinicians in this rapidly developing technological field remains critical to it reaching its full potential in improving patient care, health-care delivery in general, and return to all its stakeholders.

CLINICS CARE POINTS

- Further EHR developments targeting a balance among stakeholders are needed.
- Clinical decision support systems stand at a critical juncture in their development, and clinician involvement will likely be pivotal to their success and growing adoption.
- There exists a large disparity in access to modern EHR technology owing to financial and technological resources in underresourced environment and developing countries.

DISCLOSURE

G. Clermont is funded by the National Institutes of Health, United States and the Department of Defense, United States. He also is cofounder of NOMA AI, Inc.

REFERENCES

1. Blumenthal D. Launching HITECH. N Engl J Med 2010;362(5):382–5.
2. Federal Register. 2015 Edition Health information technology (health IT) certification criteria, 2015 edition base electronic health record (EHR) definition, and ONC health IT certification program modifications [Internet]. Available at: https://www.federalregister.gov/documents/2015/10/16/2015-25597/2015-edition-health-information-technology-health-it-certification-criteria-2015-edition-base. Accessed February 10, 2023.
3. CHPL search [Internet]. Available at: https://chpl.healthit.gov/#/search. Accessed February 10, 2023.
4. Jones SS, Rudin RS, Perry T, et al. Health information technology: an updated systematic review with a focus on meaningful use. Ann Intern Med 2014; 160(1):48–54.
5. Rathert C, Porter TH, Mittler JN, et al. Seven years after Meaningful Use: physicians' and nurses' experiences with electronic health records. Health Care Manage Rev 2019;44(1):30–40. Available at: https://journals.lww.com/hcmrjournal/Fulltext/2019/01000/Seven_years_after_Meaningful_Use__Physicians__and.5.aspx.
6. Thompson G, O'Horo JC, Pickering BW, et al. Impact of the electronic medical record on mortality, length of stay, and cost in the hospital and ICU: a systematic review and metaanalysis. Crit Care Med 2015;43(6):1276–82. Available at: https://journals.lww.com/ccmjournal/Fulltext/2015/06000/Impact_of_the_Electronic_Medical_Record_on.17.aspx.
7. Wolfstadt JI, Gurwitz JH, Field TS, et al. The effect of computerized physician order entry with clinical decision support on the rates of adverse drug events: a systematic review. J Gen Intern Med 2008;23(4):451–8.
8. Nuckols TK, Smith-Spangler C, Morton SC, et al. The effectiveness of computerized order entry at reducing preventable adverse drug events and medication errors in hospital settings: a systematic review and meta-analysis. Syst Rev 2014; 3(1):56.
9. Roumeliotis N, Sniderman J, Adams-Webber T, et al. Effect of electronic prescribing strategies on medication error and harm in hospital: a systematic review and meta-analysis. J Gen Intern Med 2019;34(10):2210–23. Available at: https://link.springer.com/article/10.1007/s11606-019-05236-8.
10. Radley DC, Wasserman MR, Olsho LEW, et al. Reduction in medication errors in hospitals due to adoption of computerized provider order entry systems. J Am Med Inform Assoc 2013;20(3):470–6.

11. Kruse CS, Bolton K, Freriks G. The effect of patient portals on quality outcomes and its implications to meaningful use: a systematic review. J Med Internet Res 2015;17(2).

12. Tapuria A, Porat T, Kalra D, et al. Impact of patient access to their electronic health record. Systematic review 2021;46(2):192–204. Available at: https://www.tandfonline.com/doi/abs/10.1080/17538157.2021.1879810.

13. Menachemi N, Rahurkar S, Harle CA, et al. The benefits of health information exchange: an updated systematic review. J Am Med Inf Assoc 2018;25(9):1259–65. Available at: https://academic.oup.com/jamia/article/25/9/1259/4990601.

14. Hersh WR, Totten AM, Eden KB, et al. Outcomes from health information exchange: systematic review and future research needs. JMIR Med Inform 2015; 3(4):e39.

15. Eftekhari S, Yaraghi N, Singh R, et al. Do health information exchanges deter repetition of medical services? ACM Trans Manag Inf Syst 2017;8(1):1–27.

16. Gardner RL, Cooper E, Haskell J, et al. Physician stress and burnout: the impact of health information technology. J Am Med Inf Assoc 2019;26(2):106–14.

17. Khairat S, Burke G, Archambault H, et al. Focus section on health IT usability: perceived burden of EHRs on physicians at different stages of their career. Appl Clin Inform 2018;9(2):336–47.

18. Harris DA, Haskell J, Cooper E, et al. Estimating the association between burnout and electronic health record-related stress among advanced practice registered nurses. Appl Nurs Res 2018;43:36–41.

19. Khairat S, Xi L, Liu S, et al. Understanding the association between electronic health record satisfaction and the well-being of nurses: survey study. JMIR Nursing 2020; 3(1):e13996 [Internet]. 2020 Jun 23 [cited 2023 Feb 10];3(1):e13996. Available at: https://nursing.jmir.org/2020/1/e13996.

20. Cyber insecurity in healthcare: cost & impact on patient care | Proofpoint US [Internet]. Available at: https://www.proofpoint.com/us/cyber-insecurity-in-healthcare. Accessed February 11, 2023.

21. Hemingway H, Asselbergs FW, Danesh J, et al. Public attitudes toward consent and data sharing in Biobank research: a large multi-site experimental survey in the US. Am J Hum Genet 2018;100(3):414–27.

22. Ballantyne A, Schaefer GO. Consent and the ethical duty to participate in health data research. J Med Ethics 2018;44(6):392–6.

23. Stockdale J, Cassell J, Ford E. Giving something back": A systematic review and ethical enquiry into public views on the use of patient data for research in the United Kingdom and the Republic of Ireland. Wellcome Open Res 2019;3:6.

24. McCradden MD, Sarker T, Paprica PA. Conditionally positive: a qualitative study of public perceptions about using health data for artificial intelligence research. BMJ Open 2020;10(10):e039798.

25. Holm S, Kristiansen TB, Ploug T. Control, trust and the sharing of health information: the limits of trust. J Med Ethics 2021;47(12):E35.

26. Kalkman S, van Delden J, Banerjee A, et al. Patients' and public views and attitudes towards the sharing of health data for research: a narrative review of the empirical evidence. J Med Ethics 2022;48(1):3–13. Available at: https://jme.bmj.com/content/48/1/3.

27. Saltz JS, Dewar N. Data science ethical considerations: a systematic literature review and proposed project framework. Ethics Inf Technol 2019;21(3):197–208. Available at: https://link.springer.com/article/10.1007/s10676-019-09502-5.

28. Cordeiro J v. Digital technologies and data science as health enablers: an outline of appealing promises and compelling ethical, legal, and social challenges. Front Med 2021;8:1028.

29. Wilkinson MD, Dumontier M, Aalbersberg IjJ, et al. The FAIR Guiding Principles for scientific data management and stewardship. Sci Data 2016;3(1):1–9 [Internet]. 2016 Mar 15 [cited 2023 Feb 10];3(1):1–9. Available at: https://www.nature.com/articles/sdata201618.

30. FAIR Principles - GO FAIR. Available at: https://www.go-fair.org/fair-principles/. Accessed February 10, 2023.

31. Pushkarna M, Zaldivar A, Kjartansson O. Data cards: purposeful and transparent dataset documentation for responsible AI. ACM International Conference Proceeding Series 2022;1776–826. Available at: https://dl.acm.org/doi/10.1145/3531146.3533231.

32. Hunt DL, Haynes RB, Hanna SE, et al. Effects of computer-based clinical decision support systems on physician performance and patient outcomes: a systematic review. JAMA 1998;280(15):1339–46. Available at: https://jamanetwork.com/journals/jama/fullarticle/188081.

33. Garg AX, Adhikari NKJ, McDonald H, et al. Effects of computerized clinical decision support systems on practitioner performance and patient outcomes: a systematic review. J Am Med Assoc 2005;293(10):1223–38.

34. Bright TJ, Wong A, Dhurjati R, et al. Effect of clinical decision-support systems: a systematic review. Ann Intern Med 2012;157(1):29–43.

35. Nieuwlaat R, Connolly SJ, Mackay JA, et al. Computerized clinical decision support systems for therapeutic drug monitoring and dosing: a decision-maker-researcher partnership systematic review. Implement Sci 2011;6(1):1–14.

36. Index - FHIR v4.3.0 [Internet]. Available at: http://www.hl7.org/fhir/. Accessed February 11, 2023.

37. Mandel JC, Kreda DA, Mandl KD, et al. SMART on FHIR: a standards-based, interoperable apps platform for electronic health records. Journal of the American Medical Informatics Association 2016;23(5):899–908. Available at: https://academic.oup.com/jamia/article/23/5/899/2379865.

38. Bender D, Sartipi K, HL7 FHIR. An agile and RESTful approach to healthcare information exchange. Proceedings of CBMS 2013 - 26th IEEE International Symposium on Computer-Based Medical Systems 2013;326–31.

39. Collaborative MAM. The impact of the NHS electronic-alert system on the recognition and management of acute kidney injury in acute medicine. Clin Med 2019;19(2):109–13.

40. Atia J, Evison F, Gallier S, et al. Does acute kidney injury alerting improve patient outcomes? BMC Nephrol 2023;24(1):1–10. Available at: https://bmcnephrol.biomedcentral.com/articles/10.1186/s12882-022-03031-y.

41. Perry Wilson F, Martin M, Yamamoto Y, et al. Electronic health record alerts for acute kidney injury: multicenter, randomized clinical trial. BMJ 2021;372. Available at: https://www.bmj.com/content/372/bmj.m4786.

42. Kashani K, Herasevich V. Utilities of electronic medical records to improve quality of care for acute kidney injury: past, present, future. Nephron 2015;131(2):92–6.

43. Al-Jaghbeer M, Dealmeida D, Bilderback A, et al. Clinical Decision Support for In-Hospital AKI. J Am Soc Nephrol 2018;29(2):654–60.

44. Kellum JA, Bihorac A. Artificial intelligence to predict AKI: is it a breakthrough? Nat Rev Nephrol 2019;15(11):663–4.

45. Kashani KB. Automated acute kidney injury alerts. Kidney Int 2018;94(3):484–90.

46. Wang L, Olson JE, Bielinski SJ, et al. Impact of diverse data sources on computational phenotyping. Front Genet 2020 Jun 3;11:556.
47. Alzoubi H, Alzubi R, Ramzan N, et al. A review of automatic phenotyping approaches using electronic health records. Electronics 2019;8:1235 [Internet]. 2019 Oct 29 [cited 2023 Feb 11];8(11):1235. Available at: https://www.mdpi.com/2079-9292/8/11/1235/htm.
48. Kirby JC, Speltz P, Rasmussen Lv, et al. PheKB: a catalog and workflow for creating electronic phenotype algorithms for transportability. J Am Med Inf Assoc 2016 Nov 1;23(6):1046–52.
49. Singer M, Deutschman CS, Seymour CW, et al. The third international consensus definitions for sepsis and septic shock (Sepsis-3). JAMA 2016;315(8):801. Available at: http://jama.jamanetwork.com/article.aspx?doi=10.1001/jama.2016.0287.
50. Seymour CW, Gesten F, Prescott HC, et al. Time to treatment and mortality during mandated emergency care for sepsis. N Engl J Med 2017;376(23):2235–44. Available at: https://www.nejm.org/doi/full/10.1056/NEJMoa1703058.
51. Nemati S, Holder A, Razmi F, et al. An interpretable machine learning model for accurate prediction of sepsis in the ICU. Crit Care Med 2018;46(4):547. Available at: http://pmc/articles/PMC5851825/.
52. Semler MW, Weavind L, Hooper MH, et al. An electronic tool for the evaluation and treatment of sepsis in the icu: a randomized controlled trial. Crit Care Med 2015;43(8):1595–602.
53. Giannini HM, Ginestra JC, Chivers C, et al. A machine learning algorithm to predict severe sepsis and septic shock: development, implementation, and impact on clinical practice. Crit Care Med 2019;47(11):1485–92.
54. Delahanty RJ, Alvarez JA, Flynn LM, et al. Development and evaluation of a machine learning model for the early identification of patients at risk for sepsis. Ann Emerg Med 2019;73(4):334–44.
55. Henry KE, Hager DN, Pronovost PJ, et al. A targeted real-time early warning score (TREWScore) for septic shock. Sci Transl Med 2015 Aug 5;(299):7.
56. Adams R, Henry KE, Sridharan A, et al. Prospective, multi-site study of patient outcomes after implementation of the TREWS machine learning-based early warning system for sepsis. Nat Med 2022;28:7 [Internet]. 2022 Jul 21 [cited 2023 Feb 11];28(7):1455–60. Available at: https://www.nature.com/articles/s41591-022-01894-0.
57. Henry KE, Adams R, Parent C, et al. Factors driving provider adoption of the TREWS machine learning-based early warning system and its effects on sepsis treatment timing. Nat Med 2022;28:7 [Internet]. 2022 Jul 21 [cited 2023 Feb 11];28(7):1447–54. Available at: https://www.nature.com/articles/s41591-022-01895-z.
58. Ginestra JC, Giannini HM, Schweickert WD, et al. Clinician perception of a machine learning–based early warning system designed to predict severe sepsis and septic shock. Crit Care Med 2019;47(11):1477–84.
59. Guidi JL, Clark K, Upton MT, et al. Clinician perception of the effectiveness of an automated early warning and response system for sepsis in an academic medical center. Ann Am Thorac Soc 2015;12(10):1514–9.
60. Wong A, Otles E, Donnelly JP, et al. External validation of a widely implemented proprietary sepsis prediction model in hospitalized patients. JAMA Intern Med 2021;181(8):1065–70. Available at: https://jamanetwork.com/journals/jamainternalmedicine/fullarticle/2781307.
61. Collins GS, Dhiman P, Andaur Navarro CL, et al. Protocol for development of a reporting guideline (TRIPOD-AI) and risk of bias tool (PROBAST-AI) for diagnostic

and prognostic prediction model studies based on artificial intelligence. BMJ Open 2021;11(7):e048008. Available at: https://bmjopen.bmj.com/content/11/7/e048008.

62. Ghassemi M, Naumann T, Schulam P, et al. Practical guidance on artificial intelligence for health-care data. Lancet Digit Health 2019;1(4):157e–9e.

63. Cruz Rivera S, Liu X, Chan AW, et al. Guidelines for clinical trial protocols for interventions involving artificial intelligence: the SPIRIT-AI extension. Lancet Digit Health 2020;2(10):e549–60. Available at: http://www.thelancet.com/article/S2589750020302193/fulltext.

64. Futoma J, Doshi-Velez F, Leo D, et al. The myth of generalisability in clinical research and machine learning in health care. Lancet Digit Health 2020;2(9):e489–92. Available at: http://www.thelancet.com/article/S2589750020301862/fulltext.

65. Caldas S, Jeanselme V, Clermont G, et al. A case for federated learning: enabling and leveraging inter-hospital collaboration. Am J Respir Crit Care Med 2020;201.

66. Rieke N, Hancox J, Li W, et al. The future of digital health with federated learning. npj Digital Medicine 2020;3(1):1–7, Internet]. 2020 Sep 14 [cited 2023 Feb 11];3(1):1–7. Available at: https://www.nature.com/articles/s41746-020-00323-1.

67. Dietvorst BJ, Simmons JP, Massey C. Algorithm aversion: people erroneously avoid algorithms after seeing them err. J Exp Psychol Gen 2015;144(1):114–26.

68. Dunning D. The dunning–kruger effect: on being ignorant of one's own ignorance. Adv Exp Soc Psychol 2011;44:247–96.

69. Chen JH, Asch SM. Machine learning and prediction in medicine—beyond the peak of inflated expectations. N Engl J Med 2017;376(26):2507–9.

70. King AJ, Cooper GF, Clermont G, et al. Leveraging eye tracking to prioritize relevant medical record data: comparative machine learning study. J Med Internet Res 2020;22(4):e15876.

71. Tajgardoon M, Cooper GF, King AJ, et al. Modeling physician variability to prioritize relevant medical record information. JAMIA Open 2021;3(4):602–10. Available at: https://academic.oup.com/jamiaopen/article/3/4/602/6056383.

72. Floridi L. Establishing the rules for building trustworthy AI. Nat Mach Intell 2019;1:6 [Internet]. 2019 May 7 [cited 2021 Jul 5];1(6):261–2. Available at: https://www.nature.com/articles/s42256-019-0055-y.

73. Lebiere C, Blaha LM, Fallon CK, et al. Adaptive cognitive mechanisms to maintain calibrated trust and reliance in automation. Front Robot AI 2021;8:652776.

74. Wu X, Xiao L, Sun Y, et al. A survey of human-in-the-loop for machine learning. Future Generat Comput Syst 2022;135:364–81.

75. Topol EJ. High-performance medicine: the convergence of human and artificial intelligence. Nat Med 2019;25(1):44–56.

76. Angus DC, Berry S, Lewis RJ, et al. The REMAP-CAP (randomized embedded multifactorial adaptive platform for community-acquired pneumonia) study. Rationale and design. Ann Am Thorac Soc 2020;17(7):879–91. Available at: https://www.ncbi.nlm.nih.gov/pubmed/32267771.

77. Upmc Remap-Covid Group on behalf of the RCAPI. Implementation of the randomized embedded multifactorial adaptive platform for COVID-19 (REMAP-COVID) trial in a US health system-lessons learned and recommendations. Trials 2021;22(1):100. Available at: https://www.ncbi.nlm.nih.gov/pubmed/33509275.

78. Hauskrecht M, Batal I, Valko M, et al. Outlier detection for patient monitoring and alerting. J Biomed Inform [Internet] 2013;46(1):47–55. Available at: http://www.ncbi.nlm.nih.gov/pubmed/22944172.

79. Hauskrecht M, Batal I, Hong C, et al. Outlier-based detection of unusual patient-management actions: an ICU study. J Biomed Inform 2016;64:211–21. Available at: http://www.ncbi.nlm.nih.gov/pubmed/27720983.

80. Odekunle FF, Odekunle RO, Shankar S. Why sub-Saharan Africa lags in electronic health record adoption and possible strategies to increase its adoption in this region. Int J Health Sci 2017;11(4):59. Available at:/pmc/articles/PMC56 54179/.

81. Piza FM de T, Celi LA, Deliberato RO, et al. Assessing team effectiveness and affective learning in a datathon. Int J Med Inform 2018;112:40–4.

82. Aboab J, Celi LA, Charlton P, et al. A "datathon" model to support cross-disciplinary collaboration. Sci Transl Med 2016;8(333). Available at: https://www.science.org/doi/10.1126/scitranslmed.aad9072.

Promise 2: Better Understanding of Critical Care Deployment and Epidemiology

The Role of Data Science in Closing the Implementation Gap

Andrew J. King, PhD[a], Jeremy M. Kahn, MD, MSc[a,b],*

KEYWORDS

- Implementation science • Data science • Evidence-based practice
- Intensive care units • Critical care • Mechanical ventilation

KEY POINTS

- Many critically ill patients fail to receive evidence-based practices proven to save lives, leading to preventable morbidity and mortality.
- By leveraging novel data sources and novel modeling approaches, data science has the potential to overcome the limitations of traditional methods for closing this implementation gap.
- Key opportunities include novel context-adaptive recommender systems that can be tailored to specific clinical situations and novel prediction tools that can support individual decision-making at the moment of need.
- These approaches will be facilitated by emerging technologies including interoperable data applications and the Internet of Things.
- Challenges remain to ensure that these efforts do not ingrain existing biases, widen health disparities, or disrupt clinical workflows.

INTRODUCTION

Recent decades have witnessed an extraordinary expansion of our understanding of how to treat patients with critical illness.[1] Now more than ever, the ways in which we provide critical care, including mechanical ventilation, sedation, renal replacement therapy, and resuscitation in shock, among others, are informed by clinical trials rather than clinical intuition. In turn, trial evidence forms the basis of numerous clinical practice guidelines, which summarize the evidence, inform treatments at the bedside, and reduce unwanted variation in critical care delivery and outcomes.

[a] Department of Critical Care Medicine, University of Pittsburgh School of Medicine, 3500 Terrace Street, Suite 600, Pittsburgh, PA 15261, USA; [b] Department of Health Policy and Management, University of Pittsburgh School of Public Health, 130 De Soto Street, Pittsburgh, PA 15261, USA
* Corresponding author.
E-mail address: jeremykahn@pitt.edu

Crit Care Clin 39 (2023) 701–716
https://doi.org/10.1016/j.ccc.2023.03.005
0749-0704/23/© 2023 Elsevier Inc. All rights reserved.

This sea change has undoubtedly led to improvements in outcomes among patients admitted to the intensive care unit (ICU).[2] Yet, it also has revealed the immense complexities inherent in providing consistent, high-quality critical care. Like elsewhere in health care, ICU clinicians frequently fail to consistently deliver evidence-based practices at the bedside, meaning that many patients do not receive treatments that are proven to save lives.[3] Closing this so-called "implementation gap" is a major priority for clinicians, policymakers, and healthcare administrators struggling to provide the best possible outcomes for patients.

Implementation science is the study of the mechanisms by which effective health care interventions are either adopted or not adopted.[2] Rather than generating new clinical evidence, implementation science is primarily concerned with how to package, distribute, prioritize, remind, motivate, or embed information such that evidence-based practices are consistently applied.[4,5] In cases of failed adoption, implementation scientists seek to understand why clinicians acted in the way they did and if their actions were justifiable.[6] This information can then form the basis of targeted interventions designed to align care with the best available evidence and improve patient outcomes.[7]

Although advances in data science are rapidly transforming health care,[8] relatively few data science applications are directly focused on closing the implementation gap.[9] Rather, most applications have focused on discovering new phenotypes,[10] measuring disease severity,[11] and prediction of adverse events.[12,13] A focus on discovery and prediction is unsurprising given that the field of biomedical data science is foremost about the afferent process of extracting knowledge from health data.[14] Yet, modern electronic clinical workflows also generate an extraordinary amount of data about clinical practice delivery at the patient and provider level. These data can provide novel insight into implementation, enabling new strategies to support consistent delivery of evidence-based practice.[15]

In this article, the authors outline the role of data science in closing critical care's implementation gap. First, the authors examine the sources of the implementation gap and discuss why existing implementation strategies often fail. Next, the authors review the ways in which data science might improve on existing approaches and help close the implementation gap. Finally, the authors identify the technologies that will be required for data science to fulfill its promise, review the limitations of data science in this domain, and highlight what challenges remain for leveraging data to improve delivery of evidence-based practice in the ICU.

THE IMPLEMENTATION GAP

Failure to consistently translate evidence into practice is pervasive in critical care. For example, the LUNG-SAFE study, an international survey of patients with acute respiratory distress syndrome, showed that only a minority of patients were receiving tidal volumes consistent with lung-protective ventilation.[16] Other studies showed that many patients with sepsis do not receive timely antibiotics and fluid resuscitation[17]; mechanically ventilated patients often do not receive daily interruptions of sedation and spontaneous breathing trials (SBTs) to facilitate liberation[18]; and extubated patients at high risk for re-intubation do not receive preventive respiratory support such as noninvasive ventilation or oxygen by high-flow nasal cannula.[19]

The sources of the implementation gap are complex and varied. Traditional implementation frameworks identify three main groups of barriers: knowledge (ie, clinicians are not aware of the evidence); attitudes (ie, clinicians are aware of the evidence but are not in agreement); and behaviors (ie, clinicians face cognitive, functional, and organizational roadblocks to evidence-based practices even when they are aware and in agreement).[20] In the ICU setting, these barriers are further complicated by the fact that critical care is provided by interprofessional teams rather than individual clinicians.[21] Teams enable division of labor and broaden the available expertise; however, they also create additional failure points, as communication breakdowns and unreliable team dynamics can lead to clinical fumbles.[22,23]

Traditional strategies for overcoming these barriers include education, audit and feedback, protocols, checklists, and automated reminders, among others (**Fig. 1**). Unfortunately, these strategies are generally ineffective, resulting in either no significant improvements or small early improvements that are not sustained.[24] For example, a 2014 cluster-randomized trial showed that rounding checklists could increase the use of lung-protective ventilation, but post-intervention use was still only 68% and there were no associated changes in mortality.[25] Another study used a combination of academic detailing and Web-based education to improve the use of lung-protective ventilation; however, post-intervention use was still only 70%.[26] These modest improvements in performance are the exception rather than the rule, with many other high-profile studies showing no changes in performance at all.[27–29] These failures underscore the urgent need to identify novel strategies for evidence-uptake in critical care so that effective treatments consistently reach patients at the bedside.

ROLE OF DATA SCIENCE

The potential for data science to close the implementation gap is based on its ability to reconcile two classic tensions in health care. First is the tension between *population health* versus *individual health*—often care that will benefit an entire group of people on average will not benefit, or may even harm, individual patients within that group.[30] Second is the tension between health care that *should be delivered* versus health care that is *practically deliverable*—often patients may benefit from many different treatments, yet actually delivering all beneficial treatments is impossible under given resource constraints.[31]

An archetypal example is the use of checklists during interprofessional rounds. Checklists have a tremendous impact in aviation and other industries due to their effectiveness and ease of use.[32] However, checklists in hospital settings such as the ICU

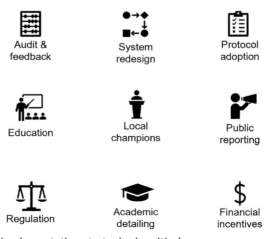

Fig. 1. Traditional implementation strategies in critical care.

often fail to affect change.[33–35] This failure is due to the temptation to fill rounding checklists with long lists of items that, if delivered, will benefit most patients.[36,37] Yet many of these items won't apply to every patient, and long checklists are onerous to complete.[38] As a result, traditional checklists, viewed by providers as redundant and disruptive, are ultimately shelved, thereby failing to achieve their intended effects.[38] One solution is parsimony when designing checklists: choose only a few critical items at a time, substituting them as uptake improves or priorities evolve. Although a shorter checklist increases completability, it also means that very important practices may be missed.

Data science offers a way to alter this calculus (**Fig. 2**). The methods of data science—harvesting, curating, analyzing, and displaying information from data—can identify the specific situation in which specific care practices are both indicated and beneficial. By selectively identifying and isolating these situations, data science can provide context-adaptive interventions that are mindful of the patients, clinicians, and clinical environments (**Box 1**). Specific opportunities, described in detail below, include dynamic checklists, customized audit and feedback, intelligent prompts for evidence-based practice, recommender systems, just-in-time evidence, and intelligent workflow design (**Table 1**).

Dynamic Checklists

A dynamic, or adaptive, checklist takes clinical context into consideration to emphasize items that are most important and remove items that are not indicated.[39–41] These types of checklists can be informed by hard-coded logic or machine learning models that assess the patient's eligibility for specific practices. For example, if the patient is not receiving invasive mechanical ventilation, then their checklist need not include prompts for SBTs or low tidal volume ventilation. Similarly, a patient might need an SBT but may be at low likelihood of receiving one because of their specific clinical characteristics or if the ICU is busy that day, as determined by an algorithm. In such a case, the SBT item can be elevated to the top of the checklist. Such a checklist would change from patient-to-patient and from day-to-day (**Fig. 3**). In this way, clinical workload can be reduced while not sacrificing evidence than may benefit individual patients.

Customized Audit and Feedback

Audit and feedback gives providers data on their past performance, affording them the insight and opportunity to improve their performance on future patients. Traditional

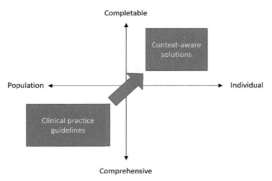

Fig. 2. Data science can enable movement from comprehensive, population-wide implementation strategies (such as clinical practice guidelines) to completable, individually tailored context-sensitive solutions.

Box 1
What comprises a situation?

Patient:
- Demographics
- Physiologic measurements
- Comorbidities
- Current therapeutics

Clinician(s):
- Training
- Experience
- Relationship with other providers
- History of evidence uptake

Environment:
- Geo-location
- Moment in time
- Concurrent patient load
- Local policies and institutional norms

Data science can enable implementation solutions that are tailored to individual situations, increasing their effectiveness. The details of each situation can relate to the individual patient, the individual provider (or groups of providers), and the clinical environment.

---

audit and feedback fails because the feedback is not timely and actionable—providers receive data after the moment of need and in ways that do not direct them on how to take action.[42] Using data science, audit and feedback can be automated and potentially gamified using Electronic Health Record (EHR) data and a record of past actions.[43,44] With automatically generated reports, feedback can be more regular, increasing the opportunities to learn from one's existing habits. Feedback can also be tailored to individual clinicians, in that a provider who needs help in one specific area can preferentially receive feedback in this area. This feedback can include comparisons to a clinician's past performance or the average performance of similar professionals (ie, peer benchmarking).[45] These approaches need not be limited to actual clinical actions but can be applied in simulation and virtual settings.[46]

Table 1
Strategies for integrating data science and implementation science

Strategy	Description
Dynamic checklists	Using rules or machine learning to adapt a checklist of evidence-based practices to a current situation, eliminating items that are not indicated.
Customized audit and feedback	Automating the generation of feedback for clinicians so that it is timelier and more actionable.
Intelligent prompts for evidence-based practice	Predicting when an indicated evidence-based practice will not be applied and thus should be prompted for.
Recommender systems	Using reinforcement learning to maximize the use of evidence-based practices.
Just-in-time evidence	Generating evidence from local data for a specific circumstance, right when it is needed.
Intelligent workflow design	Highlighting EHR variables that are pertinent to making evidence-informed decisions; precision scheduling of clinical tasks to improve adoption of evidence.

Example ICU Rounding Checklist

- ☐ Assess, prevent and manage pain?
- ☐ Both SAT and SBT?
- ☐ Choice of analgesia and sedation?
- ☐ Delirium: assess, prevent and manage?
- ☐ Early mobility?
- ☐ Family engagement?
- ☐ Central line removed?
- ☐ VTE prophylaxis?
- ☐ Stress ulcer prophylaxis?
- ☐ Nutrition per protocol?

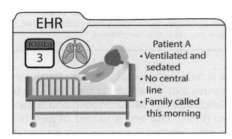

EHR

ICU day **3**

Patient A
- Ventilated and sedated
- No central line
- Family called this morning

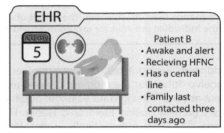

EHR

ICU day **5**

Patient B
- Awake and alert
- Recieving HFNC
- Has a central line
- Family last contacted three days ago

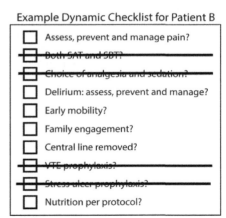

Example Dynamic Checklist for Patient A

- ☐ Assess, prevent and manage pain?
- ☐ Both SAT and SBT?
- ☐ Choice of analgesia and sedation?
- ☐ Delirium: assess, prevent and manage?
- ☐ ~~Early mobility?~~
- ☐ ~~Family engagement?~~
- ☐ ~~Central line removed?~~
- ☐ VTE prophylaxis?
- ☐ Stress ulcer prophylaxis?
- ☐ Nutrition per protocol?

Example Dynamic Checklist for Patient B

- ☐ Assess, prevent and manage pain?
- ☐ ~~Both SAT and SBT?~~
- ☐ ~~Choice of analgesia and sedation?~~
- ☐ Delirium: assess, prevent and manage?
- ☐ Early mobility?
- ☐ Family engagement?
- ☐ Central line removed?
- ☐ ~~VTE prophylaxis?~~
- ☐ ~~Stress ulcer prophylaxis?~~
- ☐ Nutrition per protocol?

Fig. 3. A demonstration of a generic ICU rounding checklist versus a dynamic checklist. A generic checklist prompts all the same items for every patient regardless of whether they are applicable. A dynamic checklist adapts its content based on EHR data, or other sources, to eliminate items that are not applicable and/or were already addressed by the care team. SAT,spontaneous awakening trial, SBT, spontaneous breathing trial, VTE, venous thromboembolism, HFNC, high-flow nasal cannula.

Intelligent Prompts for Evidence-Based Practice

Electronic prompts for evidence-based practice fail because they are agnostic to the specific situation, often firing when the practice in question is not indicated or is already being provided.[47,48] As a result, they distract from the workflow without providing new information. This problem also leads to alarm fatigue, which in turn leads providers to ignore all prompts, even those that could help.[49] Alternatively, machine learning applications can mine the EHR to predict when an evidence-based practice is applicable but not likely to be applied. Applications can then trigger alerts only when they are likely to be helpful and informative. For example, a machine learning algorithm might predict that a patient is unlikely to receive lung-protective ventilation based on factors such as the patient's characteristics, the attending physician's practice history, and the ICU census. The resulting prompts would be rarer, reducing alarm fatigue, but also more actionable, increasing impact.

An additional advance would be the ability to deliver these prompts directly at the moment of need, before a given decision is made. Part of the problem with alerts embedded in computerized order entry is that they are only triggered after the clinician has entered the medical record with a plan to place a specific order, that is, after decision is made. In this context, the alert must overcome a major barrier of changing the clinician's mind.[50] A related problem is that alerts give providers information about a diagnosis (eg, sepsis) after the provider is already aware of the diagnosis.[51] Preemptively priming a clinician toward making a higher value decision is likely to be more effective.[52]

Recommender Systems

Reinforcement learning can underpin recommender systems designed to optimize a given patient outcome. For example, the Artificial Intelligence (AI) Clinician used reinforcement learning to recommend one of 25 possible combinations of fluid and vasopressors for patients with sepsis with a goal of optimizing (ie, minimizing) 90-day mortality.[53] Although in this situation the model was trained to reduce mortality, rather than to increase the use of specific evidence, the proximal affect would be to change resuscitation practices, which in theory bringing them into alignment with evidence-based practices.[54] Similar methods might be used to train a model for directly optimizing on the use of evidence-based practices inferred by the states of the patient (which treatment decisions are most likely to get the patient to a state where they could receive the practice), the clinician (which individuals are most likely to benefit from and act on a notification), and the environment (at which point in the day and by which means will notifying the clinician likely result in the desired action).

Most experimental systems applying reinforcement learning in medicine rely on fixed, retrospective datasets.[55] For deployed systems to realize the added benefit of ongoing real-world interactions, "online" systems that efficiently update clinical recommendations as practice evolves are needed. For example, an online learning framework using a multi-armed bandits algorithm has been applied with some success to the problem of early sepsis detection.[55]

Just-In-Time Evidence Creation

Many clinical guidelines are informed by randomized controlled trials that only enroll patients that fit into strict inclusion criteria. There are many benefits to this approach, but one limitation is that real-world patients rarely look that those that are enrolled. Instead, patients possess unique clinical trajectories and combinations of comorbidities, meaning that no trial scenario exactly matches the patient's clinical situation. A novel alternative is locally sourced, just-in-time evidence that is only generated when a clinician requests it.[56] Although such evidence would be based on observational data, with resulting biases, it would be customized to the clinical needs for a specific care decision for an individual patient. Relatedly, machine learning can be applied to the EHR to detect unusual deviations from practice under the assumption that these deviations represent opportunities to improve.[57,58] Unusual treatment decisions can be flagged and reviewed by the clinician to see if it is contrary to evidence, supporting evidence-uptake in real time.

Intelligent Workflow Design

Finally, data science can be used to redesign the clinical workflow in ways that support the use of evidence-based practice. For example, EHR information that is related to an evidence-based practice could be strategically highlighted. By highlighting the information that is relevant to a practice, a clinician may be more likely to perform the practice. Researchers have used a combination of mouse clicks and eye-tracking data to capture past information access patterns and machine learning to predict what information will be accessed in a current EHR interaction, reducing information retrieval time.[59,60] Extensions of this process could optimize on showing information that leads to the use of evidence-based practices.

Similarly, data could be used to help clinicians prioritize their workdays through intelligent scheduling. For example, machine learning applications could tell providers which patients need to be seen first based on who is most likely to pass an SBT, reducing extubation delays. This approach can reduce cognitive load and time pressure on the clinical team, helping them make more evidence-informed decisions. Ultimately, it might be possible to sequence the order of patients discussed during rounds such that there is cognitive carry-over so that important practices performed on one will be fresh in the team's mind when they reach the next.

Workflow redesigns also have the potential to impact another pressing issue in health care: clinician burnout.[61] Burnout affects nurses and physicians alike and is in part due to the time spent using the EHR, poor EHR usability, documentation burden, and messaging volumes.[62–65] Streamlining workflows and reducing alert burden are strategies for addressing technological sources of burnout as they allow clinicians more time to focus on more rewarding activities that directly improve care.[66,67]

DATA SOURCES AND ENABLING TECHNOLOGIES

Although several of the ideas above are under active investigation, few are in active deployment. Moving ahead will require more efficient access to data, primarily data from the EHR. As with other research, data will likely be sourced from analytic data warehouses, which include data duplicated from a health system's primary clinical system. Problematically, these data sources often have a time delay of between a few minutes to many days. Although traditional clinical research can tolerate such delays, implementation science applications will need some aspects of data nearly instantaneously. In many cases, there will need to be a defined priority in terms of what data can be updated once a day versus what needs to be known within 15 minutes versus what needs to be known right now.

Advancements speeding this process are the evolving interoperable data standards such as Health Level 7 Fast Health Interoperability Resources (HL7 FHIR).[68] HL7 FHIR is based on common Internet standards and is meant to support the development of third-party applications, similar to app stores on a mobile phone. Applications using the FHIR standards will be capable of querying necessary data across multiple EHRs and writing data back to the EHR based on clinician interactions with the app.

Also necessary for these applications will be greater connectivity between the EHR, medical devices (eg, bedside monitors and mechanical ventilators), and personal devices (eg, mobile phones and geolocation trackers). Greater connectivity will make new types of data and more granular data available to applications in real time (**Table 2**). For example, ventilator waveform data can be harnessed to understand if a patient is eligible for and receiving an SBT, but only if those data can be processed and made available to the AI application in real time. As another example, radio frequency identification technology can be used to assess team member interaction, facilitating team-based practices.[69] This capability will be enhanced as medical devices join the Internet of Things, enabling them to communicate directly with internet applications rather than through human or electronic intermediaries.[70]

LIMITATIONS AND CHALLENGES

Numerous challenges prevent the rapid application of data science methods to implementation challenges. For one, the types of data needed are often not directly available for application development and research. When they are available, it is usually through cumbersome extract, transform, and load (ETL) procedures. To shift this paradigm, researchers and quality improvement (QI) specialists must adapt existing data interoperability technologies to the health care domain (such as HL7 FHIR), develop new ETL techniques, navigate varied institutional policies and governmental laws, and overcome hesitation from patients who have reasonable concerns about data confidentiality and privacy.

A second concern is the current ethical and regulatory environment may be insufficient to support the development of these technologies. In the United States, current regulatory frameworks make a distinction between human subjects research, which needs approval from an institutional review board (IRB), and QI, which does not.[71]

Table 2	
Examples of novel data streams that can inform efforts to implement evidence-based practice	
Strategy	**Description**
Wearables	Devices (eg, pedometer) worn by patients or providers that periodically measure and report vital signs, location, or other variables.
Internet of Things	The network of devices (including wearables) that measure and report variables such as inventory levels or equipment location and status or that can be controlled remotely.
Waveforms	The use of raw high-frequency data streams (such as continuous electrocardiogram monitoring) rather than less frequent point measurements.
Voice recordings	Much of health care involves conversations (between clinicians and between a clinician and a patient). Audio recordings are quickly becoming a viable data source with the increasing accuracy of automatic transcription software and natural language processing.
Video recordings	Like voice recordings, advances in deep learning are making it feasible to extract information from video recordings such as clinician actions, patient positions, or equipment usage.
Eye-tracking	By measuring what clinicians view within the EHR, it may be possible to infer what a clinician knows (or does not know) about a patient.

Yet, this distinction is largely artificial, and most work conducted under the rubric of implementation science can be labeled as both research and QI.[72] Developers then face a quandary: conduct the work as research which strains IRBs and creates potentially burdensome red tape or conduct the work as QI which may cause developers to forgo sufficient protections for human subjects. New regulatory frameworks are needed that transcend this distinction within the context of learning health systems that support rapid innovation.[73,74]

In addition, current regulatory frameworks are focused on protecting patients, whereas much of the data used by implementation scientists and data scientists are of health care providers. For example, meta-data from the EHR can be used to identify providers and understand their individual practice patterns[75], and voice or video data can be used to make sense of presentations on daily rounds.[76,77] The addition of these new data types introduces novel concerns about data privacy, autonomy, and the role of informed consent for health care providers.

A third concern is that the application of AI to implementation science will ingrain known biases in clinical decision-making and widen health disparities. Underrepresented minorities may be less likely to receive evidence-based practices in critical care.[78] If machine learning models are trained on biased data, then the resulting models will be biased. Importantly, even the data generating devices might lead to biased data. For example, both old and new data suggest that pulse oximeters are often inaccurate in patients with dark skin color.[79,80] If oximetry readings are used in a model to predict whether a patient should receive lung-protective ventilation, the model may help only some of the patients, widening health disparities. Care must be taken to ensure that such models enhance care delivery for all patients, in particular those most likely not to receive them.

A fourth concern is ensuring the trustworthiness of AI recommendations. Just with any area of AI in medicine, clinicians are rightfully hesitant to heed black box recommendations (ie, those that are given without an explanation for how the system came up with the decision to make the recommendation). This is particularly problematic in implementation science because the quality of recommendations from AI systems can't be immediately verified. If recommendations from the AI run counter to clinician intuition, clinicians will be naturally dismissive. To address this problem, careful attention needs to be paid to designing trustworthy systems.[81] Options can include giving an explanation of the model predictions, comparing recommended actions to past actions that were successful, directly communicating uncertainty, and performing rigorous internal and external validation.[82,83]

A fifth concern is the need to integrate these systems into existing workflows. Checklists are the classic example of an implementation science intervention that fails because it makes work harder rather than easier.[38] Application developers must be wary of adding to clinical workflow (eg, duplicate data entry, requirements to open or log into additional applications, or recommending work that was already performed). Ideally, systems will be integrated so well that task load, cognitive load, and time load are all reduced. In the ICU, this issue is particularly salient because care is team based. In the context of team-based care, applications cannot focus on a single decision maker. Rather, they need to consider multiple decision makers that dynamically interact. This requires recognizing, measuring, and analyzing how workload changes for the entire team. A helpful practice might be to imagine the AI system as another team member, one that is hyperintelligent but potentially lacking the emotional wisdom necessary to effectively relate in a fast-moving and complex environment. How we approach the "computer as a team member" will determine whether these applications succeed or fail.

SUMMARY

The field of critical care medicine is facing an implementation crisis. Many evidence-based practices fail to reach patients, leading to preventable morbidity and mortality. Data scientists can play a key role in closing the gap and ensuring that life-saving treatments are efficiently implemented at the bedside. Our understanding of disease has greatly benefited from data science-driven retrospective analyses that build the knowledge base of evidence-based practices.[84] The task of evidence adoption is highly likely to benefit from similar methods. A decade from now, we may find that integration of data science methods into the implementation science toolbox was a linchpin in closing the implementation gap.

CLINICS CARE POINTS

- Data science can enhance efforts to translate evidence into practice in critical care.
- Context-sensitive implementation strategies are tailored to individual patients, clinicians, and situations.
- Interprofessional collaboration is required to ensure that novel applications address rather than perpetuate biases in care.

DISCLOSURE

The authors have no competing commercial interests.

ACKNOWLEDGMENTS

The authors thank Dr Gregory F. Cooper for his intellectual contributions to this work. The work reported in this publication was supported in part by the National Heart, Lung, and Blood Institute of the National Institutes of Health under award number R35 HL144804.

REFERENCES

1. Cook DJ, Sibbald WJ, Vincent JL, et al. Evidence based critical care medicine. What is it and what can it do for us? Crit Care Med 1996;24(2):334–7.
2. Weiss CH, Krishnan JA, Au DH, et al. An official American Thoracic Society research statement: implementation science in pulmonary, critical care, and sleep medicine. Am J Respir Crit Care Med 2016;194(8):1015–25.
3. Institute of Medicine. Crossing the quality chasm. Washington, D.C.: National Academies Press; 2001.
4. Leeman J, Birken SA, Powell BJ, et al. Beyond "implementation strategies": classifying the full range of strategies used in implementation science and practice. Implement Sci 2017;12(1):125.
5. Handley MA, Gorukanti A, Cattamanchi A. Strategies for implementing implementation science: a methodological overview. Emerg Med J 2016;33(9):660–4.
6. Kahn JM. Bringing implementation science to the intensive care unit. Curr Opin Crit Care 2017;23(5):398–9.
7. Bero LA, Grilli R, Grimshaw JM, et al. Closing the gap between research and practice: an overview of systematic reviews of interventions to promote the implementation of research findings. The Cochrane Effective Practice and Organization of Care Review Group. BMJ 1998;317(7156):465–8.

8. Zhu L, Zheng WJ. Informatics, data science, and artificial intelligence. JAMA 2018;320(11):1103–4.

9. Nguyen D, Ngo B, VanSonnenberg E. AI in the intensive care unit: up-to-date review. J Intensive Care Med 2021;36(10):1115–23.

10. Seymour CW, Kennedy JN, Wang S, et al. Derivation, validation, and potential treatment implications of novel clinical phenotypes for sepsis. JAMA 2019; 321(20):2003–17.

11. Delahanty RJ, Kaufman D, Jones SS. Development and evaluation of an automated machine learning algorithm for in-hospital mortality risk adjustment among critical care patients. Crit Care Med 2018;46(6):e481–8.

12. Zimmerman JE, Kramer AA. A history of outcome prediction in the ICU. Curr Opin Crit Care 2014;20(5):550–6.

13. Tomašev N, Harris N, Baur S, et al. Use of deep learning to develop continuous-risk models for adverse event prediction from electronic health records. Nat Protoc 2021;16(6):2765–87.

14. Payne PRO, Bernstam E v, Starren JB. Biomedical informatics meets data science: current state and future directions for interaction. JAMIA Open 2018;1(2): 136–41.

15. Rule A, Chiang MF, Hribar MR. Using electronic health record audit logs to study clinical activity: a systematic review of aims, measures, and methods. J Am Med Inform Assoc 2020;27(3):480–90.

16. Bellani G, Laffey JG, Pham T, et al. Epidemiology, patterns of care, and mortality for patients with acute respiratory distress syndrome in intensive care units in 50 countries. JAMA 2016;315(8):788–800.

17. Seymour CW, Gesten F, Prescott HC, et al. Time to treatment and mortality during mandated emergency care for sepsis. N Engl J Med 2017;376(23):2235–44.

18. Pun BT, Balas MC, Barnes-Daly MA, et al. Caring for critically ill patients with the ABCDEF Bundle: results of the ICU Liberation Collaborative in over 15,000 adults. Crit Care Med 2019;47(1):3–14.

19. Nuzzo EA, Kahn JM, Girard TD. Provider perspectives on preventive postextubation noninvasive ventilation for high-risk intensive care unit patients. Ann Am Thorac Soc 2020;17(2):246–9.

20. Cabana MD, Rand CS, Powe NR, et al. Why don't physicians follow clinical practice guidelines? A framework for improvement. JAMA 1999;282(15):1458–65.

21. Ervin JN, Kahn JM, Cohen TR, et al. Teamwork in the intensive care unit. Am Psychol 2018;73(4):468–77.

22. Diabes MA, Ervin JN, Davis BS, et al. Psychological safety in intensive care unit rounding teams. Ann Am Thorac Soc 2021;18(6):1027–33.

23. Dietz AS, Pronovost PJ, Mendez-Tellez PA, et al. A systematic review of teamwork in the intensive care unit: what do we know about teamwork, team tasks, and improvement strategies? J Crit Care 2014;29(6):908–14.

24. Sinuff T, Muscedere J, Adhikari NKJ, et al. Knowledge translation interventions for critically ill patients: a systematic review. Crit Care Med 2013;41(11):2627–40.

25. Cavalcanti AB, Bozza FA, Machado FR, et al. Effect of a quality improvement intervention with daily round checklists, goal setting, and clinician prompting on mortality of critically ill patients: a randomized clinical trial. JAMA 2016; 315(14):1480–90.

26. Rubenfeld GD, Manoharan V, Scales DC, et al. Evaluation of a web based intervention to improve adherence to lung protective ventilation: the Lung Injury Knowledge Network (LINK). Am J Respir Crit Care Med 2017;195:A7609. Available at:

https://www.atsjournals.org/doi/abs/10.1164/ajrccm-conference.2017.195.1_MeetingAbstracts.A7609. Accessed January 2, 2023.

27. Scales DC, Dainty K, Hales B, et al. A multifaceted intervention for quality improvement in a network of intensive care units: a cluster randomized trial. JAMA 2011;305(4):363–72.

28. Bion J, Richardson A, Hibbert P, et al. Matching Michigan": a 2-year stepped interventional programme to minimise central venous catheter-blood stream infections in intensive care units in England. BMJ Qual Saf 2013;22(2):110–23.

29. Wilson FP, Shashaty M, Testani J, et al. Automated, electronic alerts for acute kidney injury: a single-blind, parallel-group, randomised controlled trial. Lancet 2015;385(9981):1966–74.

30. Iwashyna TJ, Burke JF, Sussman JB, et al. Implications of heterogeneity of treatment effect for reporting and analysis of randomized trials in critical care. Am J Respir Crit Care Med 2015;192(9):1045–51.

31. Huppert JS, Fournier AK, Bihm JL, et al. Prioritizing evidence-based interventions for dissemination and implementation investments: AHRQ's model and experience. Med Care 2019;57(10 Suppl 3):S272–7.

32. Gawande A. The checklist manifesto. Profile Books; London, England; 2011.

33. Anthes E. Hospital checklists are meant to save lives - so why do they often fail? Nature 2015;523(7562):516–8.

34. Urbach DR, Govindarajan A, Saskin R, et al. Introduction of surgical safety checklists in Ontario, Canada. N Engl J Med 2014;370(11):1029–38.

35. Reames BN, Krell RW, Campbell DAJ, et al. A checklist-based intervention to improve surgical outcomes in Michigan: evaluation of the Keystone Surgery program. JAMA Surg 2015;150(3):208–15.

36. Russ SJ, Sevdalis N, Moorthy K, et al. A qualitative evaluation of the barriers and facilitators toward implementation of the WHO surgical safety checklist across hospitals in England: lessons from the "Surgical Checklist Implementation Project". Ann Surg 2015;261(1):81–91.

37. Dixon-Woods M, Leslie M, Tarrant C, et al. Explaining Matching Michigan: an ethnographic study of a patient safety program. Implement Sci 2013;8:70.

38. Hallam BD, Kuza CC, Rak K, et al. Perceptions of rounding checklists in the intensive care unit: a qualitative study. BMJ Qual Saf 2018;27(10):836–43.

39. Geva A, Albert BD, Hamilton S, et al. eSIMPLER: a dynamic, electronic health record–integrated checklist for clinical decision support during PICU daily rounds. Pediatr Crit Care Med 2021;22(10).

40. de Bie AJR, Nan S, Vermeulen LRE, et al. Intelligent dynamic clinical checklists improved checklist compliance in the intensive care unit. Br J Addiction: Br J Anaesth 2017;119(2):231–8.

41. Lane D, Ferri M, Lemaire J, et al. A systematic review of evidence-informed practices for patient care rounds in the ICU. Crit Care Med 2013;41(8):2015–29.

42. Sinuff T, Muscedere J, Rozmovits L, et al. A qualitative study of the variable effects of audit and feedback in the ICU. BMJ Qual Saf 2015;24(6):393–9.

43. Hung AJ, Chen J, Gill IS. Automated performance metrics and machine learning algorithms to measure surgeon performance and anticipate clinical outcomes in robotic surgery. JAMA Surg 2018;153(8):770–1.

44. Hung AJ, Chen J, Che Z, et al. Utilizing machine learning and automated performance metrics to evaluate robot-assisted radical prostatectomy performance and predict outcomes. J Endourol 2018;32(5):438–44.

45. Burgon T, Casebeer L, Aasen H, et al. Measuring and improving evidence-based patient care using a web-based gamified approach in primary care (QualityIQ): randomized controlled trial. J Med Internet Res 2021;23(12):e31042.
46. Mohan D, Farris C, Fischhoff B, et al. Efficacy of educational video game versus traditional educational apps at improving physician decision making in trauma triage: randomized controlled trial. BMJ 2017;359:j5416.
47. Patterson ES, Doebbeling BN, Fung CH, et al. Identifying barriers to the effective use of clinical reminders: bootstrapping multiple methods. J Biomed Inform 2005; 38(3):189–99.
48. Holt TA, Thorogood M, Griffiths F. Changing clinical practice through patient specific reminders available at the time of the clinical encounter: systematic review and meta-analysis. J Gen Intern Med 2012;27(8):974–84.
49. Cho OM, Kim H, Lee YW, et al. Clinical alarms in intensive care units: perceived obstacles of alarm management and alarm fatigue in nurses. Healthc Inform Res 2016;22(1):46–53.
50. Olakotan OO, Yusof MM. Evaluating the alert appropriateness of clinical decision support systems in supporting clinical workflow. J Biomed Inform 2020;106: 103453.
51. Semler MW, Weavind L, Hooper MH, et al. An electronic tool for the evaluation and treatment of sepsis in the ICU: a randomized controlled trial. Crit Care Med 2015;43(8):1595–602.
52. Cialdini R. Pre-suasion: a revolutionary way to influence and persuade. Simon and Schuster; New York, NY; 2016.
53. Komorowski M, Celi LA, Badawi O, et al. The artificial intelligence clinician learns optimal treatment strategies for sepsis in intensive care. Nat Med 2018. https://doi.org/10.1038/s41591-018-0213-5.
54. Evans L, Rhodes A, Alhazzani W, et al. Surviving sepsis campaign: international guidelines for management of sepsis and septic shock 2021. Intensive Care Med 2021;47(11):1181–247.
55. Zhou A, Raheem B, Kamaleswaran R. OnAI-Comp: an online AI experts competing framework for early sepsis detection. IEEE/ACM Trans Comput Biol Bioinform 2022;19(6):3595–603.
56. Ostropolets A, Zachariah P, Ryan P, et al. Data Consult Service: can we use observational data to address immediate clinical needs? J Am Med Inform Assoc 2021;28(10):2139–46.
57. Chen J, Sun L, Guo C, et al. A fusion framework to extract typical treatment patterns from electronic medical records. Artif Intell Med 2020;103:101782.
58. Hauskrecht M, Batal I, Hong C, et al. Outlier-based detection of unusual patient-management actions: an ICU study. J Biomed Inform 2016;64:211–21.
59. King AJ, Cooper GF, Clermont G, et al. Using machine learning to selectively highlight patient information. J Biomed Inform 2019;100:103327.
60. King AJ, Cooper GF, Clermont G, et al. Leveraging eye tracking to prioritize relevant medical record data: comparative machine learning study. J Med Internet Res 2020;22(4):e15876.
61. Moss M, Good VS, Gozal D, et al. An Official Critical Care Societies Collaborative Statement: burnout syndrome in critical care healthcare professionals: a call for action. Crit Care Med 2016;44(7):1414–21.
62. Padden J. Documentation burden and cognitive burden: how much is too much information? Comput Inform Nurs 2019;37(2):60–1.
63. Embriaco N, Azoulay E, Barrau K, et al. High level of burnout in intensivists: prevalence and associated factors. Am J Respir Crit Care Med 2007;175(7):686–92.

64. Yan Q, Jiang Z, Harbin Z, et al. Exploring the relationship between electronic health records and provider burnout: a systematic review. J Am Med Inform Assoc 2021;28(5):1009–21.
65. Nguyen OT, Jenkins NJ, Khanna N, et al. A systematic review of contributing factors of and solutions to electronic health record-related impacts on physician well-being. J Am Med Inform Assoc 2021;28(5):974–84.
66. Thomas Craig KJ, Willis VC, Gruen D, et al. The burden of the digital environment: a systematic review on organization-directed workplace interventions to mitigate physician burnout. J Am Med Inform Assoc 2021;28(5):985–97.
67. McGreevey JD 3rd, Mallozzi CP, Perkins RM, et al. Reducing alert burden in electronic health records: state of the art recommendations from four health systems. Appl Clin Inform 2020;11(1):1–12.
68. Griffin AC, He L, Sunjaya AP, et al. Clinical, technical, and implementation characteristics of real-world health applications using FHIR. JAMIA Open 2022;5(4): ooac077.
69. Ito-Masui A, Kawamoto E, Nagai Y, et al. Feasibility of measuring face-to-face interactions among ICU healthcare professionals using wearable sociometric badges. Am J Respir Crit Care Med 2020;201(2):245–7.
70. Ahmed HS, Ali AA. Smart intensive care unit design based on wireless sensor network and internet of things. In: 2016 Al-Sadeq International Conference on Multidisciplinary in IT and Communication Science and Applications (AIC-MITCSA). IEEE 2016;1–6.
71. Casarett D, Karlawish JH, Sugarman J. Determining when quality improvement initiatives should be considered research: proposed criteria and potential implications. JAMA 2000;283(17):2275–80.
72. Lynn J, Baily MA, Bottrell M, et al. The ethics of using quality improvement methods in health care. Ann Intern Med 2007;146(9):666–73.
73. Asch DA, Joffe S, Bierer BE, et al. Rethinking ethical oversight in the era of the learning health system. Healthc (Amst) 2020;8(4):100462.
74. Fiscella K, Tobin JN, Carroll JK, et al. Ethical oversight in quality improvement and quality improvement research: new approaches to promote a learning health care system. BMC Med Ethics 2015;16(1):63.
75. Kahn JM, Minturn JS, Riman KA, et al. Characterizing intensive care unit rounding teams using meta-data from the electronic health record. J Crit Care 2022;72: 154143.
76. King AJ, Kahn JM, Brant EB, et al. Initial development of an automated platform for assessing trainee performance on case presentations. ATS Sch 2022;3(4): 548–60.
77. Katanami Y, Hayakawa K, Shimazaki T, et al. Adherence to contact precautions by different types of healthcare workers through video monitoring in a tertiary hospital. J Hosp Infect 2018;100(1):70–5.
78. McGowan SK, Sarigiannis KA, Fox SC, et al. Racial disparities in ICU outcomes: a systematic review. Crit Care Med 2022;50(1):1–20.
79. Jubran A, Tobin MJ. Reliability of pulse oximetry in titrating supplemental oxygen therapy in ventilator-dependent patients. Chest 1990;97(6):1420–5.
80. Sjoding MW, Dickson RP, Iwashyna TJ, et al. Racial bias in pulse oximetry measurement. N Engl J Med 2020;383(25):2477–8.
81. Markus AF, Kors JA, Rijnbeek PR. The role of explainability in creating trustworthy artificial intelligence for health care: a comprehensive survey of the terminology, design choices, and evaluation strategies. J Biomed Inform 2021;113:103655.

82. Chen H, Gomez C, Huang CM, et al. Explainable medical imaging AI needs human-centered design: guidelines and evidence from a systematic review. NPJ Digit Med 2022;5(1):156.

83. Ghassemi M, Oakden-Rayner L, Beam AL. The false hope of current approaches to explainable artificial intelligence in health care. Lancet Digit Health 2021;3(11): e745–50.

84. Vashisht R, Jung K, Schuler A, et al. Association of hemoglobin A1c levels with use of sulfonylureas, dipeptidyl peptidase 4 inhibitors, and thiazolidinediones in patients with type 2 diabetes treated with metformin: analysis from the Observational Health Data Sciences and Informatics Initiat. JAMA Netw Open 2018; 1(4):e181755.

Promise 3: More Efficient Research Practices and Strategies

Designing and Implementing "Living and Breathing" Clinical Trials

An Overview and Lessons Learned from the COVID-19 Pandemic

Christopher M. Horvat, MD, MHA[a,b,]*, Andrew J. King, PhD[b],
David T. Huang, MD, MPH[b]

KEYWORDS

- Learning health system • Pragmatic trial • Augmented intelligence
- Evidence-based medicine • Electronic health record

KEY POINTS

- "Living, breathing" trials are ushering in a new era of rapid learning, accelerating care improvements, and are providing a solution to some of the biggest challenges in health care.
- Modern health care information systems can support more efficient trial data collection and facilitate the incorporation of advanced trial analytics at the point of care, helping to realize the vision of the learning health care system.
- "Living, breathing" trials are a clinical research paradigm that is rapidly evolving, and trial teams will often need to "learn while doing."
- Leveraging the electronic record for trial workflow implementation and data collection requires health system leadership support.
- The workload associated with harmonizing data collection strategies and trial protocols is commonly underestimated; both efforts require ample planning and sufficient resources.

INTRODUCTION

The practice of medicine is characterized by uncertainty. "Life is short and the Art long; the occasion fleeting; experience fallacious; and judgement difficult," posited Hippocrates,[1] an insight reemphasized 2 millennia later by Osler, who offered

[a] UPMC Children's Hospital of Pittsburgh, Faculty Pavilion, 4401 Penn Avenue, Suite 0200, Pittsburgh, PA 15224, USA; [b] Department of Critical Care Medicine, University of Pittsburgh School of Medicine, 3550 Terrace Street, 603A, Pittsburgh, PA 15261, USA
* Corresponding author. UPMC Children's Hospital of Pittsburgh, Faculty Pavilion, 4401 Penn Avenue, Suite 0200, Pittsburgh, PA 15224.
E-mail address: Christopher.horvat@chp.edu

Crit Care Clin 39 (2023) 717–732
https://doi.org/10.1016/j.ccc.2023.02.002
0749-0704/23/© 2023 Elsevier Inc. All rights reserved.

"Medicine is a science of uncertainty and an art of probability."[2] Curbing uncertainty in medical decision making to optimize outcomes is the primary objective of clinical investigation.[3]

Randomized clinical trials (RCTs) and amalgamations of RCT findings, such as systematic reviews and meta-analyses, are stationed at the top of the hierarchy of medical evidence meant to aid clinicians in wrangling uncertainty.[4] This position at the top is earned by way of the quality of information generated through the power of randomization, which, unlike any other method, controls for both measured and unmeasured confounders. When properly executed, randomly assigning patients to prespecified treatment regimens provides data affording as close a vantage as possible to assess the effect of an intervention compared with the counterfactual scenario. Consequently, the findings of well-conducted trials constitute the bedrock of contemporary "evidence-based medicine," are especially influential in determining which recommendations are put forward in consensus guidelines, and play a large role in shaping the delivery of bedside care.

RCTs also have limitations. Conducting an RCT is a cumbersome endeavor, which many argue contributes to longer than necessary times between the identification of a potential therapeutic breakthrough and actionable clinical results. The infrastructure necessary to run a large RCT is specialized and expensive, commonly confining implementation to academic health systems with sufficient economies of scale to successfully enroll patients while reaping adequate returns to make ongoing participation sustainable.[5] However, differences between academic RCT sites and community health care settings, such as varied staffing patterns, case mixes, and trainee volumes, limit generalizability, as do extensive lists of RCT eligibility criteria. Moreover, RCT findings are traditionally analyzed using frequentist statistical comparisons of the average treatment effect of an intervention in the enrolled population, obscuring heterogenous treatment effects corresponding with substantial benefit (or harm) in patient subpopulations.

To overcome some of these limitations, new trial paradigms rooted in the origins of evidence-based medicine are beginning to disrupt the traditional mold.[6–8] These new designs recognize uncertainty permeates medical decision making and aim to capitalize on modern health system infrastructure to integrate investigation as a component of care delivery. Such designs leverage the computational capabilities of modern health care information systems, present opportunities for more efficient trial data collection and monitoring, draw from quality and performance improvement toolkits, promote greater equity in enrollment, and can enmesh dynamically with existing clinical workflows. "Living, breathing" trials represent a major movement in the direction of the National Academy of Medicine's vision of a large-scale learning health care system,[9,10] and such trials have gained equal or greater traction around the globe. The COVID-19 pandemic accelerated adoption of such "living, breathing" trials, with several successful studies demonstrating partial or almost entire integration into clinical workflows, and rapidly generating landmark treatment insights.[6,8,11,12]

Appreciating the relevance of this tectonic shift in the clinical trial landscape necessitates a brief history of the term "evidence-based medicine," a concise overview of quality improvement science, and a broad-stroke description of both the benefits and the drawbacks of relying on modern information systems for clinical investigation. The rapid evolution of this new paradigm necessitates that investigator teams must frequently "learn while doing" while looking to recent examples of "living, breathing" trials, several of which are presented in this review as guideposts.[13] Finally, investigators should be aware of anticipated developments in the space of data standards and information systems that are expected to shape how "living, breathing" trials are deployed, as well as areas of controversy regarding the ethics of intertwining clinical trials and care delivery.

"Living, BREATHING" CLINICAL TRIALS AND THE COVID-19 PANDEMIC

Apart from established supportive care measures, there were no known treatments for COVID-19 when the World Health Organization declared a pandemic in March 2020. The worldwide desperation to rapidly learn about the disease and determine effective therapies prompted innumerable investigations of varied designs. Multiple randomized trials sprouted up, although many were too small or ineffectively designed to provide meaningful findings.[14] In contrast, the COVID-19 pandemic highlighted the utility of pragmatic trials to quickly identify effective treatments that were readily translatable into real-world clinical settings. Pragmatic trials can take multiple forms but share the commonality of a design that meshes with clinical workflows. In a sentinel work defining what constitutes a pragmatic trial, French statisticians Schwartz and Lellouch[15] contrasted "normal," or the everyday clinical environment, with the "laboratory" context of a traditional clinical trial to distinguish "pragmatic" from what they called "explanatory" trials. Explanatory trials test the effects of an intervention in a select population, whereas pragmatic trials examine the effect of the intervention in real-world conditions. This model helps distinguish between pragmatic versus traditional trial designs; however, the reality is these 2 descriptions sit on opposite ends of a continuum, with no single point of demarcation.[16,17]

Master protocols are a more recent complement to pragmatic designs that allow investigators to simultaneously assess multiple interventions, multiple diseases, or both multiple diseases and multiple interventions within a single, overarching trial.[18] There are 3 types of trials that rely on a master protocol: umbrella, basket, and platform trials. An umbrella trial simultaneously studies treatment effects within subgroups of a single disease. A basket trial studies a therapy for multiple diseases within a single trial. A platform trial studies multiple therapies for a disease in perpetuity, allowing study treatments to dynamically enter and exit the platform throughout the trial's lifespan. Realizing the advantages of master protocols necessitates strategies to reduce the ostensible complexities of these trial designs so that trialists and staff responsible for day-to-day operations are not overwhelmed. Notably, although trial design and analyses can be complex, proper trial implementation should render these complexities invisible to clinical staff and end-users. Modern health care information systems, emerging clinical informatics tools, and cutting-edge bioinformatics techniques are increasingly essential to conduct these trials efficiently. Technology can be leveraged to deploy the trial within an electronic record workflow, incorporate Bayesian inference into randomization and trial analyses, facilitate secure data transfer to support adaptive updates to trial design, and support trial data collection by obviating some or all manual data abstraction. Although the vision of the learning health care system outlined by the National Academy of Medicine[10] includes a seamless integration of patient care, electronic workflows, clinical investigation, and system priorities, many COVID-19 trials have been successful by featuring some, but not necessarily all, of these ingredients. Consider the Randomised Evaluation of COVID-19 Therapy (RECOVERY) platform trial conducted in the United Kingdom, which identified dexamethasone as an effective therapy that was rapidly incorporated as standard of care for hospitalized, hypoxemic patients within weeks of the start of the pandemic.[19] RECOVERY was not fluently integrated into existing electronic record workflows at that time, but did rely on a Web service for randomization and a simple on-line case report form for minimal data collection, while leaning on the structure of the UK's National Health

System (NHS) to accommodate trial workflow within care delivery processes, as well as the NHS' data sets and national registries to complement manually collected data.[11]

Other examples of platform trials designed and implemented to address the global public health emergency of COVID-19 included the 'Investigation of Serial studies to Predict Your Therapeutic Response with Imaging and moLecular Analysis (I-SPY 2 TRIAL) for COVID-19 coordinated in the United States,[6] the Accelerating COVID-19 Therapeutic Interventions and Vaccines (ACTIV) trials coordinated in the United States,[20] the Anti-Thrombotic Therapy to Ameliorate Complications of COVID-19 (ATTACC) trial coordinated in Canada,[7] and the global Randomized, Embedded, Multi-factorial, Adaptive, Platform trial for Community Acquired Pneumonia (REMAP-CAP).[12,21] Each of these trials offers its own case study providing insight into both the promise and the challenges of the "living, breathing" paradigm of clinical trials. The present discussion centers on the authors' experience with the implementation of REMAP-CAP during the COVID-19 pandemic in the United States. To date, REMAP-CAP has provided insights regarding multiple therapies for COVID-19, including corticosteroids,[22] antivirals,[23] convalescent plasma,[24] anticoagulation,[25,26] antiplatelet medications,[27] and interleukin-6 blockade,[28] among others.

EVIDENCE-BASED MEDICINE AND BAYESIAN INFERENCE IN CLINICAL DECISION MAKING

REMAP-CAP relies on Bayesian inference to increasingly favor randomization into better performing trial arms as outcome data accrue, an approach often termed "response adaptive randomization."[12] Bayesian analyses are also used to report the primary outcomes, presented as posterior probabilities of benefit (or harm). The use of Bayesian, instead of frequentist, statistical analyses is an increasingly common design feature of new living, breathing trials. To implement response adaptive randomization in REMAP-CAP, most domains are conducted with an initial run-in period of balanced randomization. A multifactorial Bayesian inference model accounts for patient age, trial site and region, time era, tested regimen, and stratum (eg, moderate vs severe illness), as well as interactions between different interventions and strata. Monthly data updates allow the statistical analysis committee to calculate posterior probabilities for each regimen being tested by stratum and adjusted for sample size. A priori thresholds are defined for superiority (eg, >99% probability that an intervention is superior), equivalence (eg, >90% probability that odds of death for 2 interventions differ by <0.2), or inferiority (eg, <1% probability that an intervention is superior). Monte Carlo simulation is used to assess trial performance under a variety of conditions.[12]

Although seemingly novel from its application in many machine learning–based analyses,[29] the application of Bayesian inference to medical decision making is a foundational cornerstone of evidence-based medicine and can be traced back to its very inception. The term "evidence-based medicine" was first coined by Eddy[30,31] in workshops on physician decision making beginning around 1985 and published in 1990. As a concept, evidence-based medicine was borne out of increasing recognition that physician judgment frequently did not align with available objective data, or in many instances, lacked supporting data altogether. This insight coincided with breakthrough work by psychologists Kahneman and Tversky,[32] who characterized commonplace flaws in human decisions made under risk. In contrast to the long-held theory that risk-laden decisions are made in a manner that maximizes individual utility, Kahneman and Tversky demonstrated that people routinely rely on heuristic, or pattern-based, assessments in making decisions, rather than an objective assessment of available data and probabilities. One solution Eddy put forward for medical decision making required application of the centuries-old Bayes theorem, which considers the prior probability of an outcome and accounts for the objective weight of influential factors, such as the result of a diagnostic test, to calculate a posterior probability. This proposed Bayesian approach to medical decision making, also articulated by other leaders of analytical thinking at the time, such as Feinstein,[33] was accordingly installed as a cornerstone of the foundation of evidence-based medicine.

Several challenges are apparent, however, when the practicalities of applying Bayesian decision making in the real world are considered. Generating prior probability distributions can amount to a coarse, variable estimate when adequate data are not available.[34] Although the probabilistic output of Bayes theorem may represent the range of decisional uncertainty facing a clinician, the decisions themselves are commonly binary or at least discrete (eg, a treatment is administered or not, or a test is considered positive or negative). When designing a clinical trial, traditional sample size calculations are not readily applicable to a Bayesian design, lending uncertainty to both the required number of patients to enroll and the trial costs. Furthermore, calculating probabilities based on multidimensional input can be computationally intensive. Limitations to a Bayesian approach to practicing medicine have been recognized for decades and offer some explanation as to why this paradigm is not regularly used explicitly in modern practice.[33,35]

Frequentist statistics, in which parameters are considered fixed and an assertation about either accepting or rejecting a null hypothesis is made on the basis of a P value, have long dominated trial design.[36] In part, this convention arose because software has been widely available for conducting frequentist analyses. However, advances in both computer hardware and software in recent decades have overcome some of the barriers favoring the frequentist route and have made Bayesian analyses much more accessible. In addition, an advantage of using a Bayesian approach is that data can be analyzed and expressed as posterior probabilities, which is more quantitative and potentially more useful than a dichotomous frequentist analysis based on an arbitrary P-value threshold. As a result, an increasing volume of Bayesian analyses are appearing in the medical literature,[37] including a growing number of trials using a Bayesian analysis of the primary endpoint.[38] Secondary Bayesian analyses have also called into question previous conclusions of frequentist trials, such as in the study of extracorporeal membrane oxygenation for severe acute respiratory distress syndrome[39] and therapeutic hypothermia for pediatric out-of-hospital cardiac arrest.[40]

Bayesian trial designs have benefits compared with traditional frequentist designs. Berry[38] notes that by measuring uncertainty and allowing for continuous learning, Bayesian trials allow investigators to make iterative updates to a trial while it is underway. These updates, or adaptations, can include halting enrollment, adding or dropping interventions and arms, and updating prior probabilities and associated randomization weights to assign patients to better performing therapies. Given the resource-intensive computation required for Bayesian analyses, deployment of this approach currently appears best suited to occur within larger data wrangling infrastructures capable of readily gathering and curating the necessary variables to account a priori for factors that need to be incorporated into determination of posterior probabilities. With these traits in mind, learning Bayesian trials can be seen as a natural evolution of an earlier, more embryonic state of evidence-based medicine.

QUALITY AND PERFORMANCE IMPROVEMENT IN MEDICINE AND THE LEARNING HEALTH CARE SYSTEM

The overlap between increasingly rigorous, cyclical performance improvement strategies in health care, modern health care information systems, and clinical investigation has been acknowledged in the learning health care system framework.[9] In combination with skilled clinical investigators, modern quality improvement implementation, data, and scientific elements provide the necessary ingredients to launch clinical trials embedded within care delivery systems. Implementation of REMAP-CAP across the University of Pittsburgh Medical Center (UPMC) system in the United States relied heavily on supervisory structures typically dedicated to overseeing operations rather than research. For example, at the outset of the pandemic, certain medications that were possible treatments for COVID-19, such as hydroxychloroquine, could only be used within the context of the clinical trial. The UPMC pharmacy and therapeutics committee instituted this edict to simultaneously limit unwarranted variation in COVID-19 treatment practices while promoting system-level learning by relying on the REMAP-CAP platform to assess treatment effectiveness.

Health system and local culture were also shaped by relying on UPMC marketing and education teams to generate enthusiasm about the trial, by crafting reference materials and launching awareness campaigns through both internal and external media outlets.[41] Information system tools, such as near-real-time dashboards used to track COVID-19 disease burden in the health system, were accessed by clinical leaders focused on resource allocation as well as by trial teams working to identify patients for study enrollment. In some cases, separate from REMAP-CAP, the act of randomization to determine treatment allocations was performed out of necessity owing to resource scarcity. As an example, a weighted lottery system governed by the UPMC quality improvement committee determined the distribution and administration of remdesivir while promoting both equity and an opportunity for causal inference.[42] In addition, UPMC conducted a pragmatic comparative effectiveness platform trial of monoclonal antibodies, simultaneous with expanding access to these therapies across the system, yielding both new knowledge and increased treatment with these therapies.[43–46] Together, these efforts created a culture of learning and rapid improvement that was reflected in an estimated 5% lower odds of 30-day COVID-19 mortality across UPMC each month between March 2020 and June 2021.[47] In acknowledgment of the quality improvement function that REMAP-CAP played at UPMC during the COVID-19 pandemic, the American Board of Internal Medicine approved maintenance of certification quality improvement credit for physicians who played a substantial role in the conduct of the trial.[48]

LEVERAGING HEALTH CARE INFORMATION SYSTEMS TO DEPLOY RANDOMIZED, EMBEDDED, MULTIFACTORIAL, ADAPTIVE, PLATFORM TRIAL FOR COMMUNITY-ACQUIRED PNEUMONIA IN THE UNITED STATES

Modifying electronic workflows and data capture to accommodate trial design (even simple designs) often requires substantial effort on the part of health care information technology (IT) teams. At UPMC, implementation of REMAP-CAP required navigating a complex network of IT systems and governance structures across 30 hospitals in the Western and Central Pennsylvania regions. The rapidly growing clinical informatician workforce, which consists of physicians, nurses, pharmacists, and other clinicians with additional training in health information systems and human factors, proved essential to bridge the communication gap between clinical investigators and IT teams.[49,50]

Depending on trial context, existing electronic workflows may span several arenas of care and related IT systems. Implementation of REMAP-CAP in the United States leveraged IT for virtual screening, recruitment, enrollment, deploying assigned treatment regimens, direct data collection from the electronic health record (EHR), long-term follow-up, iterative submission of outcome updates to the trial statistical analysis committee, and iterative receipt of randomization weights to support adaptive randomization, as previously described.[8] Completing this effort in the midst of a pandemic was only possible with the support of top-level health system leadership, which allocated IT resources and promoted awareness of the REMAP-CAP efforts, and within a university ecosystem experienced in the execution of clinical trials. Even with such pillars in place, the US REMAP-CAP investigative team had to draft detailed blueprints for trial implementation while also building the software infrastructure for coordinating treatment assignments at the bedside and associated, automated data extraction, a process aptly named "learning while doing."[13] When implementing learning IT platforms across multicenter organizations, the act of obtaining necessary, site-level IT governance approvals can consume a plurality of deployment efforts.[51] A need for expediency, demanded by the pandemic, promoted necessary accommodations and updates to governance structures across UPMC to occur efficiently. In turn, this allowed the trial team to move quickly to intertwine trial operations as part of the system's larger efforts to address COVID-19.

Throughout the pandemic, UPMC relied on patient data sourced from multiple different EHRs across the system, including products from vendors such as Cerner and Epic. Data extracted from these installations had to be harmonized both locally and globally to integrate with REMAP-CAP data collected from around the world. **Fig. 1** displays the major steps of the associated extract, transform, and load (ETL) of data from UPMC to support trial analyses performed by the international data-coordinating center in partnership with contracted biostatistical support. Stage 1 refers to source data in their respective systems, such as the EHR production databases. To avoid negatively impacting patient care systems, portions of these databases are commonly duplicated in institutional warehouses to support business intelligence and research efforts, which is displayed as stage 2. In the case of REMAP-CAP, many international sites relied on a traditional electronic data capture system with online case report forms and an associated data dictionary. Stage 3

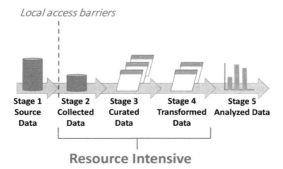

Fig. 1. The stages of data extraction, transformation, and analysis of real-world data sources, such as the EHR. The dashed red line refers to local access barriers, such as governance policies that may make it difficult for research teams to access these data sources. Stages 2 through 4 are resource-intensive and may consume as much as 90% of the time and effort associated with leveraging these types of data.

represents the curation of EHR data elements needed to fulfill the variables per a study's case report form. Stage 4 demonstrates the transformation of the curated data to achieve both the structure and the function of the final data model used for analyses. For example, several data elements, such as vital signs, laboratory values, and comorbidities, are necessary to calculate risk adjustment variables, such as the acute physiology and chronic health evaluation (APACHE) score. These elements were curated for enrolled patients in stage 3 and then organized into a composite, calculated score arranged in a format common to other data providers for the trial in stage 4.

Data derived from different systems are not readily interoperable (eg, heart rates might be stored with different variable names requiring different queries for different EHR instances within a given health system). Navigating data governance structures and transforming real-world data into a harmonized endpoint therefore requires adequate local expertise, resources for data analyst, software developer and clinical informatician time, and a secure IT infrastructure for data storage, transformation, and transfer. These ETL steps apply to all clinical investigations aiming to leverage data from the EHR and highlight steps that may be overlooked by investigators who have not previously worked with real-world data provisioned from source systems. Stages 2 to 4 should be expected to demand approximately 90% of the effort spent on acquiring and analyzing data. Each stage can be made substantially more efficient for multicenter studies by engaging clinical informaticians during trial design. With their knowledge of what patient data are available and how they are represented in EHR databases, clinical informaticians can inform the design of trial outcome measures and case report forms to reduce the difficulty of automating case reporting from real-world data. The experience of using multicenter EHR data for trial reporting during a public health emergency provided the insight to formulate a set of recommendations for future pragmatic trials aiming to leverage EHR data (**Table 1**).

Although REMAP-CAP adopted a set of practical, need-based steps to exchange data and rapidly address a global public health emergency, seamless and timely exchange of research data between different systems may one day be substantially easier because of the emergence of interoperability standards and requirements. In the United States and much of the world, health care information systems have emerged without prioritizing interoperability between health care organizations. Lack of interoperability is a major barrier to leveraging real-world data from different sources and poses a substantial challenge to achieving the vision of large-scale learning health care systems.[52] This challenge is changing by way of legislation in the United States and abroad that is enforcing adherence to common data standards. In the United States, the 21st Century Cures Act, signed in 2016 and finalized in 2020,[53] includes provisions requiring that EHR vendors support interoperable data transfer to be certified by the Office of the National Coordinator. This includes support for application programming interfaces capable of transferring data in Health Level Seven International's (HL7) Fast Healthcare Interoperability Resources (FHIR) standard,[a] which facilitates the exchange of health information using third-party applications. FHIR defines the format and syntax of data exchange based on widely used Internet standards. The Cures Act also requires mapping core data within a hospital or health system to standard terms, such as logical observations identifiers names

---

[a] The HL7 FHIR standard adheres to a community-involved, staged development cycle and is currently on its fourth released version, known as R4.

Table 1
Recommendations for leveraging electronic health record data in pragmatic trials

Recommendation	Explanation	How It Was Addressed in REMAP-CAP
Define variable labels and associated attributes	Combining multiple data sources requires harmonizing multiple databases. Each variable, such as baseline heart rate, should be assigned a reporting name (eg, "Bas_HeartRate") and the expected attributes should be clearly defined (eg, integer variable ranging from 0 to 300). Discrete fields should include value sets of acceptable responses	Early in the pandemic, the expected variable names and discrete responses for the REMAP-CAP database were shared with the US data-coordinating center team to serve as a guidepost
Define the reporting schema	The expected format of reported data should be clearly defined at trial outset, such as whether data will be captured on a single table or multiple, relational tables	See above
Establish accepted formats and methods of data transfer	Data formats, such as csv files or SQL exports, should be established, and methods of transfer, such as secure file transfer protocol servers, should be defined early in the trial	Globus secure file exchange has been used to send trial data between the regional and international data-coordinating centers
Include standard vocabulary codes in data definitions	When defining variables, value sets of acceptable standardized codes should be included. For example, the LOINC codes 2951-2, 42570-2, and 77139-4 all refer to sodium measurements and may be included in a value set of acceptable codes	In the United States, reported variables were mapped to LOINC codes where appropriate to aid in local standardization of EHR data
Do not leave logic gaps in the data dictionary	Reporting guidelines written and reviewed by clinicians may not be clear to nonclinicians who cannot fill in logic gaps that require medical knowledge and experience. For example, if methods of supplemental oxygen delivery, such as simple facemask and nonrebreather facemask, are expected to be mapped to fraction of inspired oxygen values (F_iO_2), the expected F_iO_2 values associated with each delivery device should be defined in the data dictionary	Close partnerships between programmers, biomedical informaticists, and clinical informaticists helped to ensure that any logic gaps addressed were translated appropriately into data extraction and transformation scripts

(continued on next page)

Table 1
(continued)

Recommendation	Explanation	How It Was Addressed in REMAP-CAP
Provide explicit sequence and time bounds for composite variables	Composite variables, such as P_aO_2/F_iO_2 ratios, may necessitate combining fields documented in close proximity but without identical timestamps. Consider providing guidance on the expected sequence and time bounds for programming such variables (eg, an F_iO_2 value must have been documented within 4 hours before a P_aO_2 value to calculate a ratio)	In cases of uncertainty, decisions regarding programming requirements related to composite variables were discussed between regional and international data-coordinating centers to ensure agreement
Use technology to facilitate open communication and harmonization among data providers	Online tools, such as shared word documents, spreadsheets, and GitHub repositories, can facilitate both communication and version control of data dictionaries, schemas, and reporting scripts	Shared spreadsheets containing the expected data schema were created by the international data-coordinating center to facilitate a harmonized data set and served as a guidepost for the regional data-coordinating centers. GitHub repositories were maintained by the United States data-coordinating center to aid in version control of extraction and transformation scripts

and codes (LOINC)[54] for observational data, including vital signs and laboratory test values, and RxNorm[55] for medications. Last, use of common data elements, which are clearly defined variables with specific response values common to multiple data sets and trials, such as the National Heart, Lung, and Blood Institute COVID-19 common data elements, can aid data harmonization.[56] By adopting standardized value sets and vocabularies, transmitted data can have shared understanding and meaning between source and recipient information systems. For clinical trials, adoption of these standards may eventually give way to easy-to-install applications capable of deploying a customized trial workflow in the EHR while simultaneously collecting pertinent data to support intended analyses.

Although the vision of a robust EHR app store stocked with clinical trial applications will take at least several years to materialize, of more immediate benefit is the growing number of health systems that are transforming their real-world data warehouses into a common data model that facilitates easy exchange of code for extracting and analyzing data elements of interest. The Observational Health Data Science Initiative's Observational Medical Outcomes Partnership (OMOP) common data model and related tools include a common schema for arranging health care data, adherence to standard vocabularies, and an increasingly robust, open-source toolkit for exchanging analytic code.[57] One international network participating in REMAP-CAP has developed a modular registry to promote both quality improvement and clinical investigation across several low- and middle-income countries, relying on the OMOP common data model to support participation in multicenter research.[58]

ETHICAL CONSIDERATIONS OF "LIVING, BREATHING" TRIALS

The COVID-19 pandemic highlighted the conflict intrinsic in the unresolved ethics debates surrounding the vision of large-scale learning health care systems.[59] Limited supplies of novel medications, such as vaccines and monoclonal antibodies, forced health systems to develop rationing systems relying on lotteries that incorporated inclusion and exclusion criteria. These steps were taken out of necessity but also took the form of natural experiments providing an opportunity to evaluate a given intervention's effectiveness under randomized conditions outside of a formal trial.[42,60] Similarly, reliance on therapeutic interchange became commonplace with different formulations of mechanistically identical medications substituted by pharmacists on the basis of availability.[61] Therapeutic interchange among monoclonal antibodies during the pandemic also provided the basis for a comparative effectiveness trial at UPMC.[46]

Controversy exists regarding whether informed consent processes warrant revision to support some living, breathing trial designs in the era of the learning health care system. Bioethicists Faden, Beauchamp, and Kass[62] have previously dissected whether traditional consent procedures should be uniformly required, offering that "[o]ne major question is whether informed consent should always be required for randomized comparative-effectiveness studies, particularly studies conducted in a learning health care system. Our answer to this question is no." However, this viewpoint is not unanimously shared.[63] For the last half-century, clinical care and clinical research have coexisted as related but separate enterprises. This division represents an overarching effort to ensure that patients' rights are protected in the course of both care and investigation, according to ethics principles, such as those outlined in The Belmont Report.[64] The principles of respect for persons, beneficence, and justice are unquestionably just as applicable today as they were when originally outlined by the National Commission for the Protection of Human Subjects in Biomedical and Behavioral Research in the

1970s. Less clear is where the ethical divide exists when balancing considerations, such as how to design studies to answer questions regarding existing, alternative standards of usual care with the potential need to implement consent practices more resource-intensive than would occur during the typical care delivery. Ambiguity in this area is amplified by relatively vague language in major legislation intended to protect patient rights. The Health Insurance Portability and Accountability Act (HIPAA), which includes the Privacy Rule governing protected health information (PHI), and the Common Rule, which includes regulations relating to informed consent processes, provide only broad guidance on how PHI should be accessed by research teams before consent for study participation. Uncertainty in this space has resulted in substantial variation in "cold-calling" practices, or how research teams approach patients for study participation, around the country.[65]

Although separation of research and care has helped create rigorous procedures for informed consent, assessment of risks and benefits, and selection of subjects in clinical investigations, the need for distinct, parallel infrastructures also contributes to slower investigation, increased costs, and less generalizable insights. These considerations have given rise to proposed updates to the clinical research ethics framework that include an increasing role for investigation as part of care delivery, as well as a contextualized approach to informed consent that accounts for scenarios in which individual informed consent may not be necessary despite randomization.[66] Whether examples of the learning health care system in action during the pandemic will help motivate greater consensus on an updated ethics framework for the design and conduct of living, breathing clinical trials remains to be seen.

SUMMARY

Since the first description of the learning health care system, there has been a growing number of clinical trials demonstrating increasing integration with clinical care that uses medical informatics infrastructure and analytic approaches. This phenomenon appears to have been accelerated by the COVID-19 pandemic. Weaving systematic learning into the delivery of health care is a promising approach to improve the efficiency of clinical trials and more rapidly optimize disease management; however, controversies exist in how to best protect and respect patients within the learning health care system framework. Experiences gained during the pandemic are invaluable for advancing the concept of "living, breathing" trials and can be expected to yield insights for years to come.

CLINICS CARE POINTS

- Integrating randomized clinical trials into the delivery of care has the potential to overcome many limitations of traditional clinical trials.
- Modern information systems can be leveraged to promote efficiency in trial patient identification, workflows, and data collection.
- "Living, breathing" clinical trials are woven into the fabric of health care delivery and promote rigorous, continuous learning for a range of therapies and diseases.
- More work is necessary to achieve consensus regarding clinical research ethics frameworks that promote seamless integration of research into the delivery of care.

FUNDING

C.M. Horvat is supported by K23 HD099331.

DISCLOSURE

The authors have nothing to disclose.

REFERENCES

1. Weissler AM. The Hippocratic ethic in a contemporary era of clinical uncertainty. Mayo Clin Proc 1991;66(9):966–7.
2. Lancet T. Uncertainty in medicine. Lancet 2010;375(9727):1666.
3. Rysavy M. Evidence-based medicine: a science of uncertainty and an art of probability. AMA Journal of Ethics 2013;15(1):4–8.
4. Burns PB, Rohrich RJ, Chung KC. The levels of evidence and their role in evidence-based medicine. Plast Reconstr Surg 2011;128(1):305–10.
5. Speich B, von Niederhäusern B, Schur N, et al. Systematic review on costs and resource use of randomized clinical trials shows a lack of transparent and comprehensive data. J Clin Epidemiol 2018;96:1–11.
6. Files DC, Matthay MA, Calfee CS, et al. I-SPY COVID adaptive platform trial for COVID-19 acute respiratory failure: rationale, design and operations. BMJ Open 2022;12(6):e060664.
7. Houston BL, Lawler PR, Goligher EC, et al. Anti-thrombotic therapy to ameliorate complications of COVID-19 (ATTACC): study design and methodology for an international, adaptive Bayesian randomized controlled trial. Clin Trials 2020;17(5): 491–500.
8. UPMC REMAP-COVID Group, on behalf of the REMAP-CAP Investigators. Implementation of the randomized embedded multifactorial adaptive platform for COVID-19 (REMAP-COVID) trial in a US health system-lessons learned and recommendations. Trials 2021;22(1):100.
9. Committee on the learning health care system in America, Institute of Medicine. In: Smith M, Saunders R, Stuckhardt L, et al, editors. Best care at lower cost: the path to continuously learning health care in America. National Academies Press (US); 2013. Available at: http://www.ncbi.nlm.nih.gov/books/NBK207225/. Accessed October 23, 2022.
10. Institute of Medicine (US). In: Olsen L, Aisner D, McGinnis JM, editors. Roundtable on evidence-based medicine. The learning healthcare system: workshop summary. National Academies Press (US); 2007. Available at: http://www.ncbi.nlm.nih.gov/books/NBK53494/. Accessed October 27, 2022.
11. Pessoa-Amorim G, Campbell M, Fletcher L, et al. Making trials part of good clinical care: lessons from the RECOVERY trial. Future Healthc J 2021;8(2):e243–50.
12. Angus DC, Berry S, Lewis RJ, et al. The REMAP-CAP (randomized embedded multifactorial adaptive platform for community-acquired pneumonia) study. Rationale and design. Ann Am Thorac Soc 2020;17(7):879–91.
13. Angus DC. Optimizing the trade-off between learning and doing in a pandemic. JAMA 2020;323(19):1895–6.
14. Califf RM, Cavazzoni P, Woodcock J. Benefits of streamlined point-of-care trial designs: lessons learned from the UK RECOVERY study. JAMA Intern Med 2022;182(12):1243–4.
15. Schwartz D, Lellouch J. Explanatory and pragmatic attitudes in therapeutical trials. J Chronic Dis 1967;20(8):637–48.

16. Thorpe KE, Zwarenstein M, Oxman AD, et al. A pragmatic-explanatory continuum indicator summary (PRECIS): a tool to help trial designers. J Clin Epidemiol 2009; 62(5):464–75.

17. Tuzzio L, Larson EB. The promise of pragmatic clinical trials embedded in learning health systems. EGEMS (Wash DC) 2019;7(1):10.

18. Woodcock J, LaVange LM. Master protocols to study multiple therapies, multiple diseases, or both. N Engl J Med 2017;377(1):62–70.

19. Welcome — RECOVERY trial. Available at: https://www.recoverytrial.net/. Accessed October 28, 2022.

20. COVID-19 Therapeutics prioritized for testing in clinical trials. National Institutes of Health (NIH). 2020. Available at: https://www.nih.gov/research-training/medical-research-initiatives/activ/covid-19-therapeutics-prioritized-testing-clinical-trials. Accessed October 28, 2022.

21. Response to COVID-19 pandemic. REMAP-CAP trial. Available at: https://www.remapcap.org/coronavirus. Accessed October 28, 2022.

22. Angus DC, Derde L, Al-Beidh F, et al. Effect of hydrocortisone on mortality and organ support in patients with severe COVID-19: the REMAP-CAP COVID-19 corticosteroid domain randomized clinical trial. JAMA 2020;324(13):1317–29.

23. Arabi YM, Gordon AC, Derde LPG, et al. Lopinavir-ritonavir and hydroxychloroquine for critically ill patients with COVID-19: REMAP-CAP randomized controlled trial. Intensive Care Med 2021;47(8):867–86.

24. Writing Committee for the REMAP-CAP Investigators. Effect of convalescent plasma on organ support–free days in critically ill patients with COVID-19: a randomized clinical Trial. JAMA 2021;326(17):1690–702.

25. ATTACC Investigators, ACTIV-4a Investigators, REMAP-CAP Investigators, et al. Therapeutic anticoagulation in noncritically ill patients with Covid-19. N Engl J Med 2021. https://doi.org/10.1056/NEJMoa2105911.

26. REMAP-CAP Investigators, ACTIV-4a Investigators, ATTACC Investigators, et al. Therapeutic anticoagulation with heparin in critically ill patients with Covid-19. N Engl J Med 2021. https://doi.org/10.1056/NEJMoa2103417.

27. REMAP-CAP Writing Committee for the REMAP-CAP Investigators, Bradbury CA, Lawler PR, et al. Effect of antiplatelet therapy on survival and organ support-free days in critically ill patients with COVID-19: a randomized clinical trial. JAMA 2022;327(13):1247–59.

28. REMAP-CAP Investigators, Gordon AC, Mouncey PR, et al. Interleukin-6 receptor antagonists in critically ill patients with Covid-19. N Engl J Med 2021. https://doi.org/10.1056/NEJMoa2100433.

29. How bayesian machine learning works. Open data science - your news source for ai, machine learning & more. 2020. Available at: https://opendatascience.com/how-bayesian-machine-learning-works/. Accessed January 1, 2023.

30. Eddy DM. The origins of evidence-based medicine: a personal perspective. AMA Journal of Ethics 2011;13(1):55–60.

31. Eddy DM. Practice policies: where do they come from? JAMA 1990;263(9):1265–75.

32. Kahneman D, Tversky A. Prospect theory: an analysis of decision under risk. Econometrica 1979;47(2):263–91.

33. Feinstein AR. Clinical biostatistics. XXXIX. The haze of Bayes, the aerial palaces of decision analysis, and the computerized Ouija board. Clin Pharmacol Ther 1977;21(4):482–96.

34. Bland JM, Altman DG. Bayesians and frequentists. BMJ 1998;317(7166):1151–60.

35. Winkler RL. Why Bayesian analysis hasn't caught on in healthcare decision making. Int J Technol Assess Health Care 2001;17(1):56–66.
36. Christensen R. Testing Fisher, Neyman, Pearson, and Bayes. Am Statistician 2005;59(2):121–6.
37. Hackenberger BK. Bayes or not Bayes, is this the question? Croat Med J 2019; 60(1):50–2.
38. Berry DA. Bayesian clinical trials. Nat Rev Drug Discov 2006;5(1):27–36.
39. Goligher EC, Tomlinson G, Hajage D, et al. Extracorporeal membrane oxygenation for severe acute respiratory distress syndrome and posterior probability of mortality benefit in a post hoc bayesian analysis of a randomized clinical trial. JAMA 2018;320(21):2251–9.
40. Harhay MO, Blette BS, Granholm A, et al. A Bayesian interpretation of a pediatric cardiac arrest trial (THAPCA-OH). NEJM Evidence 2022;2(1). https://doi.org/10.1056/EVIDoa2200196. EVIDoa2200196.
41. Keely SD. Marshall. UPMC launches "learning while doing" clinical trial of COVID-19 vaccine. WJAC. 2020. Available at: https://wjactv.com/news/local/upmc-launches-learning-while-doing-clinical-trial-of-covid-19-vaccine. Accessed November 17, 2022.
42. White DB, McCreary EK, Chang CCH, et al. A multicenter weighted lottery to equitably allocate scarce COVID-19 therapeutics. Am J Respir Crit Care Med 2022;206(4):503–6.
43. Huang DT, McCreary EK, Bariola JR, et al. The UPMC OPTIMISE-C19 (optimizing treatment and impact of monoclonal antIbodieS through Evaluation for COVID-19) trial: a structured summary of a study protocol for an open-label, pragmatic, comparative effectiveness platform trial with response-adaptive randomization. Trials 2021;22(1):363.
44. McCreary EK, Bariola JR, Minnier T, et al. Launching a comparative effectiveness adaptive platform trial of monoclonal antibodies for COVID-19 in 21 days. Contemp Clin Trials 2022;113:106652.
45. McCreary EK, Bariola JR, Minnier TE, et al. The comparative effectiveness of COVID-19 monoclonal antibodies: a learning health system randomized clinical trial. Contemp Clin Trials 2022;119:106822.
46. Huang DT, McCreary EK, Bariola JR, et al. Effectiveness of Casirivimab-Imdevimab and Sotrovimab during a SARS-CoV-2 delta variant surge: a cohort study and randomized comparative effectiveness trial. JAMA Netw Open 2022; 5(7):e2220957.
47. McCreary EK, Kip KE, Bariola JR, et al. A learning health system approach to the COVID-19 pandemic: system-wide changes in clinical practice and 30-day mortality among hospitalized patients. Learning Health Systems 2022;6(3):e10304.
48. QI/PI activities | ABIM.org. Available at: https://www.abim.org/maintenance-of-certification/earning-points/qi-pi-activities/?altTemplate=qipidetail&product=c1b750e9-9ce8-4f7c-bf3b-f0dd8b4bba7b. Accessed January 3, 2023.
49. Kohn MS, Topaloglu U, Kirkendall ES, et al. Creating learning health systems and the emerging role of biomedical informatics. Learn Health Syst 2022;6(1):e10259.
50. Valenta AL, Berner ES, Boren SA, et al. AMIA Board White Paper: AMIA 2017 core competencies for applied health informatics education at the master's degree level. J Am Med Inf Assoc 2018;25(12):1657–68.
51. Bradshaw RL, Kawamoto K, Kaphingst KA, et al. GARDE: a standards-based clinical decision support platform for identifying population health management cohorts. J Am Med Inf Assoc 2022;29(5):928–36.

52. NIH collaboratory rethinking clinical trials - the living textbook. Rethinking clinical trials. Available at: https://rethinkingclinicaltrials.org/. Accessed October 23, 2022.

53. 21st century Cures act: interoperability, information blocking, and the ONC health IT certification program. Federal register. 2020. Available at: https://www.federal register.gov/documents/2020/05/01/2020-07419/21st-century-cures-act-interoper ability-information-blocking-and-the-onc-health-it-certification. Accessed November 26, 2022.

54. Home. LOINC. Available at: https://loinc.org/. Accessed October 30, 2022.

55. RxNorm. Available at: https://www.nlm.nih.gov/research/umls/rxnorm/index.html. Accessed October 30, 2022.

56. Weissman A, Cheng A, Mainor A, et al. Development and implementation of the national heart, lung, and blood institute COVID-19 common data elements. Journal of Clinical and Translational Science 2022;1–25. https://doi.org/10.1017/cts.2022.466.

57. OMOP common data model – OHDSI. Available at: https://www.ohdsi.org/data-standardization/the-common-data-model/. Accessed October 30, 2022.

58. Aryal D, Beane A, Dondorp AM, et al. Operationalisation of the randomized embedded multifactorial adaptive platform for COVID-19 trials in a low and lower-middle income critical care learning health system. Wellcome Open Res 2021;6:14.

59. Casey JD, Beskow LM, Brown J, et al. Use of pragmatic and explanatory trial designs in acute care research: lessons from COVID-19. Lancet Respir Med 2022;10(7):700–14.

60. White DB, Angus DC. A proposed lottery system to allocate scarce COVID-19 medications: promoting fairness and generating knowledge. JAMA 2020;324(4):329–30.

61. Darrow JJ, Chong JE, Kesselheim AS. Reconsidering the scope of US state laws allowing pharmacist substitution of generic drugs. BMJ 2020;369:m2236.

62. Faden RR, Beauchamp TL, Kass NE. Informed consent, comparative effectiveness, and learning health care. N Engl J Med 2014;370(8):766–8.

63. Anderson JR, Schonfeld TL. Informed consent for comparative effectiveness trials. N Engl J Med 2014;370(20):1958.

64. Protections (OHRP) O for HR. Read the Belmont report. HHS.gov. 2018. Available at: https://www.hhs.gov/ohrp/regulations-and-policy/belmont-report/read-the-belmont-report/index.html. Accessed October 31, 2022.

65. McHugh KR, Swamy GK, Hernandez AF. Engaging patients throughout the health system: a landscape analysis of cold-call policies and recommendations for future policy change. J Clin Transl Sci 2019;2(6):384–92.

66. Faden RR, Kass NE, Goodman SN, et al. An ethics framework for a learning health care system: a departure from traditional research ethics and clinical ethics. Hastings Cent Rep 2013;(Spec No):S16–27. https://doi.org/10.1002/hast.134.

How Electronic Medical Record Integration Can Support More Efficient Critical Care Clinical Trials

Ankita Agarwal, MD, MSc[a], Joseph Marion, PhD[b], Paul Nagy, PhD[c,d],
Matthew Robinson, MD[e], Allan Walkey, MD, MSc[f],
Jonathan Sevransky, MD, MHS[a],*

KEYWORDS

- Data science • Critical care research • Precision medicine
- Randomized controlled trials • Adaptive trials • Platform trials

KEY POINTS

- Current challenges to interventional trials and critical care research include an inefficient trial design, heterogenous patient populations, heterogeneous treatment effects, and difficulties with patient enrollment.
- Precise phenotyping of critically ill patients may allow more targeted enrollment of patients in critical care trials and better stratification of assignment to treatment arms.
- The use of electronic surveillance systems and electronic medical record can help increase efficiency in screening and automate data collection in clinical trials.
- Platform and adaptive trials can leverage data science methods and use existing information to inform flexible trial designs testing multiple treatments.

INTRODUCTION

The increased use of monitoring and diagnostic devices in the intensive care unit (ICU) has led to greater production of complex streams of information. The growing use of

---

[a] Division of Pulmonary, Allergy, Critical Care and Sleep Medicine, Emory University School of Medicine, Emory Critical Care Center, Emory Healthcare, Atlanta, GA, USA; [b] Berry Consultants; [c] Department of Medicine, Johns Hopkins University School of Medicine, Baltimore, MD, USA; [d] Department of Biomedical Engineering, Johns Hopkins University School of Medicine, Baltimore, MD, USA; [e] Division of Infectious Diseases, Johns Hopkins University School of Medicine, Baltimore, MD, USA; [f] Department of Medicine – Section of Pulmonary, Allergy, Critical Care and Sleep Medicine, Boston University School of Medicine, Boston, MA, USA
* Corresponding author. Division of Pulmonary, Allergy, Critical Care and Sleep Medicine, 615 Michael Street, Suite 205, Atlanta, GA 30322.
E-mail address: jsevran@emory.edu

Crit Care Clin 39 (2023) 733–749
https://doi.org/10.1016/j.ccc.2023.03.006
0749-0704/23/© 2023 Elsevier Inc. All rights reserved.

data science in health care (particularly through the use of electronic health records [EHRs] and large-scale patient registries[1,2]) has increased the ability to capture, analyze, and generate new knowledge from the routine care of ICU patients in a learning health system designed to improve care for patients with life-threatening illnesses. The primary goals of clinical research trials are to assess response and effectiveness of therapies and clinical outcomes for future patients.[3] This article will review current challenges in critical care research and how data science can support more efficient research in critical care through identifying promising patient subgroups for trial enrollment, automating enrollment, trial data collection, and pilot testing interventions in virtual trials. We will also highlight the potential intersection of the use of big data and the use of adaptive platform trial (APT) designs.

CURRENT CHALLENGES IN CRITICAL CARE RESEARCH

Patients with life-threatening illnesses present a special challenge for the clinical researcher. While the number of patients with or at risk of a critical illness appears to be increasing,[4] heterogenous patient populations, syndromic definitions, difficulties in patient and surrogate consent, and the high cost of clinical trials all complicate our ability to improve care for those with a life-threatening injury or illness.[5] Advances in care for the critically ill have come primarily from performance-improvement projects and improvements in supportive care, rather than the development of novel medications or technologies to treat those with life-threatening illnesses.[6–8] A review of critical care research studies suggests that the majority of randomized controlled trials (RCTs) in critically ill patients have shown no net treatment effect,[9] and promising signals of benefit in many early trials (eg, neuromuscular blockade for acute respiratory distress syndrome [ARDS],[7] early goal directed therapy,[8,10] and recombinant activated protein c in sepsis[11,12]) were not replicated when tested in subsequent, larger, multicenter trials. The factors that make critical care unique, including life-threatening illnesses, heterogenous clinical presentations with rapidly changing trajectories, and secular trends in cares, pose significant challenges for critical care research (**Table 1**).

Others have commented on reasons for the lack of treatment effect found in most critical care clinical trials including outcome selection, power, and potential differences in treatment effect in subgroups.[9,13] Many critical care trials have used mortality as the primary outcome, but detecting differences in mortality can be challenging and requires a large amount of data.[14,15] Selection of non–mortality-based outcomes presents its own challenges due to unclear patient-centeredness, differing definitions, potential for bias, and difficulties in interpretation of results, particularly for composite outcomes.[16,17] Choosing the appropriate effect size can be difficult in intensive care, and there is limited consensus on the definition of a "clinically important difference." Most studies have to balance the desire to detect even small differences as clinically significant with the practical consideration that detecting a small mortality difference requires thousands of patients. This can result in many "negative studies" that were underpowered and, thus, limited in the ability to detect beneficial therapies.[16,18]

Clinical complexity and presence of comorbidities also make identification and enrollment of large numbers of critically ill subjects difficult. Many clinical trials have narrow selection criteria and may exclude large numbers of patients with a disease of interest to help select the subgroup of patients most likely to benefit from the particular intervention[19] and to maximize trial safety. When potential subjects are identified, recruitment and enrollment can be challenging because the patients often cannot participate in the screening, recruitment, and enrollment processes, and studies must rely on clinician referrals, EHR screening, and surrogates for consent.[19,20]

Table 1	
Challenges and potential solutions to critical care research	
Challenges	**Potential Solutions**
Heterogenous Patient Populations Critically ill patients have varying comorbidities, differing clinical presentations and trajectories even within the same critical illness syndrome (such as sepsis, or ARDS).	• Identification of disease phenotypes and trials targeted to phenotypes with the greatest potential for benefit • Varying inclusion of subjects in clinical trials based on phenotypes and treatable traits
Screening, Recruitment, Enrollment Clinical trials can have strict enrollment criteria and require time/effort-intensive screening processes. Enrollment windows can be narrow to ensure subjects are enrolled within a certain therapeutic window. Consent often requires a surrogate.	• Use of electronic surveillance systems ("sniffers") to screen and identify potential subjects. Can also be integrated with an EMR platform
Trial outcome selection and effect size Many critical care trials use mortality as an outcome and non-mortality-based outcomes may have varying definitions and are difficult to interpret for a clinically meaningful difference.	• Adaptive platform trials that allow for multiintervention and multioutcome trial designs, with interim analyses allowing for prespecified changes in trial duration, sample size, allocation, and randomization
Cost Cost can be related to effort needed to screen & enroll patients, number of patients required for a reasonable power, and researcher effort for trial data collection.	• Automated extraction of clinical data from the EHR/EMR • See also solutions to challenges in screening and outcome selection above

Traditional research methodologies do not fully address challenges to critical care research, and application of data science to health care and clinical research may provide strategies to more effectively and efficiently reach these goals (see **Table 1**). In the next sections, we discuss potential uses of data science to improve identification and enrollment of subjects in clinical trials, data collection, and alternative trial designs that minimize weaknesses of traditional RCTs.

PRECISION MEDICINE AND CRITICAL CARE RESEARCH

Precision medicine aims to identify groups of patients based on shared characteristics to provide more effective diagnoses and treatment approaches.[21] For example, tumor-marker-targeted therapies have helped to define and grow precision medicine in oncology.[22] Some may consider critical care to be a few steps behind oncology on the road for precision medicine. Diagnosis is still rooted primarily in syndrome descriptions rather than biological or physiologic underpinnings, and at present, there are limited diagnostic features such as a pathologic finding on biopsy, genetic mutation, or serologic marker that will definitively diagnose diseases of the critically ill.[5] There can be substantial variability in the trigger or cause of disease, differences in the presentation and manifestations over time, and trajectory of the disease over time.[23] For example, identification of sepsis requires recognition of a constellation of clinical findings of an abnormal host response (which itself can have various presentations) and an infection source.[6,24] While attempts have been made to standardize or protocolize diagnoses, such as the Berlin classification for ARDS,[25] the natural challenge when diagnosis is based on a combination of clinical findings is making the diagnosis.[2] However, with growing attention paid to classification and identifying the biological underpinnings of critical illnesses, precision medicine that allows targeting of biological or physiologic pathways in critical care could advance treatment similar to oncology.

Heterogeneity among critically ill patients leads to limitations not only in diagnoses but also in treatment and prognostication. "One size fits all" approaches can result in different effects among subgroups of patients,[26] leading many to suggest disease heterogeneity in critical illnesses as a major driver of uninformative clinical trials in critical care.[27] Precision medicine and more accurate prediction of response to therapy may improve subject assignment to interventions in trials, potentially leading to less ambiguity or noise in study results.[28] As an example, consider a study of an anti-inflammatory agent in ARDS. If a trial could screen and selectively enroll subjects with a specific dysregulated inflammatory pathway, such as inflammasome activation in direct lung injury,[29] then the trial is theoretically more likely to show a benefit with treatment targeted to the dysregulated pathway, if one exists (**Fig. 1**). In comparison, traditional trials would screen and potentially enroll all ARDS patients, including those with less inflammation who may show no effect, or even harm, thereby diluting any potential positive benefit of the anti-inflammatory agent.[30,31]

BIG DATA AND ITS CONTRIBUTION TO PATIENT PHENOTYPES

Phenotyping patients—whether through a pathologic inflammatory response or a similar genetic change—allows us to group patients based on shared characteristics that might reflect the underlying biological process.[23,32,33] Phenotyping also allows for incorporation of patients' comorbidities in several ways. These techniques may allow the identification of "treatable traits."[5] So far, studies of phenotypes in common critical illnesses such as sepsis[34–36] or ARDS[37] have been generally limited to retrospective analyses of RCTs or prospective observational studies. Before clinical trials can use phenotypes to preferentially enroll subjects, we must develop and validate these

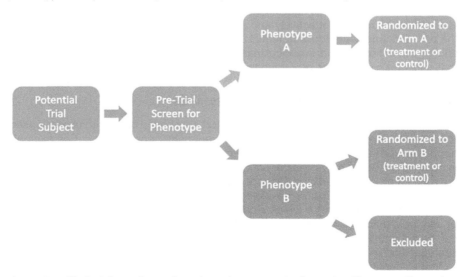

Fig. 1. Stratified trial enrollment based on phenotype. A schematic of how enrollment in a clinical trial may be stratified by subject phenotype.

phenotypes in sample populations and may also need to be able to offer multiple treatment options.[38] Big data collected on ICU patients on a daily and near minute-by-minute basis can be used to prospectively develop and evaluate phenotypes in critically ill patients.

Using precision medicine and patient phenotypes can help improve subject assignment and enhance likelihood of finding effective treatments in critical care trials, but there are some specific challenges to widespread use. Obvious barriers are the volume of data and creation of phenotype groups. Determining which and how many variables to include when phenotyping patients and how many phenotypes to create is complex. Too many variables could lead to almost as many groups as patients and results that are difficult to generalize.[39] Too few variables, while limiting costs, may compromise the ability to differentiate between distinct phenotypes and not appreciably improve the trial design and results. Additionally, some features present on a continuum (vs discrete categories), and creating cutoffs that establish presence or absence of traits may reduce the discriminative ability.[28]

Methodologically, variation in clustering techniques also poses challenges in creating phenotypes. Often phenotypes are first created based on retrospective data, and changing definitions of disease and trial enrollment criteria can lead to multiple ways to phenotype a single disease process.[33] Missingness in collected data, either because we do not know what to measure or we cannot measure what is needed, can also lead to inaccurate phenotypes. At present, there are limited data evaluating different phenotyping methods to allow for comparisons and generalizability assessments.[32]

CLUSTERING AND PRECISION MEDICINE TO IDENTIFY TREATABLE TRAITS?

Treatable traits, a form of phenotypes, are any observable traits (ie, biomarkers) that are associated with a disease state that predicts response to a particular treatment and can be monitored for a response to treatment.[40] Common examples of treatable traits include serologic markers, any observed characteristic, be a treatable trait such as genome transcriptomic features, virulence factors, imaging findings, or even heart rate variability. To be useful, treatable traits must have some generalizability and be able to be applied to a large-enough subgroup of patients with a certain disease.[23] Additionally, treatable traits are often linked to treatment response, such as eosinophils for asthma and response to biological treatments, but this may not be a necessary defining criterion for all treatable traits.

Identification of treatable traits and inclusion of subjects in trials based on these traits is a way to enrich trial enrollment (see **Fig. 1**). A secondary analysis of pediatric septic shock modeled predictive enrichment strategies and assigned 1 of two genetic endotypes to subjects to detect a subgroup with greater likelihood to benefit from corticosteroids.[41] In breast cancer, the I-SPY APT enrolls and randomizes subjects preferentially to treatment arms they are more likely to respond to based on their molecular profile.[42]

To further our identification, knowledge, and use of treatable traits, critical care needs large repositories that contain variables that can be investigated as treatable traits including biological materials, imaging data, and potentially even genetic information. It is also likely necessary, at this stage, for trials to include patients with a particular hypothesized treatable trait and those without it to specifically test whether the treatable trait truly confers a predictable response to treatment.[43]

THE USE OF ELECTRONIC "SNIFFERS" TO IDENTIFY SUBJECTS

Variations in disease diagnosis are not the only barrier to efficient identification of potential subjects for critical care trials. The variable and rapidly changing disease severity, multiple admission sources (emergency department, hospital wards, outside transfers), and generally narrow inclusion windows can make screening for potential participants a challenging, time-consuming task. A study that requires subjects be enrolled within 6 hours of presentation means trial centers must have the resources to screen, recruit, enroll, and start study procedures in a relatively small period, and many sites may not have the manpower to accomplish this. Electronic surveillance systems, or "sniffers," automatically analyze specified data from the electronic medical record (EMR) to identify potential subjects for trials. The use of electronic sniffers over traditional methods—manual screening by a research coordinator—allows for more efficient and possibly less error-prone screening.[44] EMR companies may be particularly poised to develop such systems integrated within the EMR. Epic Systems, recently launched a "Life Sciences Program," which is a program designed to do exactly this—link potential patients with clinical trials that match their profile as well as alert clinicians to possible trials their patients may be appropriate for.[45]

Several studies have evaluated the use of sniffers for identification of sepsis, acute lung injury, and acute kidney injury,[46–48] showing high sensitivity and reasonable specificity. Sniffers can be more inclusive and simply help optimize the screening process. For example, in a study of ARDS, an electronic sniffer could identify all patients on mechanical ventilation in a dashboard in the EMR for more efficient and streamlined review by a research coordinator. The electronic sniffer can also be integrated into the enrollment process by automatic inclusion (for observational studies or those not requiring informed consent), flagging the patient for clinician review and referral to research team, or even with an option for randomization once informed consent is obtained.[49] At present, the use of electronic sniffers still requires review by a human member of the research team as methods of disease identification are not perfect. Widespread use of sniffers will require validation of the tool, implementation guidance, and assessment of effect on trial enrollment.[50]

LEVERAGING THE ELECTRONIC HEALTH RECORDS TO SUPPLY CLINICAL TRIAL DATA

Critical care trials have historically required manual completion of case report forms, but much of these data are now routinely recorded in the EHR/EMR as a part of clinical care. Extraction of clinical data directly from the EHR offers to dramatically reduce the overhead of data entry into case report forms, eliminate transcription errors, and increase observation frequency. Data of interest to critical care trialists are especially suitable for automated extraction as the care of critically ill patients generates high-density structured data (ie, pulse recordings every hour, multiple hemoglobin values per day).

Clinical data from the EHR must be mapped to variables specified in the trial design. The extract, transform, load (ETL) process pulls data elements of interest from the EHR, maps source data to defined variables, and integrates these data into a specified structure. Heterogeneity of EHR installations, even among customers of the same vendor, poses a challenge to mapping source EHR data to clinical trial variables and efficient ETL deployment.

Common data models (CDMs) that use standard terminology, use mature software tools, and build on precedent in observational research offer a template for using EHR data for clinical trials. The Observational Medical Outcomes Partnership CDM offers the flexibility and broad stakeholder engagement of an open-source community.[51] Proprietary approaches such as Cosmos provide cross-institution data aggregation for research purposes for participating Epic customers.[52] However, the ETL process requires computational resources, which limits the frequency and timing of its performance. Latency in the ETL from the EHR source to research databases rarely limits the feasibility of observational research but may be too great for extracted EHR data to serve as the sole source of clinical data for some trial applications. Rapid identification of adverse events is essential for patient safety, trial management, and event reporting. For example, if a study drug were to cause hepatotoxicity, thereby meeting the criteria for participant withdrawal, and there was a 24-hour delay in the ETL for liver function test results, the clinical trial team may not be aware of the safety event in time to withdraw the patient before the next administration of study drug.

Recent regulations issued by the Centers for Medicare & Medicaid Services have incentivized health care providers to improve interoperability of EHRs.[53] The Health Level Seven International Fast Healthcare Interoperability Resources (FHIR) standard is increasingly deployed by diverse stakeholders to facilitate health record exchange.[54] The National Institutes of Health has advocated for investigators to use FHIR for research.[55,56] Although FHIR has the potential to share data to support clinical trials, it has not been widely used for this purpose to date.[57]

THE ROLE OF VIRTUAL PATIENTS AND SIMULATED CLINICAL TRIALS IN PILOT TESTING

New or repurposed therapeutic agents or devices are required to have several phases of clinical trials to test for safety and efficacy. While diagnostic tests do not have the same established regulatory phases, diagnostic tests must also undergo several trails to establish precision, reproducibility, and accuracy.[58] Patient and illness heterogeneity as well as financial and time constraints can provide significant challenges for this multiphase development, testing, and implementation of therapeutic and/or diagnostic interventions.

Simulated clinical trials, or in silico trials, use virtual patients generated by medical data and model identification to simulate different virtual protocol designs.[59] Pilot testing trial protocols in model-generated virtual patients allows for simulated trials to better account for and optimize the protocol for variability in disease and patient physiology and heterogeneity in patient response to care or behavior.[60] Generation of virtual patients and models for simulated trials requires that all clinically and physiologically relative variables to adjust treatment are included. The drug and disease models generally include endogenous pharmacokinetic properties of the drug, administration, as well as variables that may alter absorption, elimination, and effect of the drug. A simulated trial is then run, and outcomes are analyzed for performance of the intervention and safety end points (**Fig. 2**). Assessment and interpretation of in silico trial models and patient cohorts is similar to standard clinical trials—the virtual patient cohort should be diverse and representative of the entire disease spectrum, and the model should be valid for capturing clinically relevant variables.

Critical care and illness may be particularly suited for in silico trials because of the large volume of clinical data collected on patients in ICUs. There have been many simulated trials showing validation of models for glycemic control in the ICU[61,62] and results that correlate with published clinical trial results as well.[63] In addition, an in silico trial of 10,000 virtual trauma patients demonstrated that inhibition of interleukin-6 may have a small survival benefit.[64] Ventilator management and evaluation of pulmonary mechanics algorithms and assessment and management of circulatory and cardiovascular derangements represent other potentially valuable areas for simulated trials in critical care.[60,65,66] For critical care interventions, simulated clinical trials may allow for more efficient testing and decrease the number of early-phase trials required before the large late-phase RCTs.

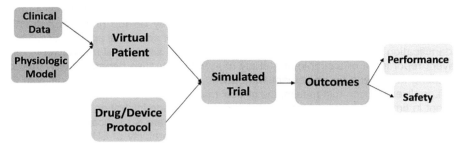

Fig. 2. Simulated clinical trial schematic. A virtual patient cohort is generated by combing through clinical data and a physiologic model for disease. A simulated trial is then conducted using the virtual patient cohort and trial protocol. Outcomes from the simulated trial are analyzed for performance and safety.

USING BIG DATA IN TRIALS TO GENERATE BIG DATA—THE USE OF ADAPTIVE PLATFORM TRIALS

As critical care research harnesses big data and data science methods to better improve identification and enrollment of subjects in clinical trials, we will benefit from more efficient trial designs. Traditional RCTs are still generally considered the gold standard for evidence in medicine. Subjects enrolled in an RCT are assigned to the experimental or control group by randomization methods not dissimilar to a "flip of a coin," which, under ideal conditions, creates an investigational intervention group and a "counterfactual" comparator group that represents the outcomes that the intervention group would have had if not assigned the intervention. Randomization minimizes the a priori effect of known and unknown confounders; thus, any differences in observed outcomes in a large, high-quality RCT can be causally attributed to the intervention tested.[58] The approval and use of new or repurposed therapeutics or diagnostic tests by regulatory bodies, such as the Food and Drug Administration (FDA) in the United States, is often supported by evidence of safety and effectiveness from RCTs.[67,68]

However, the numerous challenges discussed above limit opportunities for RCTs in the critical care setting. Classically, RCTs in critical care have compared a single intervention to control in a relatively homogenous population (**Table 2**).[58] This approach may not be the optimal trial design for critical care research. Randomizing to a solitary

Table 2	
Definitions and descriptions of clinical research terminology	
Term	**Description**
Randomized Controlled Trial	Trial design where subjects are randomly assigned to experimental or control group
Adaptive Trial	Trial allows for prespecified changes in trial characteristics while the trial is running in response to data collected in the trial.
Platform Trial	Trials focused on a single disease with multiple treatment arms, and treatment arms can be added or terminated based on interim analyses
Adaptive Platform Trial	Combination of adaptive and platform trial methodologies, allowing for an adaptive trial with multiple treatment assignments, including combination arms

treatment versus placebo is inefficient, with time and resources spent on narrowly testing a single therapy that, given past results, has a high likelihood of failing.[69] A single, rejectable null hypothesis on an intervention with a single outcome limits the conclusions drawn, as most secondary outcomes in RCTs can only be considered hypothesis-generating.[70] While some critical care RCTs do demonstrate a large difference in the primary outcome, the narrow selection of subjects can lead to a lack of external validity, or generalizability to the broader population.[71]

Addressing challenges and gaps of traditional RCTs will require a shift in clinical trial methodology to allow for smarter, more precise, and more efficient study designs. Two types of study designs—adaptive trials and platform trials—provide substantial advantages compared to the traditional RCT research paradigm. Adaptive trials are specifically designed to periodically assess study data and adapt the study design in prespecified changes in response to interim data (**Fig. 3**, see **Table 2**). Examples of changes in trial design can include sample size, study duration, treatment arms, treatment group allocation, and even study end points.[72] Platform trials focus on a specific disease or disease process and typically include multiple treatment arms, in isolation or combination, compared to each other (comparative effectiveness) or against a common control. A platform trial design also allows for investigation of multiple strata[73] and for addition or termination of treatment arms based on prespecified stopping rules (see **Table 2**).[70] APTs combine both trial methodologies and allow for an adaptive trial of multiple treatments (**Fig. 4**, see **Table 2**).[74]

APTs have greater efficiency than traditional, nonadaptive designs because they are able to test multiple interventions simultaneously and use accumulating study data to stop recruitment to treatment arms that demonstrate clear benefit or harm, or futility.[75,76] Unlike traditional RCTs, APTs can be designed to be evolving and perpetual.[74] New interventions can be added over time, allowing for the assessment and comparison of a changing set of therapies. Therapies that are determined to be futile are generally dropped from the platform. Interventions that are found to be efficacious may either graduate from the platform, to make room for new investigational arms, or may be retained within the platform, possibly replacing the control. The strata investigated within the platform may also change. The flexibility of the design is determined

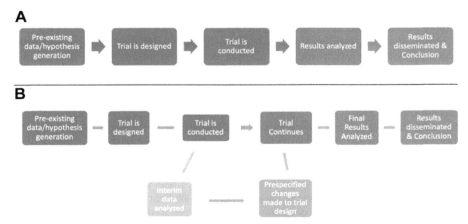

Fig. 3. Study design: randomized controlled trial versus adaptive trials. (*A*) Trial flow in a traditional RCT from the initial study design to study procedures, result analysis, and finally conclusion. (*B*) Trial flow in an adaptive trial where interim data are analyzed, while trial is ongoing, and based on interim results, prespecified changes are made to the trial design.

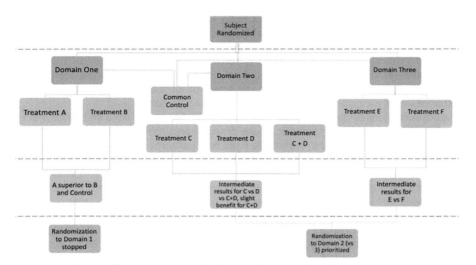

Fig. 4. Adaptive platform trial schematic. Theoretic schematic of an adaptive platform trial with 3 treatment domains (*blue boxes*) each with multiple arms (*green boxes*) and a common control. Subjects are randomized to the control arm after randomization to a domain. *Orange boxes* indicate results of interim analyses in each domain, and *purple boxes* represent changes to trial based on protocol (designed before trial initiation) and results of interim analyses.

by the master protocol and varies from platform to platform. The capability to facilitate continuous research is a core advantage of these designs. Rather than designing a trial from scratch every time a new treatment needs evaluation, platform trials provide a prebuilt infrastructure and statistical approach for assessing that intervention.[74,77]

Randomization and subject assignment can be based on subject characteristics, including phenotypes, subphenotypes or endotypes, or treatable traits. These characteristics can be used to guide randomization, preferentially assigning patients to the treatments that are expected to benefit them most. Trials even have the ability to define the characteristics at the outset of a trial or adapt them over time through an interim individualized treatment effect analysis.

Hypotheses may also be tested at the level of these strata, providing more precise characterization of which patients to treat with which intervention. To the casual reader, it may seem this is "gaming the system," but rather it is using all information available to enrich subject assignment to treatment arms—predictive enrichment.[78]

Subject assignment can also be adapted while the trial is ongoing to prioritize randomization to interventions that are showing potential benefit or an intermediate effect over those that are showing less benefit (see **Fig. 3**).[74,75] This also decreases the long-term cost of adaptive trials as fewer resources are spent on interventions that are futile or have no benefit.[69] APTs using more sophisticated subject assignment such as predictive enrichment or with multiple subject strata and/or treatment arms may also be more attractive to patients and family members and potentially improve patient safety. Depending on the design, there is a greater likelihood of allocation to an active treatment arm and/or a greater chance of assignment to better-performing interventions.[79]

The REMAP-CAP trial (randomized embedded multifactorial APT for severe community acquired pneumonia) represents a large multinational-scale APT developed to test multiple interventions for severe community-acquired pneumonia in critically ill patients.[80] REMAP-CAP was designed to study pneumonia outbreaks and incorporated a unique pandemic stratum that could be activated to respond to an emerging threat. Since the start of the coronavirus disease 2019 (COVID-19) pandemic, the trial has added domains specific to the pandemic strata including evaluation of antiviral therapies, corticosteroids, therapeutic anticoagulation, and immune modulators.[81–87] The REMAP-CAP trial, as well as other APTs,[88–94] demonstrate that these trials are feasible on a multinational, multisite scale and can lead to trials with large sample sizes and robust data.

There are some challenges in widespread use of APTs. Although these trials cost less in the long run and may provide answers in less time than traditional RCTs, the initial cost and lead time in design can be greater. APTs generally require greater research and statistical expertise to ensure study design, protocol, and adaptations are robust. Regulatory agencies are also less familiar with APTs. These challenges, primarily related to the relative unfamiliarity of the scientific community with adaptive trials, will become less important as expertise and experience with such trials grow.

The use of APTs does not necessarily mandate the use of big data or data science methodologies, but there are substantial synergies between these domains. Using electronic sniffers to identify patients and EHRs to supply clinical trial data further improves the efficiency and scalability of APTs. These techniques could also address some of the challenges associated with running APTs across multiple research institutions and countries, facilitating standardized methods for enrollment and data collection. In the other direction, APTs are well suited to testing and validating the large number of hypotheses generated by data science, including promising phenotypes or treatable traits. The "gold standard" of evidence generated by APTs will help us better understand and evaluate the results of observational data science research. Pairing these larger, more efficient clinical trials with the use of already existing information allows us to harness the power of data science and potentially provide new, large, useful quantities of data to advance the field of critical care.

SUMMARY

We collect tremendous quantities of data on critically ill patients. Leveraging these collected data to efficiently inform the design and conduct of clinical trials represents a new frontier of critical illness research. Data science may offer ways to harness the heterogeneity and complexity of critically ill subjects by more efficient identification of subjects, improved phenotyping and targeted trial group assignment for predictive enrichment, and greater use of APTs and different statistical methods. Additionally, the use of automated systems and tools embedded in the EHR may allow for faster screening and enrollment and quicker and less-error-prone data collection. The strategies discussed may provide ways to decrease cost, improve efficiency, and in some cases, provide more opportunity for patients to receive a potentially useful therapy. Some of these methods are already in use, with adaptive platform clinical trials, as well as electronic sniffers. We hope that these methods in the future will allow clinicians and researchers to help improve the care of the critically ill.

CLINICS CARE POINTS

- Traditional RCTs may be inefficient for critical care research as they test a single intervention at a time and have limited generalizability. Additionally, heterogeneity in critically ill patients can lead to diverse and contradictory responses to treatment.

- Phenotyping critical illnesses and precision medicine may allow for targeted subject enrollment and enrich the trial sample size, but better understanding of the underlying biology and pathophysiology of critical illnesses and optimal methods to create disease phenotypes is needed.
- Adaptive platform trials, such as REMAP-CAP, offer greater design flexibility and testing of multiple interventions in a single trial and have demonstrated success in critical illnesses. However, these trial designs require the use of existing large data streams and specialized research and statistical expertise to design and conduct the trial and minimize bias or error.

DISCLOSURE

The authors have nothing to disclose.

FUNDING

Dr Sevransky's has grants from the CDC foundation, the CDC, DOD, Regenron, and HHS. His insitutution also receives a stipend for his work as associate editor of Critical Care Medicine.

REFERENCES

1. Sanchez-Pinto LN, Luo Y, Churpek MM. Big data and data science in critical care. Chest 2018;154(5):1239–48.
2. Shah FA, Meyer NJ, Angus DC, et al. A research Agenda for precision medicine in sepsis and acute respiratory distress syndrome: an Official American Thoracic Society research Statement. Am J Respir Crit Care Med 2021;204(8):891–901.
3. Schneeweiss S. Learning from big health care data. N Engl J Med 2014;370(23): 2161–3.
4. Wallace DJ, Angus DC, Seymour CW, et al. Critical care bed growth in the United States. A comparison of regional and national trends. Am J Respir Crit Care Med 2015;191(4):410–6.
5. Maslove DM, Tang B, Shankar-Hari M, et al. Redefining critical illness. Nature medicine 2022;28(6):1141–8.
6. Evans L, Rhodes A, Alhazzani W, et al. Surviving sepsis campaign: international guidelines for management of sepsis and septic shock. Critical care medicine 2021;49(11):e1063–143.
7. Moss M, Huang DT, Brower RG, et al. Early neuromuscular blockade in the acute respiratory distress syndrome. N Engl J Med 2019;380(21):1997–2008.
8. Rowan KM, Angus DC, Bailey M, et al. Early, goal-directed therapy for septic shock - a patient-level meta-analysis. N Engl J Med 2017;376(23):2223–34.
9. Ospina-Tascón GA, Büchele GL, Vincent JL. Multicenter, randomized, controlled trials evaluating mortality in intensive care: doomed to fail? Crit Care Med 2008; 36(4):1311–22.
10. Rivers E, Nguyen B, Havstad S, et al. Early goal-directed therapy in the treatment of severe sepsis and septic shock. N Engl J Med 2001;345(19):1368–77.
11. Annane D, Timsit JF, Megarbane B, et al. Recombinant human activated protein C for adults with septic shock: a randomized controlled trial. Am J Respir Crit Care Med 2013;187(10):1091–7.
12. Bernard GR, Vincent JL, Laterre PF, et al. Efficacy and safety of recombinant human activated protein C for severe sepsis. N Engl J Med 2001;344(10):699–709.

13. Iwashyna TJ, Burke JF, Sussman JB, et al. Implications of heterogeneity of treatment effect for reporting and analysis of randomized trials in critical care. Am J Respir Crit Care Med 2015;192(9):1045–51.

14. Harhay MO, Wagner J, Ratcliffe SJ, et al. Outcomes and statistical power in adult critical care randomized trials. Am J Respir Crit Care Med 2014;189(12):1469–78.

15. Veldhoen RA, Howes D, Maslove DM. Is mortality a useful primary end point for critical care trials? Chest 2020;158(1):206–11.

16. Abrams D, Montesi SB, Moore SKL, et al. Powering bias and clinically important treatment effects in randomized trials of critical illness. Crit Care Med 2020; 48(12):1710–9.

17. Granholm A, Alhazzani W, Derde LPG, et al. Randomised clinical trials in critical care: past, present and future. Intensive Care Med 2022;48(2):164–78.

18. Altman DG, Bland JM. Absence of evidence is not evidence of absence. BMJ (Clinical research ed) 1995;311(7003):485.

19. Schandelmaier S, von Elm E, You JJ, et al. Premature discontinuation of randomized trials in critical and emergency care: a retrospective cohort study. Crit Care Med 2016;44(1):130–7.

20. Sole ML, Middleton A, Deaton L, et al. Enrollment challenges in critical care Nursing research. Am J Crit Care 2017;26(5):395–400.

21. Haendel MA, Chute CG, Robinson PN. Classification, ontology, and precision medicine. N Engl J Med 2018;379(15):1452–62.

22. Tsimberidou AM, Fountzilas E, Nikanjam M, et al. Review of precision cancer medicine: Evolution of the treatment paradigm. Cancer Treat Rev 2020;86: 102019.

23. Maslove DM, Lamontagne F, Marshall JC, et al. A path to precision in the ICU. Crit Care 2017;21(1):79.

24. Rhodes A, Evans LE, Alhazzani W, et al. Surviving sepsis campaign: international guidelines for management of sepsis and septic shock: 2016. Crit Care Med 2017;45(3):486–552.

25. Bellani G, Laffey JG, Pham T, et al. Epidemiology, Patterns of care, and mortality for patients with acute respiratory distress syndrome in intensive care Units in 50 countries. JAMA 2016;315(8):788–800.

26. Singer M. Sepsis: personalization v protocolization? Crit Care 2019;23(Suppl 1):127.

27. Marshall JC. Why have clinical trials in sepsis failed? Trends Mol Med 2014;20(4): 195–203.

28. Seymour CW, Gomez H, Chang CH, et al. Precision medicine for all? Challenges and opportunities for a precision medicine approach to critical illness. Crit Care 2017;21(1):257.

29. Peukert K, Fox M, Schulz S, et al. Inhibition of caspase-1 with tetracycline ameliorates acute lung injury. Am J Respir Crit Care Med 2021;204(1):53–63.

30. McNicholas BA, Rooney GM, Laffey JG. Lessons to learn from epidemiologic studies in ARDS. Curr Opin Crit Care 2018;24(1):41–8.

31. Khan YA, Fan E, Ferguson ND. Precision medicine and heterogeneity of treatment effect in therapies for ARDS. Chest 2021;160(5):1729–38.

32. Li H, Markal A, Balch JA, et al. Methods for phenotyping adult patients in sepsis and septic shock: a scoping review. Crit Care Explor 2022;4(4):e0672.

33. Loftus TJ, Shickel B, Balch JA, et al. Phenotype clustering in health care: a narrative review for clinicians. Front Artif Intell 2022;5:842306.

34. Seymour CW, Kennedy JN, Wang S, et al. Derivation, validation, and potential treatment implications of novel clinical phenotypes for sepsis. JAMA 2019; 321(20):2003–17.

35. Bhavani SV, Carey KA, Gilbert ER, et al. Identifying novel sepsis subphenotypes using temperature trajectories. Am J Respir Crit Care Med 2019;200(3):327–35.

36. Bhavani SV, Wolfe KS, Hrusch CL, et al. Temperature trajectory subphenotypes correlate with immune responses in patients with sepsis. Crit Care Med 2020; 48(11):1645–53.

37. Calfee CS, Delucchi K, Parsons PE, et al. Subphenotypes in acute respiratory distress syndrome: latent class analysis of data from two randomised controlled trials. The Lancet Respiratory medicine 2014;2(8):611–20.

38. Shankar-Hari M, Summers C, Baillie K. In Pursuit of precision medicine in the critically ill. Annual Update in Intensive Care and Emergency Medicine 2018;649–58.

39. Guyatt G, Sackett D, Taylor DW, et al. Determining optimal therapy–randomized trials in individual patients. N Engl J Med 1986;314(14):889–92.

40. Russell CD, Baillie JK. Treatable traits and therapeutic targets: goals for systems biology in infectious disease. Curr Opin Syst Biol 2017;2:140–6.

41. Wong HR, Atkinson SJ, Cvijanovich NZ, et al. Combining prognostic and predictive enrichment strategies to identify Children with septic shock responsive to corticosteroids. Crit Care Med 2016;44(10):e1000–3.

42. Park JW, Liu MC, Yee D, et al. Adaptive randomization of Neratinib in early breast cancer. N Engl J Med 2016;375(1):11–22.

43. Bos LDJ, Laffey JG, Ware LB, et al. Towards a biological definition of ARDS: are treatable traits the solution? Intensive care medicine experimental 2022;10(1):8.

44. Koenig HC, Finkel BB, Khalsa SS, et al. Performance of an automated electronic acute lung injury screening system in intensive care unit patients. Crit Care Med 2011;39(1):98–104.

45. Epic. epic launches life sciences program, unifying clinical research with care delivery. Cision US Inc. 2022, Available at: https://www.prnewswire.com/news-releases/epic-launches-life-sciences-program-unifying-clinical-research-with-care-delivery-301624287.html. Accessed December 6, 2022.

46. Herasevich V, Pieper MS, Pulido J, et al. Enrollment into a time sensitive clinical study in the critical care setting: results from computerized septic shock sniffer implementation. J Am Med Inform Assoc 2011;18(5):639–44.

47. Herasevich V, Yilmaz M, Khan H, et al. Validation of an electronic surveillance system for acute lung injury. Intensive Care Med 2009;35(6):1018–23.

48. Kashani K, Herasevich V. Sniffing out acute kidney injury in the ICU: do we have the tools? Curr Opin Crit Care 2013;19(6):531–6.

49. Fiore LD, Lavori PW. Integrating randomized comparative effectiveness research with patient care. N Engl J Med 2016;374(22):2152–8.

50. Wayne MT, Valley TS, Cooke CR, et al. Electronic "sniffer" systems to identify the acute respiratory distress syndrome. Annals of the American Thoracic Society 2019;16(4):488–95.

51. OHDSI, The book of OHDSI: observational health data sciences and Informatics, 2019, OHDSI. Available at: http:book.ohdsi.org. Accessed February 8, 2023.

52. Tarabichi Y, Frees A, Honeywell S, et al. The cosmos collaborative: a vendor-facilitated electronic health record data aggregation platform. ACI Open 2021; 5(1):e36–46.

53. Services CfMaM. Policies and technology for interoperability and burden reduction. Available at: https://www.cms.gov/Regulations-and-Guidance/Guidance/

Interoperability/index#CMS-Interoperability-and-Patient-Access-Final-Rule. Accessed November 20, 2022.

54. Griffin AC, He L, Sunjaya AP, et al. Clinical, technical, and implementation characteristics of real-world health applications using FHIR. JAMIA Open 2022;5(4). https://doi.org/10.1093/jamiaopen/ooac077.

55. Office of the Director National Institutes of Health. Fast healthcare interoperability resources (FHIR®) standard. Available at: https://grants.nih.gov/grants/guide/notice-files/NOT-OD-19-122.html. Accessed November 20, 2022.

56. Office of the Director National Institutes of Health. Accelerating clinical care and research through the Use of the United States core data for interoperability (USCDI). Available at: https://grants.nih.gov/grants/guide/notice-files/NOT-OD-20-146.html. Accessed November 20, 2022.

57. Duda SN, Kennedy N, Conway D, et al. HL7 FHIR-based tools and initiatives to support clinical research: a scoping review. J Am Med Inf Assoc 2022;29(9): 1642–53.

58. Friedman LMFC, DeMets DL, Reboussin DM, et al. Fundamentals of clinical trials. 5th edition. Cham, Switzerland: Springer International Publishing; 2015.

59. Viceconti M, Cobelli C, Haddad T, et al. In silico assessment of biomedical products: the conundrum of rare but not so rare events in two case studies. Proc Inst Mech Eng H 2017;231(5):455–66.

60. Chase JG, Preiser JC, Dickson JL, et al. Next-generation, personalised, model-based critical care medicine: a state-of-the art review of in silico virtual patient models, methods, and cohorts, and how to validation them. Biomed Eng Online 2018;17(1):24.

61. Chase JG, Suhaimi F, Penning S, et al. Validation of a model-based virtual trials method for tight glycemic control in intensive care. Biomed Eng Online 2010; 9:84.

62. Lin J, Razak NN, Pretty CG, et al. A physiological Intensive Control Insulin-Nutrition-Glucose (ICING) model validated in critically ill patients. Comput Methods Programs Biomed 2011;102(2):192–205.

63. Chase JG, Shaw GM, Lotz T, et al. Model-based insulin and nutrition administration for tight glycaemic control in critical care. Curr Drug Deliv 2007;4(4):283–96.

64. Brown D, Namas RA, Almahmoud K, et al. Trauma in silico: individual-specific mathematical models and virtual clinical populations. Sci Transl Med 2015; 7(285):285ra61.

65. Chiew YS, Chase JG, Shaw GM, et al. Model-based PEEP optimisation in mechanical ventilation. Biomed Eng Online 2011;10:111.

66. Sundaresan A, Chase JG, Shaw GM, et al. Model-based optimal PEEP in mechanically ventilated ARDS patients in the intensive care unit. Biomed Eng Online 2011;10:64.

67. Batta A, Kalra BS, Khirasaria R. Trends in FDA drug approvals over last 2 decades: an observational study. J Fam Med Prim Care 2020;9(1):105–14.

68. US Food & Drug Administration. Adaptive Designs for Medical Device Clinical Studies. Guidance for Industry and Food and Drug Administration Staff. 2018. Available at: www.fda.gov. Accessed February 10, 2023.

69. Park JJH, Sharif B, Harari O, et al. Economic evaluation of cost and time required for a platform trial vs Conventional trials. JAMA Netw Open 2022;5(7):e2221140.

70. Berry SM, Connor JT, Lewis RJ. The platform trial: an efficient strategy for evaluating multiple treatments. JAMA 2015;313(16):1619–20.

71. Frieden TR. Evidence for health Decision making — beyond randomized, controlled trials. N Engl J Med 2017;377(5):465–75.

72. Pallmann P, Bedding AW, Choodari-Oskooei B, et al. Adaptive designs in clinical trials: why use them, and how to run and report them. BMC Med 2018;16(1):29.
73. Woodcock J, LaVange LM. Master protocols to study multiple therapies, multiple diseases, or both. N Engl J Med 2017;377(1):62–70.
74. Adaptive platform trials: definition, design, conduct and reporting considerations. Nat Rev Drug Discov 2019;18(10):797–807.
75. Burnett T, Mozgunov P, Pallmann P, et al. Adding flexibility to clinical trial designs: an example-based guide to the practical use of adaptive designs. BMC Med 2020;18(1):352.
76. Saville BR, Berry SM. Efficiencies of platform clinical trials: a vision of the future. Clin Trials 2016;13(3):358–66.
77. Saville B, Berry S. Platform trials. Platform trial Designs in drug development. 1st edition. New York, NY: Chapman and Hall/CRC; 2018.
78. Simon R. Clinical trial designs for evaluating the medical utility of prognostic and predictive biomarkers in oncology. Per Med 2010;7(1):33–47.
79. Meurer WJ, Lewis RJ, Berry DA. Adaptive clinical trials: a partial remedy for the therapeutic misconception? JAMA 2012;307(22):2377–8.
80. Angus DC, Berry S, Lewis RJ, et al. The REMAP-CAP (randomized embedded multifactorial adaptive platform for community-acquired pneumonia) study. Rationale and design. Annals of the American Thoracic Society 2020;17(7):879–91.
81. Implementation of the randomized embedded multifactorial adaptive platform for COVID-19 (REMAP-COVID) trial in a US health system-lessons learned and recommendations. Trials 2021;22(1):100.
82. Angus DC, Derde L, Al-Beidh F, et al. Effect of hydrocortisone on mortality and organ support in patients with severe COVID-19: the REMAP-CAP COVID-19 corticosteroid domain randomized clinical trial. JAMA 2020;324(13):1317–29.
83. Arabi YM, Gordon AC, Derde LPG, et al. Lopinavir-ritonavir and hydroxychloroquine for critically ill patients with COVID-19: REMAP-CAP randomized controlled trial. Intensive Care Med 2021;47(8):867–86.
84. Bradbury CA, Lawler PR, Stanworth SJ, et al. Effect of Antiplatelet therapy on survival and Organ support-Free Days in critically ill patients with COVID-19: a randomized clinical trial. JAMA 2022;327(13):1247–59.
85. Estcourt LJ, Turgeon AF, McQuilten ZK, et al. Effect of Convalescent Plasma on Organ support-Free Days in critically ill patients with COVID-19: a randomized clinical trial. JAMA 2021;326(17):1690–702.
86. Goligher EC, Bradbury CA, McVerry BJ, et al. Therapeutic anticoagulation with heparin in critically ill patients with covid-19. N Engl J Med 2021;385(9):777–89.
87. Gordon AC, Mouncey PR, Al-Beidh F, et al. Interleukin-6 receptor antagonists in critically ill patients with covid-19. N Engl J Med 2021;384(16):1491–502.
88. Clinical trial design during and beyond the pandemic: the I-SPY COVID trial. Nature medicine 2022;28(1):9–11.
89. PANORAMIC platform adaptaive trial of novel antivirals for early treatment of covid-19 in the community. University of Oxford. Available at: https://www.panoramictrial.org/. Accessed November 9, 2022.
90. Casirivimab and imdevimab in patients admitted to hospital with COVID-19 (RECOVERY): a randomised, controlled, open-label, platform trial. Lancet (London, England) 2022;399(10325):665–76.
91. Alexander BM, Ba S, Berger MS, et al. Adaptive global innovative learning environment for glioblastoma: GBM AGILE. Clin Cancer Res 2018;24(4):737–43.

92. Paganoni S, Berry JD, Quintana M, et al. Adaptive platform trials to transform amyotrophic lateral sclerosis therapy development. Ann Neurol 2022;91(2): 165–75. https://doi.org/10.1002/ana.26285.
93. Picozzi VJ, Duliege A-M, Maitra A, et al. Abstract PO-050: precision Promise (PrP): an adaptive, multi-arm registration trial in metastatic pancreatic ductal adenocarcinoma (PDAC). Cancer Res 2021;81(22_Supplement). PO-050-PO-050.
94. Reis G, Dos Santos Moreira-Silva EA, Silva DCM, et al. Effect of early treatment with fluvoxamine on risk of emergency care and hospitalisation among patients with COVID-19: the TOGETHER randomised, platform clinical trial. Lancet Glob Health 2022;10(1):e42–51.

The Challenges of Integrating Data Science into Critical Care Medicine

Making the Improbable Possible: Generalizing Models Designed for a Syndrome-Based, Heterogeneous Patient Landscape

Joshua Pei Le, BS[a], Supreeth Prajwal Shashikumar, PhD[b,1],
Atul Malhotra, MD[c,1], Shamim Nemati, PhD[b,1,2],
Gabriel Wardi, MD, MPH[c,d,*,2]

KEYWORDS

- Data science • Data missingness • Machine learning • Syndrome • Sepsis
- Critical care

KEY POINTS

- Barriers to the use of machine learning in critically ill patients include challenges with recognition of syndromic conditions, data missingness, and the underlying heterogeneity of health care systems which may limit the generalizability of machine-learning algorithms.
- Recent advances in machine-learning applications, such as transfer learning and conformal prediction, can overcome barriers to improve generalizability across various institutions.
- Future studies are required to confirm the benefit of these strategies in both experimental and routine clinical care.

INTRODUCTION

Although machine learning (ML)-based clinical decision support has seen some successful implementations in radiology[1,2] and ophthalmology,[3,4] its overall presence in health care is modest when compared with its potential. This underutilization remains particularly true in the intensive care unit (ICU). A major hurdle to the widespread deployment of ML models has been their inconsistent performance as a result of several

[a] School of Medicine, University of Limerick, Castletroy, Co, Limerick V94 T9PX, Ireland;
[b] Division of Biomedical Informatics, University of California San Diego, San Diego, CA, USA;
[c] Division of Pulmonary, Critical Care and Sleep Medicine, University of California San Diego, San Diego, CA, USA; [d] Department of Emergency Medicine, University of California San Diego, 200 W Arbor Drive, San Diego, CA 92103, USA
[1] Present address: 9500 Gilman Dr, La Jolla, CA 92093, USA.
[2] Authors equally contributed.
* Corresponding author.
E-mail address: gwardi@health.ucsd.edu

Crit Care Clin 39 (2023) 751–768
https://doi.org/10.1016/j.ccc.2023.02.003
0749-0704/23/© 2023 Elsevier Inc. All rights reserved.

factors, including hospital-dependent operating procedures, patient demographics, and missing data.[5–7] These factors all contribute to data heterogeneity, so an ML prediction model (herein termed "ML model" or "model") trained on one dataset may exhibit degradation in performance when deployed on another,[8] resulting in inadequate *generalizability*. However, as noted by Futoma and colleagues, the colloquial use of the term generalizability in clinical ML literature is broad and not well-defined.[9] For clinical applications of ML models, a published hierarchy[10] describes it as a set of rules that may apply to internal, temporal, and external applications relative to the original training dataset. An internal application refers to using an ML model to the same patient cohort on which it was trained (eg, the same dataset at the same hospital). A temporal application denotes using this model at the same location but across a different time period. An external application refers to using this model at a separate location during any time period. The ideal model will be able to demonstrate similar levels of performance under any application, notably external ones.[11–14] This makes sense—it is essential to verify that a model for clinical use can provide similar results for any group of patients, especially those it was not explicitly trained on.[9] Yet due to the current nature of ML and statistics, external generalizability approaches a limit as the applicable population grows because of increasing variation in workflow practices, point-of-care measurement devices, and population characteristics. As such, the current literature suggests that it is infeasible to develop a single universal prediction model. Therefore, our focus should shift toward more clearly defining the "conditions for use" of a model while improving its external generalizability *within* the intended use population. These "conditions for use" are ideally broad enough so that a prediction model can be impactful for as many patients as possible while minding the aforementioned limitations.

Patient-focused clinical predictive modeling can be classified as diagnostic versus prognostic.[15] Diagnostic tasks rely on a patient's "true state," which are typically defined by proxy criteria and construct via laboratory values, imaging, and physical symptoms, among others, to predict a clinical development (eg, sepsis). Prognostic tasks rely on the ordered tests and their results to quantify the probability of certain patient-centered outcomes (such as in-hospital mortality).[16] Both tasks have clinical utility, albeit at varying levels. Early diagnostic tasks may be able to assist clinicians administer timely interventions for a developing condition (eg, early and appropriate antibiotics for sepsis). Within the same context, prognostic tasks may help administrators optimize resource allocation for patients who are most likely to decompensate or are at risk for other adverse outcomes, including mortality.[15,17–19] In either case, existing studies investigate such tasks in critical care environments because the nature of its routine patient monitoring makes for data-rich electronic health records (EHRs) from which models can learn and make predictions.

In this review article, the authors investigate the current challenges of integrating ML models into critical care, using studies centered on early sepsis prediction as examples. The authors (1) explore clinical challenges with syndrome-based conditions, which are commonly diagnosed in the ICU; (2) clarify data science terminology surrounding these studies; (3) examine major barriers to generalizability; and (4) illustrate how current-day ML models address such obstacles via different methods of learning. The authors conclude with a discussion on areas for future research.

CHALLENGES WITH SYNDROMES

A syndrome can be defined as a recognizable complex of findings and symptoms that indicate a specific condition with a poorly understood cause.[20] A disease refers to a condition in which a causative agent or process results in a readily identifiable clinical and biological manifestation. Yet, with increased research and study, a condition that was formerly best described as a syndrome can be referred to as a disease. Indeed, Kawasaki *disease* was initially known as mucocutaneous lymph node *syndrome* because the underlying pathophysiology was uncertain and clinical manifestations were varied.[21] An increased understanding of the disease process later described clearly identifiable diagnostic features and treatment responses.

Although this distinction between a disease and syndrome is easily understood by physicians, syndromic conditions can prove challenging for ML models to identify and predict. This is particularly true in the ICU because a multitude of prevalent syndromes (ie, sepsis and the acute respiratory distress syndrome) share similar physiologic and biological derangements. For example, a patient with decompensated heart failure can show vital signs and laboratory findings that mimic septic shock. In addition, critically ill patients are frequently comorbid for these syndromes. Clinicians use contextual clues, historical components, and physical examination findings to help differentiate between possibilities, but contemporary ML models struggle because historical context and examination findings are oftentimes not readily available[14] for such rapidly evolving patients. Complicating this further are multiple definitions for any given syndrome in sepsis, the condition can either be defined by Sepsis-3,[22] Severe Sepsis and Septic Shock Management Bundle (SEP-1),[23] or the Center for Disease Control and Prevention (CDC)[24,25] criteria.

CLARIFYING TERMS

Before we begin our review on generalizability and related ML studies, it is necessary to clarify terms and concepts that are commonly used in data science and relevant to its application in critically ill patients. Three recently published ML models, Artificial Intelligence Sepsis Expert (AISE),[11,12] Weight Uncertainty Propagation and Episodic Representation Replay (WUPERR),[13] and COnformal Multidimensional Prediction Of SEpsis Risk (COMPOSER),[14] and their respective studies are used as several examples throughout this article. **Table 1** summarizes definitions and examples of relevant vernacular.

Missingness describes the presence of missing data and how it is handled, reported. This can negatively impact the predictive accuracy of a model and decrease its clinical utility.[8] However, not all missing data are created equally. There exist three primary classifications of missing data[26]: Missing Completely At Random (MCAR), Missing At Random (MAR), and Missing Not At Random (MNAR). MCAR refers to randomly missing data that does not have any distinguishable pattern to it.[27–29] MAR refers to randomly missing data that may be associated with an underlying pattern.[27,30,31] For instance, in a hypothetical case where missing Glasgow Coma Scores (GCS) among trauma patients were more likely to be observed for older patients,[32] the mechanism is MAR. MNAR refers to the likelihood of a missing value to seem as a function of the value itself[27]—following the same hypothetical, the mechanism is MNAR if a missing GCS is known to be associated with mild brain trauma.[32] For prediction models, the MNAR mechanism is typically assumed because they use longitudinal data collection, where patterns of missingness are more likely to present (eg, healthy patients routinely have fewer tests as they are not indicated). The differences in how data go missing are key to understanding their handling,[27,31] which are more deeply explored in the section Approaches to Data Missingness.

At its core, ML consists of a set of parameters that are initialized with random weights. Training then takes place, where the model is exposed to a development cohort (eg, retrospective clinical data at Hospital A). This induces key changes in

Table 1
Definitions and examples of common terms used in data science

Term	Definition	Example
Development cohort	The dataset on which an ML model was trained	AISE[11,12] was trained on data from the Emory Healthcare System, also known as the development cohort.
Validation cohort	The dataset on which an ML model must perform a task for the first time	AISE[11,12] was validated on data from the MIMIC-III cohort collected from the Beth Israel Deaconess Medical Center in Boston, also known as the validation cohort.
Generalizability	The extent to which an ML model can achieve similar performance on external validation tasks vs internal validation tasks	AISE,[11,12] WUPERR,[13] and COMPOSER[14] demonstrated comparable performance at their respective validation hospitals, on par with their performance at their respective development hospitals.
Dimension	A characteristic of data and/or a dataset, relating to the number of variables included	EHR data are multidimensional because it includes heart rate, blood pressure, temperature, laboratory values, and so forth.
Missingness	The presence of missing clinical variables and how this is handled/reported	During Patient A's 10-d ICU stay, he/she may not have regular blood pressure measurements recorded every 4 h due to movements for scans, tests, and so forth.
Omission	A method of handling missingness where patients and/or characteristics with missing data are deleted from the dataset	As Patient A is missing blood pressure data, he/she is excluded from analysis of the dataset, which uses blood pressure.
Imputation	A method of handling missingness that determines a single or multiple value(s) to replace all missing values for a specific variable	Patient A's missing blood pressure measurements are estimated by averaging blood pressure values of other patients in the ICU taken at the same time (single imputation).

They are summarized here to provide clarity to the following sections.

the weights of different rules. The idea is to give more bearing on the final output to rules that are mathematically determined to be "more important." Prediction error (or the difference between the predicted outcome and the true patient outcome) will tell the model when it produces a correct or incorrect output, prompting changes to these rule weights, a process known as supervised learning.[33] As it is exposed to a validation cohort (eg, retrospective clinical data at Hospital B), performance usually degrades because differences in the underlying data often necessitates different weights being given to different rules; this is the basis of the barriers to generalizability.[5]

ONE SIZE DOES NOT FIT ALL: THE GENERALIZABILITY PROBLEM

Generalizability was previously described as the ability for an ML model to perform similarly well on both development and validation cohorts within a well-defined intended use population. It would ideally maintain this high level of performance as it is applied to additional institutions that fit its "conditions for use." However, in order to do so, we must acknowledge the challenges it faces at different locales. These include explicit differences between institutions and missing clinical data. The following sections detail these problems in addition to potential methods that ML models might use to overcome them.

Heterogeneity in Health Care

Despite all its regulations, health care remains an area of great heterogeneity at various levels. Shashikumar and colleagues describe these levels in a recent *Behind the Paper*[5] on Nature Portfolio Health Community, starting with EHRs: different EHR vendors currently encode information in non-standardized formats which reduce their interoperability. The data are recorded using clinical instruments from different vendors which often use proprietary data processing methods with varying necessity for clinician verification. Local guidelines vary in their frequency for specific clinical measurements to be taken, but this should not be confused with the predictive value that *missing data itself* can offer (see Approaches to Data Missingness). For diagnostic records, differences in clinical inclusion and exclusion criteria between institutions can introduce label noise and give way to label bias.[34] Shifting criteria also lay the foundation for the difficulties in managing syndrome-based conditions, which were discussed in Challenges with syndromes. Temporal changes in data might occur as care and monitoring processes transform, including the disruption of existing clinical workflows resulting from implementing ML models. Taken together, these "systemic factors" all increase the heterogeneity of a clinical dataset which can confound predictive accuracy of a model not trained to recognize and correct for them (see Machine learning-based solutions, for an introduction to such methods). Regular updates to models are necessary as institutions evolve in these respects.

Differences in patient demographics between institutions can further add to the previously described data heterogeneity. However, this aspect is more difficult to handle due to the simultaneous potential for demographics to confound and improve impact predictive accuracy. Consider the following example, recent facial recognition[35] and hiring and recruitment[36] models were found to unintentionally perpetuate discriminatory harm as a result from overrepresentation of specific racial and ethnic groups during development and validation. Although the ML models themselves were independent of any explicit racial or ethnic bias, a biased data distribution contributed to the skewed outcomes[37]; this is one of many identified mechanisms behind "unfair" models.[34] In health care, large datasets may not be representative of traditionally underrepresented minorities,[38] which may similarly lead to bias. However, a demographic-specific biological susceptibility/response might also contribute to unequal distributions of patients,[39,40] and this could help improve prediction. Recent data evaluating clinical use of ML models suggest that a significant number of them did not have any evaluation of racial bias,[41] as there is currently no standardized process to do so. Of the exceptions, studies designed to predict mortality or sepsis in critically ill patients were shown to be free of any bias.[42] Further investigation into this field is therefore indicated, and careful attention must be given to precisely delineate between the two effects and their degrees of impact on patient data.

Approaches to Data Missingness

A common theme to the obstacles of generalizability thus far is data heterogeneity.[8] Missingness similarly contributes another dimension to the data, increasing its heterogeneity. Several methods have been proposed and implemented in the clinical prediction models to handle this challenge, including omission, imputation, and physiology-focused solutions. These are applied depending on the type of missingness that is present in each problem. It should also be noted that existing studies on the clinical uses of ML do not agree on a universal practice, even for the same missingness mechanism. Our goal for this section is to therefore present the prominent techniques for handling missingness to provide clarity to the existing literature.

Of the methods that can handle missing data, omission is the simplest and least computationally demanding, an important consideration for processing large health care datasets.[43] The most reported process of omission for studies of prediction models that use ML is complete case analysis (CCA).[6] As its name suggests, CCA only includes patient cases that are not missing any data on the variables of interest.[44,45] However, its use is limited to datasets with MCAR data, as applying CCA to MAR or MNAR studies can introduce bias from nonrandom deletion of patients.[46–48] Consider a dataset with MAR data, younger diabetic patients have a higher rate of missing self-reported blood sugar data versus older diabetic patients as a result from only beginning the recording regimen. If CCA is applied here, we will disproportionately delete data from younger patients, so an ML model trained on this data will be biased toward making predictions for older diabetic patients. Nevertheless, even if CCA is correctly used for MCAR data, it still suffers from decreasing statistical power,[49] a flaw inherent to data omission.

More complex than methods of omission are those of imputation. Unlike omission, imputation requires added computation to produce more complete datasets, typically with less bias.[50] Three broad subtypes of imputation can achieve this with varying degrees of success: simple, hot deck, and multiple imputation.[45] Simple imputation replaces all missing values of a particular parameter with a single value computed from the present data. Hot deck imputation replaces a patient's missing value with one computed from a subset of patients with similar characteristics. This is repeated for each patient with missing data. Multiple imputation involves multiple rounds of simple imputation with minor changes; for a missing patient value, one is computed from a *random subset* of the existing dataset. Additional values are then computed from different random subsets, resulting in multiple possible replacement values. An aggregate of these values is taken (eg, mean), which ultimately replaces the missing one. Although imputation usually results in decreased bias of the dataset when compared with methods of omission on MAR or MNAR data, simple imputation may increase bias.[27] Specifically, for a large subset of missing data, imputation with a single value can artificially decrease the variability of the dataset.

Models trained on such data may subsequently have decreased generalizability to patient data from external cohorts. Hot deck and multiple imputations do not share this immediate weakness and generally result in more balanced datasets. Yet unlike simple imputation, they are more computationally expensive to perform.

Simple, hot deck, and multiple imputation methods provide a collective foundation for increasingly sophisticated variations of imputation. These should be thoughtfully used for predictive tasks because careless estimation of missing values can introduce artifacts that impact model accuracy. Specific factors that influence the type of imputation method used include study objectives, importance of missing data to these objectives, the amount of missing data, and the learning method used in an ML model.[51] As such, **Table 2** summarizes major studies of ML use in clinical contexts and their imputation and learning methods.

We have thus far discussed statistical methods of handling classic mechanisms of missingness. Although these are useful for completing datasets with minimal bias,[44] predictive models may actually find additional physiologic value in the missing data itself, a process known as the missing indicator method (MIM).[55,56] A critical distinction must be made here, as omission and imputation methods are advantageous at completing datasets with minimal bias, they optimize for parameter estimation.[57] Alternatively, MIM may be more suitable for clinical prediction because it encompasses implicit factors that may be relevant to patient outcomes.[58,59] To clarify this concept, consider a dataset where all patients had a white blood count (WBC) ordered but at different times (4 AM and 4 PM). Agniel and colleagues demonstrated that patients with a normal 4 AM WBC were associated with a greater mortality rate than those with an abnormally high or low 4 PM WBC. Here, missingness of the 4 AM WBC is associated with an improved patient outcome, which is likely due to the fact that higher acuity patients require closer monitoring throughout the day and night.[16] As this example demonstrates, the *type* of missing data should be factored into its missingness pattern because the frequency of clinical and laboratory measurements are dictated by different guidelines and indications—not all missing data are of equal importance. Importantly, caution should be used with MIM approaches as this relies heavily on local practices and behaviors and this may lead to poor generalizability. Although MIM might introduce bias in estimation of causal relationships,[60] this can effectively improve predictive performance, a phenomenon termed "Stein's Paradox."[7,61]

When it comes to missingness, the prediction models benefit from statistical methods and MIM. MIM can provide additional insight into the state of the patient. However, it may decrease model generalizability because it strongly assumes that both the validation and development cohorts exhibit the same missingness mechanism. This is likely not the case, as missingness can be highly dependent on context. Over-reliance on MIM also limits the utility of a model as it considers information encoded in ordering clinical tests; they are consequently geared toward quantifying physician thinking instead of suggesting previously unconsidered diagnoses.[15] On the other hand, causal information in predictive models permits counterfactual prediction, a crucial component of models that provide the basis of a clinical decision.[62] How a prediction model handles missingness accordingly depends on its purpose. A focus on generalizability and counterfactual prediction should prioritize statistical methods (ie, omission/imputation), and attention to a specific environment and risk assessment should prioritize MIM.[63,64] Being that each method has its own use case, many studied models use a combination of the two rather than complete reliance on either. Still, recent reviews of ML models have frequently demonstrated an insufficient or ignored method of handling missing data.[65–70]

Table 2
Major studies of clinical applications of machine learning, method of imputation for handling missingness and learning method used

Study	Missingness Method Used	Learning Method Used
Development and validation of an ICU mortality prediction model (Davoodi et al, 2018)[52]	Gaussian Imputation by Chained Equation	Deep rule-based fuzzy model
Development and validation of an in-hospital mortality prediction model for AKI (Lin et al, 2019)[53]	Mean Imputation	Random forest
Derivation and validation of novel sepsis phenotypes (Seymour et al, 2019)[54]	Multiple Imputation with Chained Equations	Latent class analysis
Development and validation of a volume responsiveness prediction model in oliguric AKI (Zhang et al, 2019)[97]	Multivariate Imputation by Chained Equation	XGBoost
Sepsis predictive model designed to identify instances of ML prediction uncertainty (Shashikumar, et al 2021)[14]	Mean Imputation and Sample-and-Hold with a weighted input layer to learn the "hold" duration	Conformal prediction

Abbreviation: AKI, acute kidney injury.

MACHINE LEARNING-BASED SOLUTIONS

There exist various ML methods which may improve generalizability of predictive models for commonly encountered syndromic conditions in the ICU. They factor in the systemic differences between institutions described in Heterogeneity in Health Care. We focus on three approaches which critical care physicians may encounter when evaluating an ML model: transfer learning, continual learning, and conformal prediction. Each of these approaches has distinct methodologies and benefits which can yield improved performance under various situations.

Transfer Learning

Transfer learning is a technique in ML which has seen select use in health care. The current applications have been largely limited to oncology[71] and medical imaging,[72] with only recent applications into critical care. Conceptually, understanding transfer learning can be illustrated as follows: a prediction model (eg, to predict delayed septic shock) is developed and validated at a single institution. Although it can immediately be applied to a second institution, subtle differences between the locales (see Heterogeneity in Health Care) often dictate that the ML model's performance will be inferior to that of the original development institution. The initial development and validation of the ML model on a larger dataset may alleviate this drop in predictive ability, but this is not always possible. Transfer learning offers a solution to these subtle differences by using a small and representative dataset from the new location to optimize model parameters for it[73] (**Fig. 1**). Importantly, this bypasses the significant cost and data required for development and validation of a novel ML model per

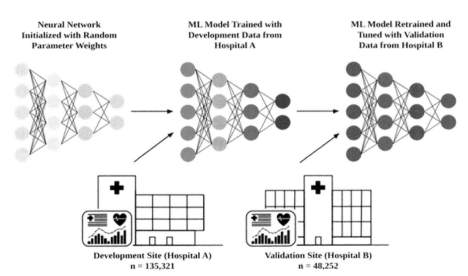

Neural Network Initialized with Random Parameter Weights

ML Model Trained with Development Data from Hospital A

ML Model Retrained and Tuned with Validation Data from Hospital B

Development Site (Hospital A)
n = 135,321

Validation Site (Hospital B)
n = 48,252

Fig. 1. Example of applying transfer learning to a delayed septic shock prediction model. The initial ML model was fine-tuned using data at a second site. The use of transfer learning significantly increased test characteristics (AUCroc) of the delayed septic shock model at the validation site. AUCroc, area under the curve of the receiver operating characteristic curve. (*From* Wardi, G. et al Predicting Progression to Septic Shock in the Emergency Department Using an Externally Generalizable Machine-Learning Algorithm. Ann. Emerg. Med. 77, 395–406 (2021); with permission.)

distinct institution to achieve similar performance. The utilization of a smaller dataset for retraining and fine-tuning of the original model is more computationally efficient and allows smaller hospitals to use such tools. However, being that the model must undergo retraining at each unique location, regulatory concerns arise as novel variants of the original model accumulate on a large scale. Nevertheless, examples of transfer learning applications in critical care include (1) fine-tuning a tracheal intubation prediction model for patients with COVID-19 pneumonia,[74] (2) adapting a delayed septic shock prediction model for use at various external institutions,[11] (3) predicting mortality in patients with end-stage renal disease,[75] (4) predicting acute kidney injury,[76] and (5) predicting acute respiratory distress syndrome on radiographs.[77] Test characteristics in these scenarios were significantly improved with the use of transfer learning.

Continual Learning

Continual learning (also referred to as lifelong learning, incremental learning, or sequential learning) describes a model that continuously learns and evolves based on increasing data, fed over time, with retention of previously gained knowledge.[78–81] In this way, it is intuitively appealing and like human cognition. One well-known use of continual learning is found in recommender systems of companies such as Amazon and Netflix—the model is continually updated with labeled data from interactions with the end-user to reflect changes in personal preference over time.[82] Yet unlike transfer learning, research into its clinical applications has been meager in the critical care domain, and no implementations currently exist[83] because of the considerable potential for "catastrophic forgetting." This describes a phenomenon in which new information interferes with previously learned patterns, resulting in a paradoxic decrease in model performance. There also exist privacy concerns as the single model is continuously fed sensitive clinical data from various institutions. Observational data suggest this approach *may* improve predictive models over time, such as in the early prediction of sepsis,[84] medication dosing,[85] or augmentation of imaging studies performed in critically ill patients.[86] Nevertheless, these have not yet been translated into clinical tools.

Conformal Prediction

Conformal prediction refers to a model's assessment of the uncertainty of a prediction based on the past experience. Intuitively, when a model encounters a scenario like its training dataset, the confidence in prediction is high. However, when a model encounters a scenario where input data are significantly different (non-conformal) from training data, the utility and confidence of the prediction are uncertain. Conformal prediction is therefore a mathematical approach that quantifies the uncertainty of an ML prediction. In effect, this allows the model to say "I don't know" for inputs that are foreign from training data.[87–90] Applications of conformal prediction have been used in various nonmedical fields, including facial recognition, financial risk, and language recognition. In health care, it has been used to augment breast cancer diagnosis[91] and prediction assessment of stroke risk,[92] albeit primarily under research applications. Conformal prediction has more recently been described to assist in sepsis prediction, as shown in **Fig. 2**.[14] In this example, potential sepsis cases in which an ML model had low certainty in prediction were identified and resulted in a significant decrease in false alarms. The ideal application of conformal prediction in the ICU would follow a similar pattern: alerting clinicians to scenarios in which a predictive model has low certainty of a prediction may increase their trust in ML predictive scores.

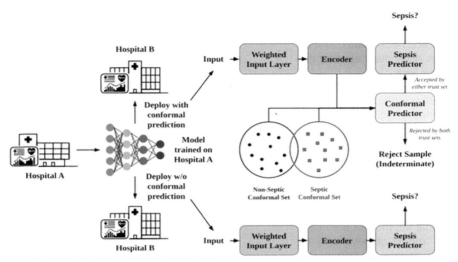

Fig. 2. Example of applying conformal prediction to a sepsis prediction model. If the model does not recognize the input data from a patient, the conformal prediction layer "rejects" the data, and the sepsis prediction layer alerts the end-user that there exists a high degree of uncertainty. This resulted in a significant decrease in false alarms. (*From* Shashikumar SP, Wardi G, Malhotra A, Nemati S. Artificial intelligence sepsis prediction algorithm learns to say "I don't know". NPJ Digit Med. 2021;4(1):134. Published 2021 Sep 9. doi:10.1038/s41746-021-00504-6.)

DISCUSSION

ML models have the potential to significantly improve care of critically ill patients by leveraging the data-rich nature of the ICU. However, despite promising research, their real-world implementations in critical care are presently scant; this unfortunately growing chasm between what has been developed and what has been implemented is a phenomenon referred to as the "implementation gap."[93] Although there are various reasons behind this discrepancy, inherent challenges with generalizability in a syndrome-based, heterogeneous patient landscape have significantly limited the utility of ML models in critical care. Our review explores many of these obstacles. Various syndrome-based conditions with overlapping clinical characteristics are difficult for ML models to delineate due to a critical delay in patient information availability and ambiguity in syndrome diagnosis. These effects are especially pronounced in the ICU, where syndrome-based conditions are common, and patients rapidly evolve. Compounding the challenge is heterogeneity in health care data itself. Data recording and storage, local health care guidelines, and temporal shifts in data necessitate correction in models themselves. Although patient demographics and missing data can further contribute heterogenous dimensions, they can also convey valuable information that might help improve prediction model accuracy.

Prevailing research on ML models use novel methods of learning to overcome these challenges and ultimately maximize external validity: transfer learning, continual learning, and conformal prediction.[11–14] Transfer learning involves retraining a model with limited data at a new deployment site so that it learns the specific nuances of that particular location.[73] Continual learning describes a central model that constantly adjusts its set of rules as it is applied to more data all while maintaining acceptable performance on prior applications.[79–81] Conformal prediction will only allow the model to predict from data that it deems "conformant" with the training data—that is, if it detects dissimilar data that may result in poor performance, it will refrain from making predictions.[87–90]

It is important to note that although we primarily demonstrate these in the context of sepsis prediction, ML models have been similarly studied for a variety of other prediction tasks, including respiratory failure in COVID-19 patients,[74,94–96] complications for critically ill patients,[76,77,97–99] and in-hospital mortality risk.[75,100–105] Other uses for clinical ML models outside of *predictive* tasks include identification of health factors related to patient outcomes, novel intervention design, and allocation of resources.[106] Future research into the applications of ML for critically ill patients should focus on *prospective* implementations across multiple centers to demonstrate clinical value. Many studies thus far are retrospective, and only a few of them undergo prospective validation; an even fewer number undertake randomized ML trials.[107] Indeed, many clinical ML models are currently developed and validated to collect dust only then in the "model graveyard."[93] Other deployed models, such as the Epic Sepsis Score (ESS), paint a cautionary tale to hospital systems that fail to perform rigorous testing and optimization during development: researchers at the University of Michigan described a significant performance drop and increased rate of false alarms of the ESS when implemented at their institution.[108] To conduct the multi-center trials necessary for demonstrating clinical value, models may therefore undergo local optimization. This can be accomplished via transfer learning or continual learning and further improved through conformal prediction or similar methods. Such approaches may help alleviate the problem of generalizability and improve test characteristics. To our knowledge, this has not yet been done and should thus be emphasized in future trial designs involving prospective validation of ML models.

SUMMARY

We believe that clinicians must understand the basics of ML and its major challenges to evaluate current and future models. This is a vital step for their successful implementation into clinical practice. Likewise, we believe that data scientists interested in the health care applications of ML must understand its unique clinical challenges; the barriers to generalizability can presently be overcome with solutions offered by transfer learning, continual learning, and conformal prediction. With increased attention, we are optimistic that a future with accurate and fair ML-based clinical aids is not far.

CLINICS CARE POINTS

- Syndromic conditions in the ICU are easy for clinicians to grasp, but many challenges exist for machine-learning models, which has thus far limited generalizability.

- Recent advances in machine-learning approaches may alleviate these concerns, although we still lack large, prospective trials demonstrating benefit in critically ill patients.

DISCLOSURE

G. Wardi is funded by the NIH (R35GM143121 and K23GM146092). A Malhotra is funded by the NIH. He reports income related to medical education from Livanova,

Eli Lilly, Jazz. ResMed, Inc provided a philanthropic donation to UC San Diego in support of a sleep center. S. Nemati is funded by the National Institutes of Health (#R56LM013517, #R35GM143121, #R01EB031539) and the Gordon and Betty Moore Foundation (#GBMF9052). S. Nemati, S.P. Shashikumar, and A. Malhotra are cofounders and hold equity in Healcisio, although unrelated to this work. The terms of this arrangement have been reviewed and approved by the University of California, San Diego in accordance with its conflict-of-interest policies. The remaining authors have no disclosures to report.

REFERENCES

1. Choy G, et al. Current applications and future impact of machine learning in radiology. Radiology 2018;288:318–28.
2. Chatterjee A, Somayaji NR, Kabakis IM. Abstract WMP16: artificial intelligence detection of cerebrovascular large vessel occlusion - nine month, 650 patient evaluation of the diagnostic accuracy and performance of the Viz.ai LVO algorithm. Stroke 2019;50. AWMP16-AWMP16.
3. van der Heijden A.A., Abramoff M.D., Verbraak F. et al., Validation of automated screening for referable diabetic retinopathy with the IDx-DR device in the Hoorn Diabetes Care System, *Acta Ophthalmol*, 96, 2018, 63–68.
4. Ratner M. FDA backs clinician-free AI imaging diagnostic tools. Nat Biotechnol 2018;36:673–4.
5. Shashikumar S., Making AI algorithms safer. Nature Portfolio health community, Available at: http://healthcommunity.nature.com/posts/dddd. Accessed September 10, 2021.
6. Nijman S, et al. Missing data is poorly handled and reported in prediction model studies using machine learning: a literature review. J Clin Epidemiol 2022;142: 218–29.
7. van Smeden M, Groenwold RHH, Moons KG. A cautionary note on the use of the missing indicator method for handling missing data in prediction research. J Clin Epidemiol 2020;125:188–90.
8. Luijken K, Groenwold RHH, Van Calster B, et al. Impact of predictor measurement heterogeneity across settings on the performance of prediction models: a measurement error perspective. Stat Med 2019;38:3444–59.
9. Futoma J, Simons M, Panch T, et al. The myth of generalisability in clinical research and machine learning in health care. Lancet Digit. Health 2020;2: e489–92.
10. Altman DG, Royston P. What do we mean by validating a prognostic model? Stat Med 2000;19:453–73.
11. Wardi G., Carlile M., Holder, A. et al., Predicting progression to septic shock in the emergency department using an externally generalizable machine-learning algorithm, *Ann Emerg Med*, 77, 2021, 395–406.
12. Holder AL, Shashikumar SP, Wardi G, et al. A locally optimized data-driven tool to predict sepsis-associated vasopressor use in the ICU. Crit Care Med 2021; 49:e1196.
13. Amrollahi F, Shashikumar SP, Holder AL, et al. Leveraging clinical data across healthcare institutions for continual learning of predictive risk models. Sci Rep 2022;12:8380.
14. Shashikumar SP, Wardi G, Malhotra A, et al. Artificial intelligence sepsis prediction algorithm learns to say "I don't know". Npj Digit. Med. 2021;4:1–9.

15. Beaulieu-Jones B., Yuan W., Brat G.A., et al., Machine learning for patient risk stratification: standing on, or looking over, the shoulders of clinicians?, *npj Digital Medicine*, 4 (1), 2021, 62.

16. Agniel D, Kohane I, Weber G. Biases in electronic health record data due to processes within the healthcare system: retrospective observational study. BMJ 2018;361:k1479.

17. Brüggemann S, Chan T, Wardi G, et al. Decision support tool for hospital resource allocation during the COVID-19 pandemic. Inform Med Unlocked 2021;24:100618.

18. Ye J, Yao L, Shen J, et al. Predicting mortality in critically ill patients with diabetes using machine learning and clinical notes. BMC Med Inf Decis Making 2020;20:295.

19. Hu C.-A., Chen C.M., Fang Y.C., et al., Using a machine learning approach to predict mortality in critically ill influenza patients: a cross-sectional retrospective multicentre study in Taiwan, BMJ Open, 10 (2020), e033898.

20. Calvo F, Karras BT, Phillips R, et al. Diagnoses, syndromes, and diseases: a knowledge representation problem. AMIA Annu. Symp. Proc. AMIA Symp. 2003;802.

21. Kawasaki T, Kosaki F, Okawa S, et al. A new infantile acute febrile mucocutaneous lymph node syndrome (MLNS) prevailing in Japan. Pediatrics 1974;54: 271–6.

22. Singer M, Deutschman CS, Seymour CW, et al. The third international consensus definitions for sepsis and septic shock (Sepsis-3). JAMA 2016; 315:801–10.

23. Hospital inpatient specifications manuals sepsis resources, Available at: https:// qualitynet.cms.gov/inpatient/specifications-manuals/sepsis-resources. Accessed June 12, 2022.

24. Rhee C., Zhang Z., Kadri S.S., et al., Sepsis surveillance using adult sepsis events simplified eSOFA criteria versus sepsis-3 sequential organ failure assessment criteria, *Crit Care Med*, 47, 2019, 307–314.

25. Seymour CW, Deutschman CS, Iwashyna TJ, et al. Assessment of clinical criteria for sepsis: for the third international consensus definitions for sepsis and septic shock (Sepsis-3). JAMA 2016;315:762–74.

26. Rubin DB. Inference and missing data. Biometrika 1976;63:581–92.

27. Fielding S, Fayers PM, McDonald A, et al. Simple imputation methods were inadequate for missing not at random (MNAR) quality of life data. Health Qual Life Outcome 2008;6:57.

28. Troxel AB, Fairclough DL, Curran D, et al. Statistical analysis of quality of life with missing data in cancer clinical trials. Stat Med 1998;17:653–66.

29. Li C. Little's test of missing completely at random. STATA J 2013;13:795–809.

30. Seaman S, Galati J, Jackson D, et al. What is meant by "missing at random". Stat Sci 2013;28:257–68.

31. Bhaskaran K, Smeeth L. What is the difference between missing completely at random and missing at random? Int J Epidemiol 2014;43:1336–9.

32. Rue T, Thompson HJ, Rivara FP, et al. Managing the common problem of missing data in trauma studies. J. Nurs. Scholarsh 2008;40:373–8.

33. Jordan MI, Mitchell TM. Machine learning: trends, perspectives, and prospects. Science 2015;349:255–60.

34. Rajkomar A, Hardt M, Howell MD, et al. Ensuring fairness in machine learning to advance health equity. Ann Intern Med 2018;169:866–72.

35. Shellenbarger S.A., Crucial step for averting AI disasters. WSJ, Available at: https://www.wsj.com/articles/a-crucial-step-for-avoiding-ai-disasters-11550069865. Accessed February 13, 2019.
36. Fawcett A., Understanding racial bias in machine learning algorithms. Educative: interactive Courses for Software Developers, Available at: https://www.educative.io/blog/racial-bias-machine-learning-algorithms. Accessed July 8, 2020.
37. Ferryman K, Pitcan M. Fairness in precision medicine. Data & society. Accessed February 26, 2018. Available at: https://datasociety.net/library/fairness-in-precision-medicine/.
38. Kamiran F, Calders T. Data preprocessing techniques for classification without discrimination. Knowl Inf Syst 2012;33:1–33.
39. Institute of Medicine (US). Committee on understanding and eliminating racial and ethnic disparities in health care. Unequal treatment: confronting racial and ethnic disparities in health care. National Academies Press: Washington DC (US); 2003.
40. Barnato AE, Alexander SL, Linde-Zwirble WT, et al. Racial variation in the incidence, care, and outcomes of severe sepsis. Am J Respir Crit Care Med 2008;177:279–84.
41. Huang J, Galal G, Etemadi M, et al. Evaluation and mitigation of racial bias in clinical machine learning models: scoping review. JMIR Med. Inform. 2022;10: e36388.
42. Allen A, Mataraso S, Siefkas A, et al. A racially unbiased, machine learning approach to prediction of mortality: algorithm development study. JMIR Public Health Surveill 2020;6:e22400.
43. Fang R, Pouyanfar S, Yang Y, et al. Computational health informatics in the big data age: a survey. ACM Comput Surv 2016;49. 12:1–12:36.
44. Donders ART, van der Heijden GJMG, Stijnen T, et al. Review: a gentle introduction to imputation of missing values. J Clin Epidemiol 2006;59:1087–91.
45. Little RJA, Rubin DB. Statistical analysis with missing data. Hoboken, NJ: John Wiley & Sons; 2019.
46. Buuren S. van, Flexible imputation of missing data, Second Edition, 2018, CRC Press: Boca Raton, FL.
47. Harel O, Mitchell EM, Perkins NJ, et al. Multiple imputation for incomplete data in epidemiologic studies. Am J Epidemiol 2018;187:576–84.
48. Sterne JAC, White IR, Carlin JB, et al. Multiple imputation for missing data in epidemiological and clinical research: potential and pitfalls. BMJ 2009;338: b2393.
49. Knol MJ, Janssen KJ, Donders AR, et al. Unpredictable bias when using the missing indicator method or complete case analysis for missing confounder values: an empirical example. J Clin Epidemiol 2010;63:728–36.
50. Liu D, Oberman HI, Muñoz J, et al. Quality control, data cleaning, imputation. https://doi.org/10.48550/ARXIV.2110.15877.
51. Syed M, Syed S, Sexton K, et al. Application of machine learning in intensive care unit (ICU) settings using MIMIC dataset: systematic review. Inform. MDPI 2021;8:16.
52. Davoodi R, Moradi MH. Mortality prediction in intensive care units (ICUs) using a deep rule-based fuzzy classifier. J. Biomed. Inform. 2018;79:48–59.
53. Lin K, Hu Y, Kong G. Predicting in-hospital mortality of patients with acute kidney injury in the ICU using random forest model. Int J Med Inf 2019;125:55–61.

54. Seymour CW, Kennedy JN, Wang S, et al. Derivation, validation, and potential treatment implications of novel clinical phenotypes for sepsis. JAMA 2019; 321:2003–17.
55. Sperrin M, Martin GP, Sisk R, et al. Missing data should be handled differently for prediction than for description or causal explanation. J Clin Epidemiol 2020;125:183–7.
56. Shmueli Galit. To explain or to predict? Stat Sci 2010;25:289–310.
57. Steyerberg EW, van Veen M. Imputation is beneficial for handling missing data in predictive models. J Clin Epidemiol 2007;60:979.
58. Choi J, Dekkers OM, le Cessie S. A comparison of different methods to handle missing data in the context of propensity score analysis. Eur J Epidemiol 2019; 34:23–36.
59. Ding Y, Simonoff JS. An investigation of missing data methods for classification trees applied to binary response data. J Mach Learn Res 2010;11:131–70.
60. Groenwold RHH, et al. Missing covariate data in clinical research: when and when not to use the missing-indicator method for analysis. Can Med Assoc J 2012;184:1265.
61. Efron B, Morris C. Stein's paradox stat. Sci Am 1977;236:119–27.
62. Lin L, Sperrin M, Jenkins DA, et al. A scoping review of causal methods enabling predictions under hypothetical interventions. Diagn. Progn. Res. 2021;5:3.
63. Sisk R., Lin L., Sperrin M., et al., Informative presence and observation in routine health data: a review of methodology for clinical risk prediction, *J Am Med Inform Assoc*, 28, 2021, 155–166.
64. Groenwold RHH. Informative missingness in electronic health record systems: the curse of knowing. Diagn. Progn. Res. 2020;4:8.
65. Collins GS, Omar O, Shanyinde M, et al. A systematic review finds prediction models for chronic kidney disease were poorly reported and often developed using inappropriate methods. J Clin Epidemiol 2013;66:268–77.
66. Tsvetanova A., Sperrin M., Peek N., et al., Missing data was handled inconsistently in UK prediction models: a review of method used, J Clin Epidemiol, 140, 2021, 149–158.
67. Dhiman P, et al. Reporting of prognostic clinical prediction models based on machine learning methods in oncology needs to be improved. J Clin Epidemiol 2021;138:60–72.
68. Galbete A, Tamayo I, Librero J, et al. Cardiovascular risk in patients with type 2 diabetes: a systematic review of prediction models. Diabetes Res Clin Pract 2022;184:109089.
69. Hayati Rezvan P, Lee KJ, Simpson JA. The rise of multiple imputation: a review of the reporting and implementation of the method in medical research. BMC Med Res Methodol 2015;15:30.
70. Karahalios A, Baglietto L, Carlin JB, et al. A review of the reporting and handling of missing data in cohort studies with repeated assessment of exposure measures. BMC Med Res Methodol 2012;12:96.
71. Kim Y-G, et al. Effectiveness of transfer learning for enhancing tumor classification with a convolutional neural network on frozen sections. Sci Rep 2020;10: 21899.
72. Alzubaidi L, Al-Amidie M, Al-Asadi A, et al. Novel transfer learning approach for medical imaging with limited labeled data. Cancers 2021;13:1590.
73. Kermany DS, Goldbaum M, Cai W, et al. Identifying medical diagnoses and treatable diseases by image-based deep learning. Cell 2018;172:1122–31.e9.

74. Bendavid I, Statlender L, Shvartser L, et al. A novel machine learning model to predict respiratory failure and invasive mechanical ventilation in critically ill patients suffering from COVID-19. Sci Rep 2022;12:10573.

75. Macias E, Morell A, Serrano J, et al. Mortality prediction enhancement in end-stage renal disease: a machine learning approach. Inform Med Unlocked 2020;19:100351.

76. Liu K, et al. Development and validation of a personalized model with transfer learning for acute kidney injury risk estimation using electronic health records. JAMA Netw Open 2022;5:e2219776.

77. Sjoding MW, Taylor D, Motyka J, et al. Deep learning to detect acute respiratory distress syndrome on chest radiographs: a retrospective study with external validation. Lancet Digit. Health 2021;3:e340–8.

78. Thrun S, Mitchell TM. Lifelong robot learning. Robot. Auton. Syst. 1995;15: 25–46.

79. Goodfellow I.J., Mirza M., Xiao D., et al., An Empirical Investigation of Catastrophic Forgetting in Gradient-Based Neural Networks. 2013. doi: 10.48550/ARXIV.1312.6211.

80. Zenke, F., Poole, B. & Ganguli, S. Continual Learning Through Synaptic Intelligence. in Proceedings of the 34th International Conference on Machine Learning 3987–3995 (PMLR, 2017).

81. van de Ven, G. M. & Tolias, A. S. Three scenarios for continual learning. (2019) doi:10.48550/arXiv.1904.07734.

82. Portugal I, Alencar P, Cowan D. The use of machine learning algorithms in recommender systems: A systematic review. Expert Syst Appl 2018;97:205–27.

83. Lee CS, Lee AY. Clinical applications of continual learning machine learning. Lancet Digit. Health 2020;2:e279–81.

84. French null. Catastrophic forgetting in connectionist networks. Trends Cogn. Sci. 1999;3:128–35.

85. Ghassemi M.M., Alhanai T., Westover M.B., et al., Personalized medication dosing using volatile data streams. In AAAI Workshops AAAI press, 2018, Available at: https://aaai.org/ocs/index.php/WS/AAAIW18/paper/view/17234.

86. Carlile M, et al. Deployment of artificial intelligence for radiographic diagnosis of COVID-19 pneumonia in the emergency department. J. Am. Coll. Emerg. Physicians Open 2020;1:1459–64.

87. Saunders C, Gammerman A, Vovk V. Transduction with confidence and credibility. Int Jt. Conf Artif. Intell. IJCAI 1999;16.

88. Vovk, V., Gammerman, A., & Saunders, C. (1999). Machine-Learning Applications of Algorithmic Randomness. International Conference on Machine Learning.

89. Papadopoulos, H., Vovk, V. & Gammerman, A. Conformal prediction with neural networks. in 19th IEEE International Conference on Tools with Artificial Intelligence(ICTAI 2007) vol. 2 388–395 (2007).

90. Shafer G., Vovk V., A tutorial on conformal prediction. 2007. Available at: http://arxiv.org/abs/0706.3188. Accessed March 10, 2023.

91. Lambrou, A., Papadopoulos, H. & Gammerman, A. Evolutionary Conformal Prediction for Breast Cancer Diagnosis. in 2009 9th International Conference on Information Technology and Applications in Biomedicine 1–4 (2009). doi:10.1109/ITAB.2009.5394447.

92. Papadopoulos H, Andreou A, Bramer M. Artificial intelligence applications and innovations. Springer: Larnaca, Cyprus.; 2010.

93. Seneviratne MG, Shah NH, Chu L. Bridging the implementation gap of machine learning in healthcare. BMJ Innov 2020;6:45–7.
94. Bolourani S, et al. A machine learning prediction model of respiratory failure within 48 hours of patient admission for COVID-19: model development and validation (preprint). 2020. Available at: http://preprints.jmir.org/preprint/24246.
95. Ferrari D, Milic J, Tonelli R, et al. Machine learning in predicting respiratory failure in patients with COVID-19 pneumonia—challenges, strengths, and opportunities in a global health emergency. PLoS One 2020;15:e0239172.
96. Assaf D, Gutman Y, Neuman Y, et al. Utilization of machine-learning models to accurately predict the risk for critical COVID-19. Intern. Emerg. Med. 2020;15: 1435–43.
97. Zhang Z, Ho KM, Hong Y. Machine learning for the prediction of volume responsiveness in patients with oliguric acute kidney injury in critical care. Crit Care 2019;23:112.
98. Hyland S.L., Faltys M., Hüser M., et al., Early prediction of circulatory failure in the intensive care unit using machine learning, Nat. Med., 26, 2020, 364–373.
99. Meyer A., Zverinski D., Pfahringer B., et al., Machine learning for real-time prediction of complications in critical care: a retrospective study, Lancet Respir Med, 6, 2018, 905–914.
100. Nanayakkara S, Fogarty S, Tremeer M, et al. Characterising risk of in-hospital mortality following cardiac arrest using machine learning: a retrospective international registry study. PLoS Med 2018;15:e1002709.
101. Di Castelnuovo A, Bonaccio M, Costanzo A, et al. Common cardiovascular risk factors and in-hospital mortality in 3,894 patients with COVID-19: survival analysis and machine learning-based findings from the multicentre Italian CORIST Study. Nutr. Metab. Cardiovasc. Dis. 2020;30:1899–913.
102. Tezza F, Lorenzoni G, Azzolina D, et al. Predicting in-hospital mortality of patients with COVID-19 using machine learning techniques. J Pers Med 2021; 11:343.
103. Du X, Min J, Shah CP, et al. Predicting in-hospital mortality of patients with febrile neutropenia using machine learning models. Int J Med Inf 2020;139:104140.
104. Kong G, Lin K, Hu Y. Using machine learning methods to predict in-hospital mortality of sepsis patients in the ICU. BMC Med Inf Decis Making 2020;20:251.
105. Brajer N, Cozzi B, Gao M, et al. Prospective and external evaluation of a machine learning model to predict in-hospital mortality of adults at time of admission. JAMA Netw Open 2020;3:e1920733.
106. Mhasawade V, Zhao Y, Chunara R. Machine learning and algorithmic fairness in public and population health. Nat Mach Intell 2021;3:659–66.
107. Fleuren L.M., Klausch T.L.T., Zwager C.L., et al., Machine learning for the prediction of sepsis: a systematic review and meta-analysis of diagnostic test accuracy, Intensive Care Med, 46, 2020, 383–400.
108. Wong A, Otles E, Donnelly JP, et al. External validation of a widely implemented proprietary sepsis prediction model in hospitalized patients. JAMA Intern Med 2021;181:1065–70.

Clinician Trust in Artificial Intelligence

What is Known and How Trust Can Be Facilitated

Juan C. Rojas, MD, MS[a],*, Mario Teran, MD[b],
Craig A. Umscheid, MD, MS[b]

KEYWORDS

- Artificial intelligence • Machine learning • Algorithms
- Clinical decision support systems • Trust • Health-care delivery

KEY POINTS

- Artificial Intelligence (AI) involves the application of mathematical algorithms to large quantities of data to derive insights.
- AI approaches commonly used in health care include machine learning, neural networks, and natural language processing.
- AI can make more accurate predictions than human decision-making.
- Many barriers exist to facilitating trust between clinicians and AI-based tools.
- Potential solutions to facilitate trust are available at both the local and national level.

A MOTIVATING CASE

Sepsis remains a leading cause of death in hospitalized patients,[1] despite evidence-based strategies to reduce mortality.[2] Given that timely recognition and treatment increase survival,[3] and that electronic data necessary for early recognition is available in real time for many hospitalized patients, early detection of sepsis has become a popular target for predictive analytics. The use case is simple enough—apply an algorithm to streams of data from hospitalized patients to estimate sepsis risk. If the risk is high enough, an alert can trigger a multidisciplinary team to the bedside to assess the risk and implement a response. However, what happens if a patient who triggers the alert

[a] Department of Internal Medicine, Rush University, 1725 West Harrison Street, Suite 010, Chicago, IL 60612, USA; [b] Agency for Healthcare Research and Quality, 5600 Fishers Lane, Mail Stop 06E53A, Rockville, MD 20857, USA
* Corresponding author.
E-mail address: juan_rojas@rush.edu

Crit Care Clin 39 (2023) 769–782
https://doi.org/10.1016/j.ccc.2023.02.004
0749-0704/23/© 2023 Elsevier Inc. All rights reserved.

does not fit the clinical teams' mental model for a patient at high risk of sepsis? Moreover, what happens if *most* patients who trigger the alert do not seem high risk to the clinical team responding? Moreover, how might this happen given our modern approach to algorithm development?

This may seem like a fantastical scenario but many of us have experienced this in our clinical roles—algorithm warnings that diverge from our clinical suspicions. In 2019, Giannini and colleagues described the development, implementation, and evaluation of an algorithm designed to predict severe sepsis or septic shock.[4] The machine learning (ML) algorithm had promising test characteristics, including an area under the curve (AUC) of 0.88, a positive predictive value of 29%, and likelihood ratio of 13, meaning that almost a third of patients who triggered the alert would ultimately have severe sepsis or septic shock, and that those triggering the alert were 13 times more likely to be diagnosed with severe sepsis or septic shock than those who did not trigger the alert. However, the impact of the alert on patient care was modest at best—small increases in ordering of laboratory tests and intravenous fluids but no significant increases in antibiotic prescribing or transfers to intensive care. An assessment of clinicians' perceptions that occurred alongside the alert suggested that most had clinical impressions that were unchanged by the alert—their patients may have been sick but likely no worse than before and not by enough to institute any changes in clinical management.

Clinician reactions to this alert that *predicted* severe sepsis and septic shock were different from their reactions to an alert used in the same health-care system years before that *detected* clinical deterioration. The alert that *detected* clinical deterioration resulted in approximately 2-fold increases in ordering of intravenous fluids, antibiotics, and lactate and blood culture measurements, and increased transfers to intensive care.[5] A survey implemented alongside the alert suggested that about a third found it helpful, and a quarter thought it improved patient care.[5]

There are many potential reasons for the differences in impact between the 2 alert types described above. For example, the newer alert was *predicting* what was to come, whereas the older alert was *detecting* what was already present. This difference can greatly affect the utility of an alert, as clinicians may have an array of tools available to address clinical deterioration detected early but may be less certain about what to do for deterioration that may occur at some future point. The alerts were also trained on different outcomes, and the practical differences between these outcome definitions likely resulted in differences in clinical utility between the 2 algorithms. The older algorithm was trained on clinical deterioration defined as an "ICU transfer, rapid response team call, or death," and the newer algorithm was trained on a nuanced definition of severe sepsis or septic shock that included diagnostic codes and blood culture results. There were also differences in the transparency of the algorithms described. The older algorithm was based on a relatively simple rule—4 or more concurrent abnormalities in any of 6 monitored measures resulted in an alert. The newer tool was based on an ML algorithm with hundreds of inputs, where the logic leading to the alert was less transparent. Regardless of the exact cause for the differences in impact between these 2 alert types, it is clear that one alert provided additional helpful information to the clinical team at a time when they were receptive to such information and willing to change the course of management, resulting in a clinical impact, and the other did not.

In this article, we reflect on provider trust in predictive analytics, and offer a roadmap to facilitate such trust. To begin, we review the different types of clinical algorithms in use, and the literature examining how provider predictions and predictions based on artificial intelligence (AI) compare, using examples relevant to intensivists.

REVIEW OF ARTIFICIAL INTELLIGENCE IN HEALTHCARE

The notion of automated ML has been around since at least the 1950s with Alan Turing's classic reference to the "learning machine."[6] However, with exponential advances in technology, AI has grown from basic algorithmic tasks to an entire field that includes intelligent machines that can achieve goals akin to human learning. Given how well developed these systems are outside of medicine, there is increasing effort to extrapolate these technologies to transform health care, including to improve diagnosis, optimize treatment, reduce provider burden, and increase the health-care system's efficiency. Due to the breadth of the field and its rapid expansion, it is important for all clinicians to understand how AI and its subdisciplines are being applied to health care today. This section will briefly review the AI subdisciplines of ML, deep learning, and natural language processing (NLP) because they relate to health care (**Table 1**).

Machine Learning

Considered a type of AI, ML can be described as a computer's ability to "learn" or infer relationships from large datasets without being explicitly programmed through predefined, rules-based methods.[7]

In supervised learning, ML algorithms learn from example with the goal of identifying a known output.[8] For instance, in automated electrocardiography (EKG) interpretation, an algorithm has been trained using sets of EKG images and related diagnoses.[8] The model created by the algorithm is then validated against a different set of related data known as the testing set.[9] Several iterations of training and testing may be performed with additional data to optimize the algorithmic model, which when sufficiently accurate can be applied to real data.

Table 1 Glossary of terms	
Term	**Definition**
AI	The science and engineering of creating machines that mimic intelligent human behaviors
Deep learning	A subset of AI involving complex algorithms that allow a computer to train itself by processing data through neural networks analogous to the human brain
ML	A subset of AI using algorithms that allows a computer the ability to learn from data and examples without being explicitly programmed by predefined, rules-based methods
Machine learning spectrum	Range of ML with complete human guidance learning on one extreme and complete machine guided learning on the other
NLP	A form of AI, which incorporates deep learning, structured learning, and linguistics to create algorithmic models that can "understand" and create speech or written language
Neural network	A software created network of interconnected nodes forming layers. Mathematical computations carried out at each layer increase the amount of information available
Supervised learning	ML process of training an algorithm using a train-test system that uses labeled data and compares correct outputs to allow the algorithm to identify patterns or make predictions
Unsupervised learning	ML process where unlabeled datasets are provided to the algorithm with no outputs to predict. The algorithm is then free to find hidden connections within the data or separate the data into groups

In unsupervised learning, unlabeled datasets are given to the algorithm with no outputs to predict.[8,9] Instead, the algorithm is free to create models to find hidden structure in the data and/or separate the data into clusters or groups as it sees fit. Although exciting new patterns or clinically unrecognized phenotypes may be identified, it is often initially difficult to determine the value of this type of ML until the model is evaluated by subsequent supervised learning algorithms (eg, how are these patterns actually useful?).[8] Currently in health care, the most compelling opportunity for this methodology is in identifying complex multifactorial diseases such as sepsis or acute respiratory distress syndrome.[10,11]

Deep Learning and Neural Networks

Inspired by the neuron networks of the human brain, deep learning involves complex algorithms that permit a computer to train itself by processing data through a network of multiple interconnected hierarchical layers.[7,9] As the data input descends "deeper" into each layer, it carries an increasingly complex level of information that allows for an increasing understanding of the input. The existing algorithm is then able to refine itself as new data is presented or new connections are made.[12]

These neural networks can be a particularly powerful tool because they can sift through large amounts of input data and can make connections on an exponential scale. This is especially relevant to image recognition.[12] For example, researchers have demonstrated a deep learning algorithm capable of detecting diabetic retinopathy from retinal photographs at a sensitivity equal to or greater than that of ophthalmologists.[13]

Natural Language Processing

NLP is a form of AI, which incorporates linguistics to create algorithmic models that can "understand" and create written language or speech.[14] These models aim to codify text or speech not only as a sequence of characters and sentences but also as a complex piece of data that can extract concept or meaning.[15]

The applications of NLP in medicine are diverse but are especially attractive in analyzing electronic health records (EHR) to improve patient outcomes. Because most clinician notes in EHRs contain a large free text element, NLP can be used to process and analyze the text to identify patients eligible for clinical trials or evaluate the effectiveness of treatments.[15] For example, a study conducted using an NLP-based electronic triage system was able to accurately identify patients who had a substantially increased risk of hospitalization or critical care admission across multiple EDs.[16]

Despite all the advancement, AI algorithms are not yet able to transform all data into medical miracles. They are, at their core, natural extensions of traditional mathematical methods that have been greatly enhanced by the power of computers. However, due to their complex and evolving nature, AI use in clinical practice has raised appropriate concern and questions. Subsequent sections of this article will outline these issues and their implications for clinical practice.

HOW DO CLINICIAN AND ARTIFICIAL INTELLIGENCE PREDICTIONS COMPARE?

Clinical decision-making can range from fast, intuitive, or heuristic decisions to well-reasoned, analytical, evidence-based decisions that drive patient care.[17] Ideally, AI would be used in situations where making incrementally more accurate predictions could meaningfully enhance decision-making for front-line clinicians. Most of the hype that surrounds the use of AI in clinical decision support is caused by expectations of advances that can flawlessly detect patients at risk of cancer, sepsis, and readmission.[18] Surprisingly, there is little literature comparing how these models perform against human clinical decision-making. This is an important gap in the field because one way to promote trust and adoption of AI is to demonstrate that an AI-informed tool can provide prognostic value meaningfully better than clinician judgment alone. In this section, we will review the existing literature comparing AI models to clinician judgment for conditions and outcomes relevant to intensivists.

Sepsis

Mortality rates of sepsis can be as high as 16% and increase to as high as 40% when patients suffer shock.[19] Given the importance of early and appropriate antibiotic therapy in sepsis outcomes,[20] there has been an increased interest in using AI to identify those at risk for sepsis and initiating appropriate treatment as soon as possible, particularly in the emergency department (ED), where many patients present with undifferentiated symptoms.[21]

A variety of clinical risk scores are used in routine clinical care to facilitate risk stratification of patients with sepsis,[22] ranging from simple scores such as the quick sequential organ failure assessment (qSOFA)[19] to more complex scores such as the abbreviated Mortality in Emergency Department Sepsis.[23] Perhaps, the most used clinical risk score is a clinician's own judgment of short-term and medium-term mortality for patients in the ED. The judgment of physicians was found to be a moderate-to-good predictor (AUC of 0.68–0.81) of short-term mortality risk for patients in the ED.[24,25] Due to the promise of AI technology, many have developed more complex prediction models to predict risk of sepsis or mortality for those patients with suspected sepsis.[26] These models outperformed commonly used disease severity scores such as Systemic Inflammatory Response Syndrome (SIRS), Modified Early Warning Score (MEWS), and Sequential Organ Failure Assessment (SOFA) Score for the screening of sepsis, severe sepsis, and septic shock.[26] However, it was not known if an AI model could outperform clinical judgment on sepsis or mortality risk. Van Doorn and colleagues were the first to compare the performance of an ML model predicting 31-day mortality in patients presenting to the ED with sepsis to the judgment of physicians.[21] The model had higher diagnostic accuracy with an AUC of 0.85 (95%CI: 0.78–0.92) compared with internal medicine physicians (AUC 0.74, CI 0.65–0.82).[21] The authors found that the ML algorithm was more sensitive compared with simpler risk scores and internal medicine physicians while retaining identical or slightly higher specificity. These findings support the development and implementation of ML models as clinical decision support tools for patients with suspected sepsis in the ED and likely in other acute care settings in the hospital.

Mortality Prediction

Patients and families rely on clinicians to provide accurate prognostic information to make the most informed choices about end-of-life care.[27] Studies have shown that physicians often overestimate survival or are reticent to discuss prognosis and end-of-life preferences owing to perceived patient distress, rapidly progressive science, and lack of prognostic confidence.[28] Within the oncology population, there remains high use of intensive care admission and underuse of hospice care near the end of life.[29] Given the increasing amount of granular patient level data, many have hope that AI models can improve prognostic confidence so that patients, caregivers, and clinicians can all have the most accurate prognostic information to discuss advanced care planning.

A widely and easily implemented prognostic tool is the surprise question (SQ), which asks clinicians whether it would surprise them if a patient died within a particular time frame. The SQ has been used most with a 1-year time frame but also with time frames between 1 week and 6 months with varying performance.[30] The SQ has performed better in oncology populations compared with those in heart or renal failure.[30] Yet, overall the SQ performs modestly to poorly as a predictive tool for death in patients with or without cancer.[30] Because the SQ has at best fair accuracy and is not widely adopted into clinical workflows consistently, health-care organizations have used ML to identify patients at high risk of mortality to facilitate goals-of-care discussions and engage palliative care consultants.[31]

As with sepsis, despite the development of multiple highly accurate mortality models, it was unknown whether these models would outperform clinician judgment alone. Zachariah and colleagues were the first to compare the prognostic performance of medical oncologists using the SQ with a supervised ML model trained to predict the risk of mortality in 3 months.[32] The authors believed such an evaluation would improve acceptability of the ML mortality predictions when the developed model was implemented at their hospital.[32] The study cohort had a 15% prevalence of 3-month mortality, with 30% sensitivity for both oncologists and the model, meaning that both the oncologists and the model could only accurately identify 30% of the patients who ultimately died in 3 months. However, the PPV for the oncologists was only 34.8% (95% CI, 30.1%–39.5%) compared with the PPV of the model at 60.0% (95% CI, 53.6%–66.3%),[32] meaning that only about a third of those identified by the oncologists as high risk of mortality died within 3 months, compared with about two-thirds of those predicted by the model. The ML model predictions were about twice as good as the oncologists.[32] These findings need further validation but suggest that ML mortality models for patients with advanced cancer could increase prognostic confidence for clinicians, thereby potentially improving discussions about goals of care between patients, families, and clinicians.

EXAMINING TRUST IN ARTIFICIAL INTELLIGENCE

In human relationships, benevolence, integrity, ability, and reliability are cornerstones for establishing trust. Such attributes may be critical for the development of trust between humans and machines as well. For example, users may want some assurance that a technology is fair, which can serve as a marker for benevolence. Similarly, transparency of a technology provides an opportunity for assuring its integrity.[33,34] Unsupervised algorithms that predict future events using phenotyping techniques not transparent to clinicians may result in limited trust and ultimately limited use.[35] However, transparency of tools may not be enough.[36] The ability or performance of a tool is also fundamental to trust. Even if an AI tool is fair and transparent, it will not be trusted if its predictive performance is poor. Reliability of that performance over time and across populations may be critical as well.

Why might it matter whether AI engenders trust? Simply put, trust in technology affects its adoption.[37] It is not the only factor; for example, adoption may also be related to the amount of effort required to use the tool, or whether respected colleagues use the tool.[38] Nevertheless, trust is essential.

Studies examining how much clinicians trust AI and how trust might differ by clinician type (eg, physicians vs nurses) and setting of AI use (eg, professional vs personal) are not available. However, there is some evidence to suggest that the use of AI may be trusted less in health care than elsewhere. This is particularly the case for patients, especially when there is a perception that AI is used without the interpretation by trusted clinicians.[39]

Placing too much trust in a technology can also be problematic, particularly if there is limited knowledge about the technology, or the technology is operating autonomously outside of its limits. Instead of blind trust, the optimal approach may be calibrated or value-based trust,[33,40] informed by the fairness, transparency, and performance of a tool. Some suggest that trust as a concept is less applicable for AI, given that AI is not a moral agent acting autonomously,[41,42] and merely provides augmented intelligence, at least in the near term.[43] Thus, the focus should more be on the technical performance of the technology, and the infrastructure and processes that ensure technical performance and safety, which can ultimately lead to trust.[44]

FACILITATING TRUSTWORTHY ARTIFICIAL INTELLIGENCE

To facilitate trust in AI, and ultimately the adoption and use of fair, effective, and safe AI, there needs to be an understanding of the barriers to trust and ways to overcome them. **Table 2** provides a list of current barriers along with potential solutions to providing the infrastructure and approaches needed to facilitate trust and adoption of AI-informed clinical decision support. The barriers are organized by those general domains described above, which are essential to establishing trust in human relationships.[33] The potential solutions highlight that health systems, vendors, and policymakers broadly need to ensure that the right clinical problems are targeted by AI; useful, robust, and transparent AI tools are embedded in the correct clinical workflows; and there is support for the creation and maintenance of the necessary local and national infrastructure, processes and teams to ensure safe, effective, and transparent model development, deployment, and evaluation. These solutions are consistent with other recommendations that have been developed for building and maintaining trust in clinical decision support tools more generally.[45]

SUPPORTING AN ENVIRONMENT CONDUCIVE TO TRUST LOCALLY AND NATIONALLY

Significant investments in local and national infrastructure are required to support the trustworthiness of AI, and by extension clinician trust in AI.[46] Below, we highlight some of the potential investments suggested in the literature.

What Can Be Done Locally to Facilitate Trust?

Health-care system leaders can ensure that the predictive health solutions deployed within their local environment are safe, effective, and equitable for both front-line clinicians and the patients they serve. One potential solution is to dedicate resources to organize and manage predictive analytics at the hospital or system level, similar to the infrastructure, standards, and processes established in health-care systems nationally to manage laboratory testing (**Fig. 1**). When a test is performed in a medical laboratory, there are standards that dictate the quality needed for a given specimen. In addition, the tests used to examine specimens are routinely calibrated. This results in laboratory findings that can reliably be used by clinicians to make informed decisions. This is often not true of "algorithmic tests" run on patient data "specimens." There may not be a quality standard for the data "specimen" used by an "algorithmic test." In addition, there may be no validation or "calibration" of the "algorithmic test" used to examine the data "specimen." This can result in algorithmic findings that provide limited incremental value in clinical decision-making and negatively impact decision-making.

Currently, less information is known about how health-care systems organize and manage predictive analytics locally. In one recent national survey of all nonacademic health-care system member sites of The Scottsdale Institute (SI), only 64% of

Table 2
Barriers to clinician trust and potential solutions, organized by key determinants of trust

Barrier	Potential Solution
Fairness	
Potential for bias	Examine disparities between less and more socially advantaged populations across model performance metrics (eg, accuracy, positive predictive value), patient outcomes, and resource allocation, and then identify root causes of the disparities (eg, biased data, interpretation) and brainstorm solutions to address the disparities before the wide-spread implementation of models in clinical practice[48]
Transparency	
Perception that risk scores are a "black box"	AI model developers need to focus on explainability. This is the extent to which the internal mechanics of a machine or deep learning system can be explained in human terms
Transparency in model development	The "Model Facts" label was designed for clinicians who make decisions supported by a AI model and its purpose is to collate relevant, actionable information in one page, which could be cited by the tool[53]
Lack of education on data science for most front-line clinicians	Undergraduate and graduate medical education currently has little to no focus on data science. Preparing future clinicians to not only use AI in care delivery and research but also critically evaluate its applicability and limitations is essential
Lack of health system infrastructure for quality assurance for predictive analytics using AI	Health systems should create infrastructure, processes and multidisciplinary teams to ensure the safe, effective, and equitable deployment of predictive models in health care that can improve clinical outcomes and advance health equity
Performance	
Targeting the right clinical problems	Select clinical problems or population health measures that are valued by front-line clinicians
Lack of provider engagement in selection, development, and implementation of predictive health solutions	Predictive health solutions are often designed and developed with little or no input from front-line clinicians. In order to build trust and increase adoption, health systems, and vendors need to meet the needs of the end-users of clinical decision support tools
Lack of evidence of clinical utility showing that the model can improve clinical decision-making above and beyond routine clinician judgment	Developers of AI models should ensure their model offers meaningfully improved predictions above and beyond clinicians intending to use it

(continued on next page)

Table 2 (continued)	
Barrier	Potential Solution
Usability	Use existing best practices for effective clinical decision support (CDS). These CDS 5 rights can be used as a framework when planning to implement CDS interventions within a facility or practice, or when creating an extensive CDS program. The 5 rights include providing: the right information, to the right person, in the right intervention format, through the right channel, at the right time in workflow[54]

respondents reported having a team or individual accountable for the clinical application of predictive algorithms.[47] This estimate is likely overly optimistic because the health-care systems who are members of the SI are those with a specific interest in health-care innovation. Most notably, health-care leaders in this survey viewed lack of acceptance by clinical teams as the most significant threat to the adoption of AI in medicine.[47] As noted recently by Roski and colleagues, local governance models established by health-care systems need to address all phases of the AI lifecycle as described by the National Academy of Medicine,[43] namely[46] identifying the priorities

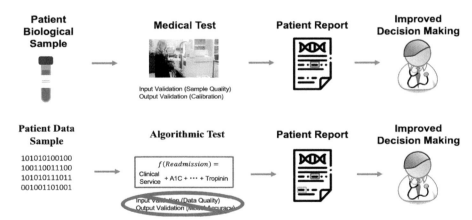

Fig. 1. Why does AI need local governance? When a test is performed in a medical laboratory, there are standards that dictate the quality needed for a given specimen, and the tests used to examine the specimen are routinely calibrated. This results in laboratory findings that can reliably be used by clinicians to inform decision-making. This is often not true of "algorithmic tests" run on patient data "specimens." There may not be a quality standard for the data "specimen" used by an "algorithmic test." Moreover, there may be no validation or "calibration" of the "algorithmic test" used to examine the data "specimen." This can result in algorithmic findings that provide limited incremental value in clinical decision-making and negatively impact decision-making. To address this challenge, similar infrastructure, standards, and processes used to manage local laboratory testing could be considered for "algorithmic" tests.

addressed by AI; understanding how AI solutions might fit into existing workflows; acquiring or designing the most appropriate models; training, validating and deploying models in the local setting; and monitoring model performance and revising models as appropriate.[48] To facilitate trustworthy AI, health-care systems must invest in the leadership, infrastructure, processes, and multidisciplinary teams needed to ensure the safe, effective, and equitable deployment of predictive models in health care that can improve clinical outcomes and advance health equity. Fostering trust will require transparency of these approaches for clinicians who will be end-users of these novel predictive health solutions, including regular and open communication about how such initiatives have strengthened care, as well as where they have fallen short and required revision or deimplementation.

What Can Be Done Nationally to Facilitate Trust?

Federal agencies, such as those in the Department of Health and Human Services, can use various levers to promote trustworthy AI in health care.[46] For example, the Office of the National Coordinator for Health Information Technology provides certification of EHRs. Such certification could include reviews of the fairness, transparency, and performance of AI-based health solutions available in EHRs, balancing the need for innovation with the necessary data and patient protections. The US Food and Drug Administration has traditionally regulated software that informs clinical devices, such as those implanted into patients, as well as medical imaging systems. Although EHR software has not typically met the criteria for such regulation, that could change as EHRs evolve to include increasingly sophisticated AI-based predictive health-care solutions that use streams of big data to estimate patient risk and make clinical recommendations in real time.[49,50]

Nonfederal organizations can also promote trustworthy AI nationally. For example, the Joint Commission could use their certification process to ensure that management of predictive health-care solutions across health-care systems meets minimum standards to increase the safety and maximize the value of such solutions. Such certification processes are particularly potent levers for health-care system leaders because reimbursement for care provided to patients covered by the Centers for Medicare and Medicaid Services is conditioned on such certification. Similarly, organizations responsible for accrediting undergraduate, graduate, and continuing clinical education programs could support minimum standards for training in data science for those clinicians who are most frequently the end-users of such tools to not only strengthen their ability to use such tools more effectively but also their ability to be more effective partners to developers, implementers, and evaluators of such tools, and more effective role models for trainees. Such education need not be limited to clinicians but could be available to patient communities as well, to increase their effectiveness as partners and advocates.

Many other groups can also facilitate trustworthy AI tools nationally, including researchers and funders, who can conduct and support the publication of rigorous evaluations of such tools to ensure their safety and effectiveness.[51] Currently, there is limited research assessing the impact of AI-based tools across health-care systems, and even fewer studies of high rigor.[52]

SUMMARY

Despite current distrust of AI in medicine, we remain optimistic that this technology can strengthen patient care. For this to occur, clinicians will need to trust, or at least value, these solutions. Although many barriers to facilitating such trust exist, potential solutions are available at both the local and national levels. It will likely take a broad and diverse coalition of relevant stakeholders, from health-care systems, vendors, and clinical educators to regulators, researchers, and the patient community, to help facilitate this trust so that we can realize the promise of AI in health and health care.

CLINICS CARE POINTS

- AI should be used n situations where making incrementally more accurate predictions could meaningfully enhance decision-making for front-line clinicians.
- Instead of blind trust, the optimal approach may be calibrated or value-based trust informed by fiarness and transparen for health care applications of AI.

FUNDING

Dr Rojas was supported by the National Center for Advancing Translational Sciences (NCATS) of the National Institutes of Health (NIH) through Grant Number 5KL2TR002387-05 that funds the Institute for Translational Medicine (ITM). The content is solely the responsibility of the authors and does not necessarily represent the official views of the NIH.

DISCLAIMER

The findings and conclusions in this document are those of the authors, who are responsible for its content, and do not necessarily represent the views of the Agency for Healthcare Research and Quality (AHRQ) or the U.S. Department of Health and Human Services (HHS). No statement in this report should be construed as an official position of AHRQ or HHS.

CONFLICTS OF INTEREST AND SOURCE OF FUNDING

None reported.

ACKNOWLEDGMENTS

We would like to acknowledge John Fahrenbach, PhD and Stephen Konya for their early contributions to this article, and Edwin A. Lomotan, MD and Michael I. Harrison, PhD for their review of a draft of this article.

REFERENCES

1. Rhee C, Jones TM, Hamad Y, et al. Prevalence, Underlying causes, and Preventability of sepsis-associated mortality in US acute care hospitals. JAMA Netw Open 2019;2(2):e187571.
2. Machado FR, Nsutebu E, AbDulaziz S, et al. Sepsis 3 from the perspective of clinicians and quality improvement initiatives. J Crit Care 2017;40:315–7.
3. Rivers E, Nguyen B, Havstad S, et al. Early goal-directed therapy in the treatment of severe sepsis and septic shock. N Engl J Med 2001;345(19):1368–77.
4. Giannini HM, Ginestra JC, Chivers C, et al. A machine learning algorithm to predict severe sepsis and septic shock: development, implementation, and impact on clinical practice. Crit Care Med 2019;47(11):1485–92.

5. Guidi JL, Clark K, Upton MT, et al. Clinician perception of the effectiveness of an automated early warning and response system for sepsis in an academic medical Center. Ann Am Thorac Soc 2015;12(10):1514–9.

6. Muggleton S. Alan Turing and the development of artificial intelligence. AI communications 2014;27(1):3–10.

7. Beam AL, Kohane IS. Big data and machine learning in health care. JAMA 2018; 319(13):1317–8.

8. Deo RC. Machine learning in medicine. Circulation 2015;132(20):1920–30.

9. Makhni S, Chin MH, Fahrenbach J, et al. Equity challenges for artificial intelligence algorithms in health care. Chest 2022;161(5):1343–6.

10. Le S, Pellegrini E, Green-Saxena A, et al. Supervised machine learning for the early prediction of acute respiratory distress syndrome (ARDS). J Crit Care 2020;60:96–102.

11. Nemati S, Holder A, Razmi F, et al. An interpretable machine learning model for accurate prediction of sepsis in the ICU. Crit Care Med 2018;46(4):547.

12. Helm JM, Swiergosz AM, Haeberle HS, et al. Machine learning and artificial intelligence: definitions, applications, and future directions. Current Reviews in Musculoskeletal Medicine 2020;13(1):69–76.

13. Krause J, Gulshan V, Rahimy E, et al. Grader variability and the importance of reference standards for evaluating machine learning models for diabetic retinopathy. Ophthalmology 2018;125(8):1264–72.

14. Nadkarni PM, Ohno-Machado L, Chapman WW. Natural language processing: an introduction. J Am Med Inf Assoc 2011;18(5):544–51.

15. Locke S, Bashall A, Al-Adely S, et al. Natural language processing in medicine: a review. Trends in Anaesthesia and Critical Care 2021;38:4–9.

16. Klang E, Kummer BR, Dangayach NS, et al. Predicting adult neuroscience intensive care unit admission from emergency department triage using a retrospective, tabular-free text machine learning approach. Sci Rep 2021;11(1):1–9.

17. Banning M. A review of clinical decision making: models and current research. J Clin Nurs 2008;17(2):187–95.

18. Jiang L, Wu Z, Xu X, et al. Opportunities and challenges of artificial intelligence in the medical field: current application, emerging problems, and problem-solving strategies. J Int Med Res 2021;49(3). 3000605211000157.

19. Singer M, Deutschman CS, Seymour CW, et al. The third international consensus definitions for sepsis and septic shock (Sepsis-3). JAMA 2016;315(8):801–10.

20. Seymour CW, Gesten F, Prescott HC, et al. Time to treatment and mortality during Mandated emergency care for sepsis. N Engl J Med 2017;376(23):2235–44.

21. van Doorn W, Stassen PM, Borggreve HF, et al. A comparison of machine learning models versus clinical evaluation for mortality prediction in patients with sepsis. PLoS One 2021;16(1):e0245157.

22. McLymont N, Glover GW. Scoring systems for the characterization of sepsis and associated outcomes. Ann Transl Med 2016;4(24).

23. Roest AA, Tegtmeier J, Heyligen JJ, et al. Risk stratification by abbMEDS and CURB-65 in relation to treatment and clinical disposition of the septic patient at the emergency department: a cohort study. BMC Emerg Med 2015;15(1):1–8.

24. Zelis N, Mauritz AN, Kuijpers LI, et al. Short-term mortality in older medical emergency patients can be predicted using clinical intuition: a prospective study. PLoS One 2019;14(1):e0208741.

25. Rohacek M, Nickel CH, Dietrich M, et al. Clinical intuition ratings are associated with morbidity and hospitalisation. Int J Clin Pract 2015;69(6):710–7.

26. Mao Q, Jay M, Hoffman JL, et al. Multicentre validation of a sepsis prediction algorithm using only vital sign data in the emergency department, general ward and ICU. BMJ Open 2018;8(1):e017833.
27. Bjørk E, Thompson W, Ryg J, et al. Patient preferences for discussing life expectancy: a systematic review. J Gen Intern Med 2021;36(10):3136–47.
28. White N, Kupeli N, Vickerstaff V, et al. How accurate is the 'Surprise Question'at identifying patients at the end of life? A systematic review and meta-analysis. BMC Med 2017;15(1):1–14.
29. Miccinesi G, Bianchi E, Brunelli C, et al. End-of-life preferences in advanced cancer patients willing to discuss issues surrounding their terminal condition. Eur J Cancer Care 2012;21(5):623–33.
30. Downar J, Goldman R, Pinto R, et al. The "surprise question" for predicting death in seriously ill patients: a systematic review and meta-analysis. CMAJ (Can Med Assoc J) 2017;189(13):E484–93.
31. Manz CR, Parikh RB, Small DS, et al. Effect of integrating machine learning mortality estimates with behavioral nudges to clinicians on serious illness conversations among patients with cancer: a stepped-wedge cluster randomized clinical trial. JAMA Oncol 2020;6(12):e204759.
32. Zachariah FJ, Rossi LA, Roberts LM, et al. Prospective comparison of medical oncologists and a machine learning model to predict 3-month mortality in patients with Metastatic Solid Tumors. JAMA Netw Open 2022;5(5):e2214514.
33. Asan O, Bayrak AE, Choudhury A. Artificial intelligence and human trust in healthcare: focus on clinicians. J Med Internet Res 2020;22(6):e15154.
34. Nagy M. and Sisk B. How will artificial intelligence affect patient-clinician relationships?, *AMA journal of ethics*, 22 (5), 2020, E395–E400, Available at: https://journalofethics.ama-assn.org/article/how-will-artificial-intelligence-affect-patient-clinician-relationships/2020-05. Accessed December 29, 2022.
35. Quinn TP, Jacobs S, Senadeera M, et al. The three ghosts of medical AI: can the black-box present deliver? Artif Intell Med 2022;124:102158.
36. Ghassemi M, Oakden-Rayner L, Beam AL. The false hope of current approaches to explainable artificial intelligence in health care. Lancet Digit Health 2021;3(11):e745–50.
37. Choudhury A, Asan O, Medow JE. Effect of risk, expectancy, and trust on clinicians' intent to use an artificial intelligence system – Blood Utilization Calculator. Appl Ergon 2022;101:103708.
38. Cheng M, Li X, Xu J. Promoting healthcare Workers' adoption Intention of artificial-intelligence-Assisted diagnosis and treatment: the Chain Mediation of Social Influence and human-computer trust. Int J Environ Res Public Health 2022;19(20). https://doi.org/10.3390/ijerph192013311.
39. Yakar D, Ongena YP, Kwee TC, et al. Do People Favor artificial intelligence over physicians? A survey among the general population and their view on artificial intelligence in medicine. Value Health 2022;25(3):374–81.
40. Pellikka PA, Hamza I, Carter RE. What is needed for artificial intelligence to Be trusted? Am J Med 2022;135(4):421–3.
41. DeCamp M, Tilburt JC. Why we cannot trust artificial intelligence in medicine. Lancet Digit Health 2019;1(8):e390.
42. Hatherley JJ. Limits of trust in medical AI. J Med Ethics 2020;46(7):478–81.
43. Matheny ME, Whicher D, Thadaney Israni S. Artificial intelligence in health care: a report from the national Academy of medicine. JAMA 2020;323(6):509–10.
44. Kerasidou CX, Kerasidou A, Buscher M, et al. Before and beyond trust: reliance in medical AI. J Med Ethics 2022;48(11):852–6.

45. Richardson JE, Middleton B, Platt JE, et al. Building and maintaining trust in clinical decision support: recommendations from the Patient-Centered CDS Learning Network. Learn Health Syst 2020;4(2):e10208.
46. Roski J, Maier EJ, Vigilante K, et al. Enhancing trust in AI through industry self-governance. J Am Med Inform Assoc 2021;28(7):1582–90.
47. Rojas JC, Rohweder G, Guptill J, et al. Predictive analytics programs at large healthcare systems in the USA: a national survey. J Gen Intern Med 2022; 37(15):4015–7. https://doi.org/10.1007/s11606-022-07517-1.
48. Rojas JC, Fahrenbach J, Makhni S, et al. Framework for integrating equity into machine learning models: a case study. Chest 2022;161(6):1621–7.
49. Weissman GE. FDA regulation of predictive clinical decision-support tools: what does it mean for hospitals? J Hosp Med 2021;16(4):244–6.
50. FDA. Clinical decision support software: guidance for industry and Food and Drug Administration Staff, Available at: https://www.fda.gov/regulatory-information/search-fda-guidance-documents/clinical-decision-support-software. Accessed December 29, 2022.
51. Wong A, Otles E, Donnelly JP, et al. External validation of a widely implemented Proprietary sepsis prediction model in hospitalized patients. JAMA Intern Med 2021;181(8):1065–70.
52. Quinn TP, Senadeera M, Jacobs S, et al. Trust and medical AI: the challenges we face and the expertise needed to overcome them. J Am Med Inform Assoc 2021; 28(4):890–4.
53. Sendak MP, Gao M, Brajer N, et al. Presenting machine learning model information to clinical end users with model facts labels. NPJ Digit Med 2020;3:41.
54. Osheroff JA, Teich JM, Levick D, et al. Improving outcomes with clinical decision support: an implementer's guide, HIMSS Publishing, 2nd edition, 2012, Chicago, IL.

Bioethical Dilemmas with Data Science in Critical Care

Implementing Artificial Intelligence

Assessing the Cost and Benefits of Algorithmic Decision-Making in Critical Care

Pier Francesco Caruso, MD[a,b], Massimiliano Greco, MD[a,b],*,
Claudia Ebm, MD[a], Giovanni Angelotti, MSc[c],
Maurizio Cecconi, MD[a,b]

KEYWORDS

• Artificial intelligence • Algorithmic decision-making • Cost and benefit • Critical care
• Intensive care unit

KEY POINTS

• The exponentially increasing quantity and quality of clinical data in intensive care units is a major driver to effectively develop artificial intelligence (AI) algorithms.
• Artificial Intelligence implementation will support clinicians in the decision-making processes. Benefits comprehend earlier diagnoses, detection of subclinical deteriorations and generation of new medical knowledge.
• Healthcare providers need to guarantee digital infrastructures, protection to patients' data, and the introduction of data scientists alongside the clinical personnel.
• Healthcare workers will always play a crucial role, but AI algorithms will provide new methods to increase the quality of care.

INTRODUCTION

Mortality in critically ill patients decreased over the last decades and standards of care are constantly evolving to achieve further reductions.[1] Despite these progressions, critical care practices still have room for improvement in comprehension of patient acuity, in addressing the heterogeneity of individual cases, and in providing early treatment strategies before clinical deterioration.[2]

[a] Department of Biomedical Sciences, Humanitas University, Via Rita Levi Montalcini 4, Pieve Emanuele, Milan 20072, Italy; [b] Department of Anesthesiology and Intensive Care, IRCCS Humanitas Research Hospital, Via Manzoni 56, Rozzano, Milan 20089, Italy; [c] Artificial Intelligence Center, IRCCS Humanitas Research Hospital, Via Manzoni 56, Rozzano, Milan 20089, Italy
* Corresponding author. Department of Anesthesiology and Intensive Care, IRCCS Humanitas Research Hospital, Via Manzoni 56, Rozzano, Milan 20089, Italy.
E-mail address: massimiliano.greco@hunimed.eu

Crit Care Clin 39 (2023) 783–793
https://doi.org/10.1016/j.ccc.2023.03.007
criticalcare.theclinics.com

In the last decade, intensive care units (ICUs), with the assistance of health care providers, gathered a growing quantity of clinical data, and this enormous source of information is resulting in a more organized availability, albeit one that is frequently underused. Simultaneously, with the exponentially increasing computational power, new research methods based on artificial intelligence (AI) have been developed.

AI is a field of studies on computer systems able to perform automatically tasks that normally require human intelligence, such as visual perception, speech recognition, decision-making, and translation between languages.[3] The AI breakthrough switched the paradigm from traditional programming, where a programmer needed to formulate or code rules manually, to a new data-driven approach where an algorithm automatically formulates rules, and assesses characteristics and relationships from data.[4]

Consequently, researchers were allowed to explore new relationships and patterns in complex diseases, such as sepsis and septic shock, where several papers have demonstrated a possible increase in timing and quality of diagnosis.[5] Clinical decision support systems (CDSS) have the potential to be the next step by supporting the health care providers to make more informed, accurate, and efficient decisions.[6,7] Especially in critical care, where patients' lives are at stake, AI can help to improve patients' outcomes and reduce health care costs. Nevertheless, implementation of AI algorithms in clinical practice is a slow and careful process that must reduce disparities and inequalities while providing better quality of care to patients.[8]

In this review, we provide an overview of the most useful AI algorithms developed in critical care, followed by a comprehensive outline of the benefits and limitations: starting bedside, we begin by describing how nurses and physicians might be aided by these new technologies that can monitor patients 24 hours per day. We then move to the possible changes in clinical guidelines with personalized medicine that will allow tailored therapies and probably will increase the quality of the care provided to patients. Finally, we describe how AI models can unleash researchers' minds by proposing new strategies, by increasing the quality of clinical practice, and by questioning current knowledge and understanding.

ARTIFICIAL INTELLIGENCE APPLICATIONS IN CRITICAL CARE

Modern medicine is able to generate enormous amount of data, especially when considering the critical care setting. Monitors with dozens of waveforms, ventilators, renal-replacement therapy devices, and syringe-pumps incessantly generate high-resolution data for each patient admitted to the ICU.[4]

In recent years, several applications have been developed to aid physicians in critical care, on the diagnostics and on the therapeutic side. Some of these are complex; however, the first step that we should consider in this article is how data visualization techniques can be used to summarize and make a large quantity of data interpretable for humans, data that would otherwise be lost. We previously described how heatmaps can be used to summarize vital data across multiple wards, thereby depicting a multidimensional space in a single figure.[9] These strategies are part of what is known as multidimensional scaling, a technique that depicts data as points in a multidimensional space to convey similarity between objects as spatial distance (ie, similar data are represented as close data). Consequently, multidimensional scaling lowers a dataset with a large number of dimensions to a two- or three-dimensional image, enabling the detection of similarities that may not otherwise be readable by humans. The benefits can be applied to phenotyping and precision medicine, which has been an increasingly significant objective in recent years. Latent class analysis is another type of algorithm that has been proposed to identify subgroups of patients with sepsis at risk of mortality.[10,11] The combination of different algorithms is promising too (eg, principal component analysis followed by unsupervised hierarchical clustering were proposed to identify clinically distinct phenotypes of trauma patients based on their systemic inflammatory response).[12]

AI techniques have also been used to combine large public databases of environmental and mobility data with clinical data, a valuable option in the context of the COVID pandemic.[13] AI algorithms can also be useful in COVID-19 to identify early predictors of patient outcomes from emergency and operational data from regional health care networks, hence enhancing ICU resource use throughout the pandemic's surge phases.[14]

Waveform analysis is another fascinating possibility, especially for critical care. AI may be useful for assessing data from waveform analysis, a task previously performed primarily by physicians and requiring specialized knowledge. For instance, AI has been proposed to automatically detect seizures through continuous electroencephalography waveform analysis, a challenging process that normally requires substantial training.[15]

Numerous apps have been created to assist physicians in interpreting radiologic images and in stratifying patients by combining clinical and radiologic data, hence assisting doctors in prognostication and in clinical decisions. For instance, data from MRI of patients with severe traumatic brain injury may be used for early definition of 12-month patient prognosis.[16] The integration between clinical data and radiologic images can be taken further, to build a CDSS for specific patient subtypes. CDSS are computer-based systems that aid clinicians' decision-making by providing them high-quality information they need to make informed choices. AI can be used to evaluate computed tomography scans of patients with ischemic stroke and integrate them with clinical data, to give a decision support system.[17] This may be effective in smaller centers with reduced resources, where expertise on stroke may not be readily available.

Computer vision can also be used to standardize patient monitoring in difficult-to-define conditions, such as delirium in the ICU. In a recent research, computer vision and AI were used to detect patient facial expressions and movements, and evaluate light and noise levels in the environment, to assess and monitor delirium in ICUs, a task previously performed by clinical staff only.[18]

Will AI ever be capable of providing patient care? In a landmark article on patients with sepsis, AI was trained through deep reinforcement learning (RL) to identify data patterns and suggest treatment strategies that were found to be effective in improving patient outcomes. The study showed that the trained algorithm, named the AI physician, was able to recommend treatment strategies that were similar to those recommended by human experts, and that the use of the algorithm could lead to improved patient outcomes.[19] Despite some interesting data, actual clinical data on the use of AI as support for patient therapy are lacking, and this possibility still needs further verification.

Finally, AI can be applied to scientific education and dissemination: we challenged an AI program capable of generating images from textual description, and we requested the AI to "display an intensive care physician at bedside of a monitored and ventilated patient in the intensive care unit, using a computer to analyze waveforms and take decisions." The results reported in **Fig. 1** were created using Midjourney (https://midjourney.com). Although suboptimal in some details, these images were obtained in a few seconds and completely free of costs. One small step for us as authors, a giant leap for science dissemination.

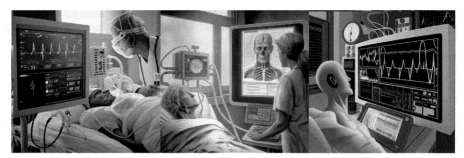

Fig. 1. Three AI-created images of a physician in intensive care, analyzing waveforms with the help of a computer. (Created using Midjourney (https://midjourney.com).)

BENEFITS

As shown by the possible applications, the benefits of AI in critical care might be disruptive. As seen in the next paragraphs, AI has the potential to increase the accuracy of diagnosis and care delivery: an early detection reduces the risk of clinical deterioration because diseases are treated preventively and not reactively, resulting in a better clinical outcome, reduced number of complications, and a shorter length of stay, whereas a tailored therapeutic strategy improves quality of care provided, reduces unnecessary side effects, and might reduce therapy escalation. AI might be beneficial to health care spending by reducing inefficiencies, waste, and cost while, at the same time, increasing the quality of care.[20]

Improving Clinical Outcomes and Precision Medicine

Roggeveen and colleagues[21] recently published the results of a two-center randomized clinical trial evaluating a model named AutoKinetics (performing bedside real-time antibiotics dosing) against standard care in patients with sepsis and septic shock. Unfortunately, the trial was stopped early because of the COVID-19 pandemic, but the results concluded that a CDSS for precision dosing for antibiotics is feasible, safe, and can improve dosing in patients with sepsis and septic shock. In addition, the doses of ciprofloxacin suggested by AutoKinetics to attain the pharmacokinetic target were significantly higher than standard care, in particular in the first 24 hours after randomization, suggesting bigger loading dosages to attain the concentration required at infections sites more rapidly. Because the AutoKinetics model was a CDSS, the doses suggested by the algorithm were validated by a clinical team, which rejected the AI output in less than 2% of cases only.

Precision medicine is defined as an individualized approach to every patient based on genetic, physiologic, and/or environmental information. The goal is to provide personalized targeted treatments for each patient, rather than a one-size-fits-all approach, leading to better outcomes at reduced health care costs. Although precision medicine originally developed in oncology, where cancer genetics analyses allowed tailored treatments, resulting in better patients' outcomes,[22] in recent years there were also important advances in intensive care where researchers identified promising genetic components in several common conditions affecting ICU patients. Hernández-Beeftink and coworkers[23] summarized more than 10 genomic approaches in acute respiratory distress syndrome that are currently under study (eg, genome-wide association studies and transcriptomics). The main goal is to better identify susceptible populations, and/or identify subgroups at increased risk of mortality. In addition to the complexity of these new techniques, which are now helped by AI-technologies, there is a more complex role of genetic, proteomic, or metabolomic tests in critical care, because clinical conditions are rapidly evolving and heterogeneous (eg, patient physiology might change dramatically within a few hours). Thus, these tests also need to be fast, repeatable, and cost-effective.[24]

Oncology showed the importance of multidisciplinary teams to achieve precision medicine.[25] In contrast, ICUs have an abundancy of physiologic data ranging from multiparametric monitors to ventilator settings that are still understudied and might have not revealed their clinical potential yet. A close collaboration among clinicians, pharmacologists, biologists, and biotechnologists is required to achieve prognosis-changing results, and this approach is starting to be introduced in some ICUs. In these units, clinicians have started to collaborate with data scientists, statisticians, and engineers specialized in analysis of signals, waveforms, and clinical data, to achieve new and personalized levels of care.[26]

Continuous Surveillance

Butler and colleagues[27] measured that, during daytime, physicians in the ICU spend less than 20% of their shift within patients' rooms, whereas for nurses the percentage sets lower than 35%. Physicians spend more than twice as much of their time in the work room to write electronic health records, to plan examinations, to review documentation, and to discuss clinical cases among colleagues. In a multicenter observational study involving eight different ICUs, Neuraz and colleagues[28] showed that mortality risk was increased when the patient-to-physician ratio exceeded 14, and when the patient-to-nurse ratio was greater than 2.5. The highest ratios discrepancy occurred during the weekends for nurses and during nights shift for physicians.

At the same time, most ICU patients are continuously monitored by multiparametric machines that gather data about their health condition across the whole hospitalization period. Checking all those data is time consuming and health care personnel do not have the feasible time to validate all of them, apart from very few moments at bedside observing the clinical monitor and ventilator's data and waveforms. But an AI-algorithm is an ideal solution to continuously filter which data are most valuable for the decision-making process. An AI-solution might also alert the health care personnel in case some specific threshold, maybe tailored to the specific patient, is reached (eg, increased risk of clinical decompensation). A hypothetical CDSS focused on continuous surveillance would not substitute the physicians in the decision-making process, but it would act as an extra eye on the patient that might also help in distributing the attention and the time of the health care personnel by highlighting patients at increased risk and by selecting informative data to faster acknowledge the actual clinical condition. A possible application of CDSS in clinical practice is reported in **Fig. 2**.

Generating Knowledge: Artificial Intelligence Suggesting Hypotheses or New Possible Strategies

One of the pillars in AI-research in intensive care is represented by the AI clinician by Komorowski and colleagues.[29] RL is a special class of algorithm family that optimized the treatment strategies for sepsis. More specifically, RL models are based on "agents" that can perform a set of actions defined by the researcher within a simulated environment. In this specific case, the group created a simulated environment based on a database of anonymized patients (MIMIC-III[30]) and asked the model to learn the best combination of vasopressors and intravenous fluids dose. Without furthering too much into technical details, the model, through cycles of simulations (in the training phase), tries to find the optimal combination of actions (in the optimization of the

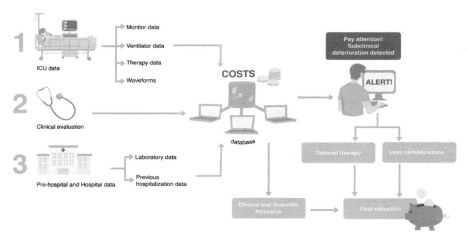

Fig. 2. Implementation of AI: different data sources need to be integrated in a centralized database. After that, AI models are tested and deployed to deliver medical value. In this example a subclinical, otherwise unnoticed, deterioration is detected by an AI algorithm. In addition, the data are resourceful for researchers to increase quality of care for patients.

reward function) to decrease the mortality of the analyzed patients. In a final step it was tested on new patients that were never presented to the model and compared its strategy and results with the clinical strategy and results actually achieved by clinicians.

RL models have an enormous potential in medicine: imagine having a playground where researchers can safely test new and different strategies or develop AI models that might hint at strategies that were never thought about. It might sound futuristic, but it has already happened in other fields, such as in a chess game where RL models developed new strategies that were studied and integrated by human players too.

On the opposite side, RL models have several limitations: in the simulated environment, representations of the natural history of patients with sepsis are not depicted, because no hospitalized patients in an ICU follow the natural history of the disease without prompt clinical intervention. Accordingly, the model needs to recreate those extreme situations based on bits of reality (eg, delay in antimicrobial therapy), and this might lead to incorrect representations. Similarly, when an agent opts for a different strategy, the clinical evolution in the simulation might differ from reality, even if it cannot be tested retrospectively. Referring to the cited paper, the vasopressor strategy chosen by AI was more aggressive than that of physicians (physicians administered fewer vasopressors 75% of the times). Similarly, in only one-third of cases did doctors and AI prescribe the same volume of fluids. In the remaining cases, the volume of fluid delivered was evenly distributed between greater and lesser amounts. Independently from the precision medicine aspect, because doses were tailored for each patient according to their specific physiology, this article elucidated another pivotal benefit of AI: instill doubt and give new insights to clinical experts. An AI algorithm questioned our vasopressor strategy: should we consider a more aggressive approach? Can we integrate in the algorithm design why we think the model is wrong in the simulated environment so that it can be trained again and propose a new strategy?

CHALLENGES

The economic challenge to implement AI algorithms in clinical practice is still unclear and impossible to anticipate. Costs will increase in the initial years of implementation, and then progressively balance as more efficient and tailored treatments are delivered. The early expenses involve structural organization to create a safe and functional information technology system where patients' privacy is protected according to laws, one of the fundamental limits to current AI application in several countries. Once the data infrastructure is up and running, AI algorithms can be enclosed in the system. Except for technical and organizational costs for implementing, maintaining, and updating the information technology system, expenses should be related to the education of the health care personnel: it requires time to train health care professionals to work side-by-side with data scientists to effectively implement these new technologies and to have them trusted by all stakeholders.[31,32]

Costs in Hospital Settings and Critical Care

Implementation of AI models in clinical practice might present high initial costs, a barrier to implementation in smaller centers or in low- and middle-income countries. Collection of data streams from medical devices might result in expensive processes that could potentially exclude many health systems, impeding data collection and deployment of AI systems in these low resource settings.[33]

The volume of data is rapidly exploding as the granularity and the quality of machines that support data extraction are increasing at a fast pace, thus a tradeoff between quality and quantity is a central point in discussions. National health systems investments in AI might vary widely. The richest systems are interested in investing in these new technologies, because the quality of their health care providers is sufficiently good, but for low- and middle-income countries the same reasoning might not hold true. This might result in the development of algorithms based on technologically biased datasets developed using data from some countries only, thus leading to inequality of care in the hospitalized population. Algorithms' transparency, defined as availability in sharing the code from design documentation to deployment, is consequently a pivotal aspect for implementation: it does not necessarily imply public disclosure of software and it can be limited to specific actors, such as for audit or certification. AI algorithms need to be guaranteed as every other clinical device in health care: the responsibility of influencing decision makers, such as physicians and nurses, is a crucial role that cannot be ignored. The role of algorithmic decision-making was the central topic of a recent paper published by the European Parliament Research Service[34]: the study reviewed opportunities and risks in every sector involved in algorithmic decision systems, focusing on technical, legal, ethical, and social aspects of AI.

Data Protection, Ownership, and Cybersecurity

The European Data Protection Supervisor defined health care in the General Data Protection Regulation as a special data category that required specific protection measures. Privacy by design and prohibition of discriminatory profiling remain a cornerstone in health data, with the addition of special safeguards for personal health data addressed by the new innovative principles of the General Data Protection Regulation.[34,35]

In 2021, the World Health Organization released guidelines on ethics and governance of AI for health, underlining the pivotal roles of privacy, transparency, informed consent, and regulation of the data protection frameworks.[36] In general, an individual should always be able to control their personal data but, specifically for health care, regulations and control must be tight. Currently, the value generated by big data is largely beneficial for researchers that adhere to data protection regulations. Because data are ubiquitously collected from many different sources that were unthinkable 20 years ago (eg, monitors, sensors, wearables), it is clear that data protection and ownership should be addressed by methods and processes able to handle every major concern.[37]

The importance of cybersecurity, a computer science field specialized in identifying and preventing criminal use of electronic data, cannot be underestimated. A malicious actor could always perform a criminal attack to steal or manipulate clinical data, or to change the decision-making algorithms. For example, a specific typology of cyberattacks, called adversarial attacks, modify clinical data in an imperceptible way to human eyes, but those specific patterns could force the AI system to make incorrect diagnoses.[38] Mirsky and colleagues[39] demonstrated that an attacker could modify a full-resolution three-dimensional computed tomography scan by introducing or removing a malignant mass in the lung parenchyma. These types of problems are independent from AI models, because they have existed since the introduction of computers, but the complexity of systems involving computer-based strategies is increasing, requiring specialized personnel to create secure systems and to prevent malicious interventions.

Filling the Translational Gap from Technical Knowledge to Solid Trust

Implementation of AI algorithms requires the acknowledgment of new specific terminologies that are already positively contaminating the medical literature as the conjunction between medicine and data science proceeds.[4,7,37,40] Medical universities are introducing lectures and courses on these topics to answers the needs expressed by students, to better understand the AI world.[41] However, familiarity with metrics and types of models is only a part of the educational process; the whole relationship between application and users must be carefully considered. At the end of the 1990s, the most common concerns raised around AI were linked to a general distrust: applications do not actually save time, the quality of algorithmic outputs is too low, or they require too much time in critical and time-sensitive circumstances.[42] Twenty-five years later, these problems are under the spotlight, because a more complete analysis of the relationship between AI and human beings is desirable for the effective use of AI in medicine. The digital experience of physicians and nurses is pivotal, and researchers are now understanding it: successful AI applications must be practical, fast, and easy-to-use. Principles of statistics, linear algebra, and model design will guarantee a competitive advantage to health care workers, because they would be more grounded in the technology per se, and more confident in acknowledging its benefits and limitations.[43] In addition, involvement of health care personnel in developing new AI algorithms is contributing to vanquish the distrust and frustration that have been often ignored while implementing informatics technologies.[44] Finally, clinicians will always play a crucial role in the digital world, serving as a safety net whenever these technologies fail,[45] and, most importantly, emotionally assisting ill patients to make complex, uncertain, and personal decisions because it requires a profound connection among human beings that cannot be replicated by AI technology.

SUMMARY

Implementation of AI algorithms will support clinicians in the decision-making processes in critical care. The amount of data acquired in ICUs will keep increasing steeply and will require systematic processes and methods to organize information efficiently and effectively. Continuous surveillance, precision medicine, and advances in clinical research are potentially disruptors of clinical practice that might lead to better care at a reduced cost. Despite all the challenges present today, the potential benefits outweigh the initial and maintenance costs. Still, case-by-case perspectives should be performed to assess the effective advantages in clinical practice. The collaboration among health care providers, professionals, patients, and researchers is essential to create a transparent environment where these new technologies can be robustly developed and safely tested. Finally, physicians and nurses will need to learn how to use the AI algorithms but will not be replaced by them. In reverse, the health care personnel will have more time to deepen the emotional connection with patients and their family, and to better understand their psychological and social perspective, resulting in a further gain in quality of care.

REFERENCES

1. Zimmerman JE, Kramer AA, Knaus WA. Changes in hospital mortality for United States intensive care unit admissions from 1988 to 2012. Crit Care 2013;17(2). https://doi.org/10.1186/cc12695.
2. Gutierrez G. Artificial Intelligence in the Intensive Care Unit. Crit Care 2020; 24(1):101.
3. Knowles E. The Oxford dictionary of phrase and fable. Oxford University Press; 2006. https://doi.org/10.1093/acref/9780198609810.001.0001.
4. Greco M, Caruso PF, Cecconi M. Artificial intelligence in the intensive care unit. Semin Respir Crit Care Med 2021;42(1):2–9.
5. Fleuren LM, Klausch TLT, Zwager CL, et al. Machine learning for the prediction of sepsis : a systematic review and meta-analysis of diagnostic test accuracy. Intensive Care Med 2020;46(3):383–400.
6. Lysaght T, Lim HY, Xafis V, et al. AI-assisted decision-making in healthcare: the application of an ethics framework for big data in health and research. Asian Bioeth Rev 2019;11(3):299–314.
7. MONTOMOLI J, HILTY MP, INCE C. Artificial intelligence in intensive care: moving towards clinical decision support systems. Minerva Anestesiol 2022. https://doi.org/10.23736/s0375-9393.22.16739-8.
8. Fleuren LM, Thoral P, Shillan D, et al. Machine learning in intensive care medicine: ready for take-off. Intensive Care Med 2020. https://doi.org/10.1007/s00134-020-06045-y.
9. Caruso PF, Angelotti G, Greco M, et al. The effect of COVID-19 epidemic on vital signs in hospitalized patients: a pre-post heat-map study from a large teaching hospital. J Clin Monit Comput 2022;36(3):829–37.
10. Soussi S, Sharma D, Jüni P, et al. Identifying clinical subtypes in sepsis-survivors with different one-year outcomes: a secondary latent class analysis of the FROG-ICU cohort. Crit Care 2022;26(1). https://doi.org/10.1186/S13054-022-03972-8.
11. Dahmer MK, Yang G, Zhang M, et al. Identification of phenotypes in paediatric patients with acute respiratory distress syndrome: a latent class analysis. Lancet Respir Med 2022;10(3):289–97.
12. Schimunek L, Lindberg H, Cohen M, et al. Computational derivation of core, dynamic human blunt trauma inflammatory endotypes. Front Immunol 2021;11. https://doi.org/10.3389/FIMMU.2020.589304.
13. Caruso PF, Angelotti G, Greco M, et al. Early prediction of SARS-CoV-2 reproductive number from environmental, atmospheric and mobility data: a supervised

machine learning approach. Int J Med Inf 2022;162. https://doi.org/10.1016/J.IJMEDINF.2022.104755.

14. Greco M, Angelotti G, Caruso PF, et al. Outcome prediction during an ICU surge using a purely data-driven approach: a supervised machine learning case-study in critically ill patients from COVID-19 Lombardy outbreak. Int J Med Inform 2022; 164:104807.

15. Fergus P, Hignett D, Hussain A, et al. Automatic epileptic seizure detection using scalp EEG and advanced artificial intelligence techniques. BioMed Res Int 2015; 2015. https://doi.org/10.1155/2015/986736.

16. Puybasset L, Perlbarg V, Unrug J, et al. Prognostic value of global deep white matter DTI metrics for 1-year outcome prediction in ICU traumatic brain injury patients: an MRI-COMA and CENTER-TBI combined study. Intensive Care Med 2022;48(2):201–12.

17. Bivard A, Churilov L, Parsons M. Artificial intelligence for decision support in acute stroke: current roles and potential. Nat Rev Neurol 2020;16(10):575–85.

18. Davoudi A, Malhotra KR, Shickel B, et al. Intelligent ICU for autonomous patient monitoring using pervasive sensing and deep learning. Sci Rep 2019;9(1). https://doi.org/10.1038/S41598-019-44004-W.

19. Liu S, See KC, NKY and CLA and SX and FM. Reinforcement learning for clinical decision support in critical care: comprehensive review. J Med Internet Res 2020; 22(7):e18477.

20. Lewkowicz D, Wohlbrandt A, Boettinger E. Economic impact of clinical decision support interventions based on electronic health records. BMC Health Serv Res 2020;20(1). https://doi.org/10.1186/s12913-020-05688-3.

21. Roggeveen LF, Guo T, Fleuren LM, et al. Right dose, right now: bedside, real-time, data-driven, and personalised antibiotic dosing in critically ill patients with sepsis or septic shock: a two-centre randomised clinical trial. Crit Care 2022; 26(1). https://doi.org/10.1186/s13054-022-04098-7.

22. Krzyszczyk P, Acevedo A, Davidoff EJ, et al. The growing role of precision and personalized medicine for cancer treatment HHS Public Access. Technology (Singap World Sci) 2018;6(4):79–100.

23. Hernández-Beeftink T, Guillen-Guio B, Villar J, et al. Genomics and the acute respiratory distress syndrome: current and future directions. Int J Mol Sci 2019; 20(16). https://doi.org/10.3390/ijms20164004.

24. Vincent JL. The coming era of precision medicine for intensive care. Crit Care 2017;21. https://doi.org/10.1186/s13054-017-1910-z.

25. Mateo J, Steuten L, Aftimos P, et al. Delivering precision oncology to patients with cancer. Nat Med 2022;28(4):658–65.

26. Tang R, Zhang S, Ding C, et al. Artificial intelligence in intensive care medicine: bibliometric analysis (Preprint). J Med Internet Res 2022. https://doi.org/10.2196/42185.

27. Butler R, Monsalve M, Thomas GW, et al. Estimating time physicians and other health care workers spend with patients in an intensive care unit using a sensor network. Am J Med 2018;131(8). 972.e9-972.e15.

28. Neuraz A, Guérin C, Payet C, et al. Patient Mortality Is Associated With Staff Resources and Workload in the ICU: A Multicenter Observational Study. Crit Care Med 2015;43(8):1587–94.

29. Komorowski M, Celi LA, Badawi O, et al. The artificial intelligence clinician learns optimal treatment strategies for sepsis in intensive care. Nat Med 2018;24(11): 1716–20.

30. Johnson AEW, Pollard TJ, Shen L, et al. MIMIC-III, a freely accessible critical care database. Sci Data 2016;3. https://doi.org/10.1038/sdata.2016.35.
31. Komorowski M. Clinical management of sepsis can be improved by artificial intelligence: yes. Intensive Care Med 2020;46:375–7.
32. Garnacho-Montero J, Martín-Loeches I. Clinical management of sepsis can be improved by artificial intelligence: no. Intensive Care Med 2020;46:378–80.
33. Rajpurkar P, Chen E, Banerjee O, et al. AI in health and medicine. Nat Med 2022; 28(1):31–8.
34. Castelluccia Claude, le Métayer Daniel, European Parliament. European Parliamentary Research Service. Scientific Foresight Unit. Understanding Algorithmic Decision-Making : Opportunities and Challenges. Available at: https://www.europarl.europa.eu/RegData/etudes/STUD/2019/624261/EPRS_STU(2019) 624261_EN.pdf. Accessed January 27, 2023.
35. Available at: https://edps.europa.eu/data-protection/our-work/subjects/health_ en. Accessed January 27, 2023.
36. Ethics and governance of artificial intelligence for health ethics and governance of artificial intelligence for health 2.; 2021. Available at: http://apps.who.int/ bookorders. Accessed January 27, 2023.
37. Ghassemi M, Celi LA, Stone DJ. State of the art review: the data revolution in critical care. Crit Care 2015;19(1). https://doi.org/10.1186/s13054-015-0801-4.
38. Finlayson SG, Bowers JD, Ito J, et al. Adversarial attacks on medical machine learning. Science (1979) 2019;363(6433):1287–9.
39. Mirsky Y, Mahler T, Shelef I, et al: Malicious tampering of 3D medical imagery using deep learning, 2019. Available at: http://arxiv.org/abs/1901.03597. Accessed January 27, 2023.
40. Topol EJ. High-performance medicine: the convergence of human and artificial intelligence. Nat Med 2019;25(1):44–56.
41. Civaner MM, Uncu Y, Bulut F, et al. Artificial intelligence in medical education: a cross-sectional needs assessment. BMC Med Educ 2022;22(1). https://doi.org/ 10.1186/s12909-022-03852-3.
42. Lillehaug SI, Lajoie SP. AI in medical education: another grand challenge for medical informatics. Artif Intell Med 1998;12(3):197–225.
43. Coiera E. The fate of medicine in the time of AI. Lancet 2018;392(10162):2331–2.
44. Friedberg MW, Chen PG, van Busum KR, et al. Factors affecting physician professional satisfaction and their implications for patient care, health systems, and health policy. Available at: www.rand.org. Accessed January 27, 2023.
45. Kim MO, Coiera E, Magrabi F. Problems with health information technology and their effects on care delivery and patient outcomes: a systematic review. J Am Med Inform Assoc 2017;24(2):246–50.

Critical Bias in Critical Care Devices

Marie-Laure Charpignon, MSc[a],*, Joseph Byers[b], Stephanie Cabral, MD[c],
Leo Anthony Celi, MD, MSc, MPH[d,e,f], Chrystinne Fernandes, PhD[d], Jack Gallifant[g],
Mary E. Lough, PhD, RN, CCNS, FCCM, FAHA, FCNS, FAAN[h], Donald Mlombwa[i,j,k],
Lama Moukheiber, MSc[l], Bradley Ashley Ong, MD[m], Anupol Panitchote, MD[n],
Wasswa William[o], An-Kwok Ian Wong, MD, PhD[p], Lama Nazer, PharmD, BCPS, FCCM[q]

KEYWORDS

• Artificial intelligence • Bias • Medical devices • Critical care

Continued

INTRODUCTION

Critical care data reflect the most physiologically unstable patients in a hospital. These patients are heavily monitored and may undergo complex treatment regimens to manage multiple organ failure. The intensive care unit (ICU) demands a rich volume of information continuously collected from the patient so that physicians can decide on immediate interventions and clinical responses to be measured, possibly triggering

---

All authors contributed equally to the article.
[a] Institute for Data, Systems, and Society (IDSS), E18-407A, 50 Ames Street, Cambridge, MA 02142, USA; [b] Respiratory Therapy, Beth Israel Deaconess Medical Center, 330 Brookline Avenue, Boston, MA 02215, USA; [c] Department of Medicine, Beth Israel Deaconess Medical Center, 330 Brookline Avenue, Boston, MA 02215, USA; [d] Laboratory for Computational Physiology, Massachusetts Institute of Technology, 77 Massachusetts Avenue, Cambridge, MA 02139, USA; [e] Division of Pulmonary, Critical Care and Sleep Medicine, Beth Israel Deaconess Medical Center, Boston, MA, USA; [f] Department of Biostatistics, Harvard T.H. Chan School of Public Health, Boston, MA, USA; [g] Imperial College London NHS Trust, St Thomas' Hospital, Westminster Bridge Road, London SE1 7EH, UK; [h] Stanford Health Care, Stanford University, 300 Pasteur Drive, Stanford, CA 94305, USA; [i] Zomba Central Hospital, 8th Avenue, Zomba, Malawi; [j] Kamuzu College of Health Sciences, Blantyre, Malawi; [k] St. Luke's College of Health Sciences, Chilema-Zomba, Malawi; [l] Institute for Medical Engineering and Science, Massachusetts Institute of Technology, 77 Massachusetts Avenue, E25-330, Cambridge, MA 02139, USA; [m] College of Medicine, University of the Philippines Manila, Calderon hall, UP College of Medicine, 547 Pedro Gil Street, Ermita Manila, Philippines; [n] Faculty of Medicine, Khon Kaen University, 123 Mittraparp Highway, Muang District, Khon Kaen 40002, Thailand; [o] Mbarara University of Science and Technology, P.O. Box 1410, Mbarara, Uganda; [p] Duke University Medical Center, 2424 Erwin Road, Suite 1102, Hock Plaza Box 2721, Durham, NC 27710, USA; [q] King Hussein Cancer Center, Queen Rania Street 202, Amman, Jordan
* Corresponding author. Institute for Data, Systems, and Society (IDSS), E18-407A, 50 Ames Street, Cambridge, MA 02142.
E-mail address: mcharpig@mit.edu

Crit Care Clin 39 (2023) 795–813
https://doi.org/10.1016/j.ccc.2023.02.005
0749-0704/23/© 2023 Elsevier Inc. All rights reserved.

criticalcare.theclinics.com

Continued

KEY POINTS

- The continuous and automated capture of physiologic information in the intensive care unit produces high-resolution and large-scale electronic health record datasets. Although this wealth of data can enable widespread data-driven applications in critical care, the generalizability of models trained on clinical data may be limited in part by inherent short-comings in the measurements generated by medical devices, differences in device and data access, and bias in data acquisition and measurement practices.
- Differences in the performance of medical devices can encode biases in clinical data that artificial intelligence may perpetuate, where measurement bias in one hospital's dataset can propagate to other health systems if models are inappropriately deployed.
- Prior studies have demonstrated the differential calibration of commonly used medical devices, such as pulse oximeters, thermometers, and sphygmomanometers, among patient subpopulations.
- Greater transparency regarding data collection, improved regulation of medical devices, increased sharing of clinical data, and improved data annotation are all necessary to identify and mitigate measurement bias in health care.

adjustments to existing treatment plans. In particular, clinical responses are obtained through repeated measurements of vital signs and laboratory results. Although also commonly measured elsewhere in the hospital, these signals are available at a much greater frequency in the ICU. Current practice and guidance rely heavily on various types of data generated by advanced medical technologies such as electro-cardiography (ECG) and electroencephalography (EEG). However, the clinical pictures these data paint are often framed by the methods used to measure patients' physiology.

In the twentieth century, physicists encountered a similar problem wherein the process of measuring quantum states seemed to affect observed classical results.[1–3] This finding created a paradigm shift best coined by Werner Heisenberg: "what we observe is not nature herself, but nature exposed to our method of questioning".[4] In critical care, the increased sophistication of medical technology and ease of measuring clinical signs with high frequency have resulted in an overreliance on medical devices and excessive trust in their outputs. Students and trainees no longer learn the physical principles underlying the measurement processes embedded in medical devices; they just learn how to use them. The measurement process has thus become a black box, where inputs are selected by clinical teams, and outputs are sometimes trusted with limited evaluation of the intermediary steps.

The increased technological capabilities of modern medical devices can leave clinical teams blind to potential measurement biases affecting data collected in the ICU. Being aware of the contexts in which data are generated and understanding the pitfalls of data collection (eg, device miscalibration, insufficient diversity in patient samples, heterogeneity in patient monitoring frequency, or errors in data entry) are key to the development of predictive models that can effectively inform clinical care and practice.[5–7] Fairness in clinical algorithms is determined partly by the sufficient representation of patient subgroups and the overall quality of data used for model development. Although some post-hoc adjustments to the outputs of medical devices or clinical algorithms can be made, it is impossible to expect artificial intelligence (AI) to fully account for measurement biases after the fact. Therefore, we must examine the measurement processes underlying medical devices commonly used in the ICU and characterize potential sources of bias—from patient selection to measurement errors—that may affect critical care data before model development begins.

This paper provides an overview of the existing literature on biases from medical devices that are commonly used in the critical care setting and their clinical impact. In particular, the following patient measurements are discussed: oxygen saturation, body temperature, and blood pressure (**Fig. 1**). Furthermore, the authors explore common mistakes in patient selection, which can introduce bias that compounds with measurement inaccuracies before patient data reach the warehouse. Finally, they comment on the limitations of post-hoc calibration of medical devices and propose key principles for mitigating their biases and ultimately improving equity in health care delivery.

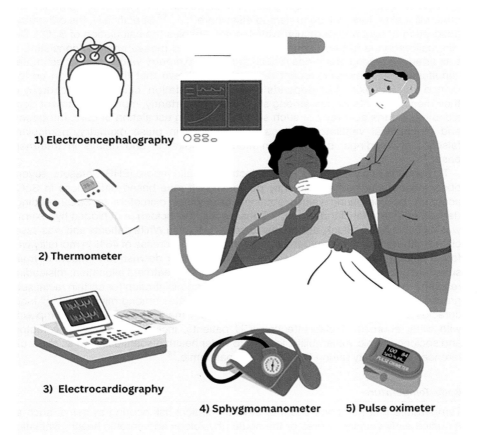

1) Electroencephalography

2) Thermometer

3) Electrocardiography

4) Sphygmomanometer   5) Pulse oximeter

Fig. 1. To inform clinical decision-making, the status of patients admitted to critical care units is frequently monitored through the following medical devices or techniques: (1) electroencephalography, (2) thermometers, (3) electrocardiography, (4) sphygmomanometers, and (5) pulse oximeters. All may suffer from measurement inaccuracies, which can compound with differences in sampling frequency and sociodemographic disparities. The article reviews previously documented discrepancies associated with medical device miscalibration for certain patient subpopulations.

CRITICAL MEASUREMENTS
Oxygen Saturation

Frequently measured peripheral oxygen saturations (SpO2) are essential to patient care in critical care settings and beyond. Although not as physiologically relevant in critical care as partial pressures of arterial oxygen, they offer a noninvasive and near-continuous evaluation of blood oxygenation.[8] First developed in 1972, pulse oximeters use the difference in red and near-infrared light absorption between oxygenated and deoxygenated hemoglobin to provide a mean saturation value.[9,10] This value can be calculated in real-time, thus providing clinical teams with an alarm signal indicating desaturation. The relative affordability of pulse oximeters, coupled with the ease of data collection, has made them staple measurements in critical care. Consequently, SpO2 has been incorporated into clinical guidelines worldwide since the 1990s.[11]

Pulse oximeters rely on the consistency of blood flow, the type of hemoglobin, and other clinical factors well documented elsewhere.[10,12,13] Specifically, the differential absorption of light at 2 particular wavelengths enables the calculation of SpO2. Device calibration is further accomplished using paired measurements, consisting of true arterial oxygen saturations (SaO2) and pulse oximetry values (SpO2) estimated simultaneously. However, recent research has shown that the calibration performance of pulse oximeters depends on skin pigmentation, causing the accuracy of their measurements to vary among skin tones. Importantly, multiple treatment decisions rely on the accuracy of such signals, including escalation of care, intubation, and mechanical ventilator settings. Inaccuracies in pulse oximetry, particularly falsely high readings, can result in hidden hypoxemia and delays in treatment onset.[14]

Through the analysis of large-scale electronic health record (EHR) datasets, several observational studies have recently demonstrated race-based differences in SpO2 accuracy by comparing values obtained from pulse oximeters to SaO2 readings derived from arterial blood gases.[15] Consistently, the incidence of hidden hypoxemia was higher in Asian, Black, and Hispanic patients than in White patients and was associated with worse patient outcomes.[14,16] Critically, an increase of 46% in mortality was found among patients with hidden hypoxemia.[14] Other downstream effects of measurement bias in pulse oximetry include differences in treatment allocation: misleading readings may result in less supplemental oxygen administration for certain racial subgroups, potentially contributing to higher mortality rates among minorities.[17,18] Inaccuracies in the key measurements obtained from medical devices can compound with other sources of bias affecting ICU patients, including demographic factors and socioeconomic vulnerability, leading to wider health disparities, such as racial differences in mortality during the COVID-19 pandemic.[19]

Body Temperature

Temperature is a key component of several medical risk scoring systems, such as modified early warning scores or the acute physiology and chronic health evaluation (APACHE) scores. These scores predict a patient's likelihood of deterioration and help guide treatment plans in clinical practice. Although methods used to measure body temperature vary across settings, institutions, and countries, core body temperature is often estimated via peripheral temperature measurements, through the use of oral, tympanic, axillary, and temporal artery thermometers.[20] Notably, cost-effective solutions are particularly needed in low- and middle-income countries[21-23]—for assessing body temperature and other vital signs alike.

Infrared technology used in temporal artery thermometers has yielded issues similar to the case of pulse oximetry: in Black patients, temporal measurements were significantly lower than oral temperature measurements. In contrast, this discrepancy was not present in White patients.[24] Such inaccuracy could delay the detection and treatment of infections if the clinician relies primarily on the measurement of temporal temperature—with a higher likelihood among darker-skinned individuals. This second example highlights the risks of miscalibration associated with medical tools relying on infrared technology to the detriment of populations with darker skin tones.

Notably, prior work suggests that discrepancies in body temperature assessment do not affect healthy subjects: using the Fitzpatrick system to categorize skin tone, one study reported no difference between temporal and oral temperature measurements in healthy volunteers.[25] This fact reinforces the importance of testing clinical devices across settings (eg, home, hospital, ICU) and in a wide variety of patient populations, as differences may appear only in specific settings or subgroups.

Sex-based differences in temperature measurements are also physiologically common, with significant variation in basal body temperature in women, which is affected by oral contraception and throughout the menstrual cycle.[26] Heterogeneity in baseline temperature is also evident among postmenopausal women on different hormone replacement therapy (HRT) regimes, as well as between women treated with HRT compared with those untreated.[27] These differences underscore the importance of considering inter- and within-group distributions when designing new thermometers, rather than relying solely on the "normal" temperature ranges attributed to the general population. The composition of groups used to determine "normal" ranges may itself suffer from selection bias. Because clinical decision-making often relies on thresholds for treatment escalation, these should be determined for specific subgroups based on the known information about differential measurement accuracy.

Blood Pressure

Blood pressure measurement via sphygmomanometers uses an inflatable cuff to temporarily occlude blood flow and measure the pressure level required to overcome this occlusion.[28] Varying performances in sphygmomanometers are acknowledged by the medical community, leading to the development of blood pressure cuffs in multiple sizes to account for patient size-based differences. However, the availability and use of appropriate cuff sizes vary across medical sites and clinicians, resulting in some patients being assessed with inappropriate cuffs, particularly those at the extremes of the weight scale. Using cuffs that are not tailored to the patient can amplify measurement bias. Inappropriate use of standard cuffs can lead to higher systolic readings than those obtained with larger and more appropriate cuffs, with discrepancies going over 9 mm Hg.[29,30] This issue can and has resulted in the inappropriate diagnosis of hypertension, with patients either not receiving the medications they need or being prescribed inappropriate treatments.[31] Notably, the reverse is also true, as inappropriately large cuffs can yield falsely lower values than those obtained with well-sized cuffs.[32]

In addition to standard blood pressure measurement with sphygmomanometers, invasive blood pressure monitoring—including arterial lines—may be available in critical care settings. Despite providing another potentially complementary source of information, invasive blood pressure monitoring is associated with increased complications and may be cost-prohibitive, particularly in low-resource settings.[33] Moreover, the budget and personnel needed to manage arterial lines may not be equally allocated within or across regions, thus contributing to unequal representation in patient data.

Electrocardiography and Electroencephalography

The issues of measurement bias and miscalibration are not unique to the medical devices described earlier. Other tools used in clinical practice and of foremost importance in critical care settings have shown differential performances across patient subgroups. Namely, miscalibrated ECG machines can underperform in obese populations, resulting in reduced sensitivity of abnormalities.[34] Similarly, the distance between EEG electrodes and the patient's scalp influences the quality of EEG signals. However, the adherence of electrodes depends on hair type and thickness, which varies across racial-ethnic subgroups and cultures. Commonly used electrodes may not stick as well to hair types of patients from the African diaspora compared with hair types present among White populations, resulting in increased noise on EEG traces.[35] These artifacts attest to the potential implications of a lack of consideration for human factors and inclusive design when manufacturing medical devices as well as downstream effects on clinical data quality.

Health Care Access, Device Allocation, and Measurement Frequency

The frequency of clinical measurements is positively associated with factors that increase patient complexity or illness severity, such as age, simplified acute physiology score, and comorbidities.[36] In addition to underlying heterogeneity in sampling frequency determined by the patient's clinical status, other factors such as biological sex, racial and ethnic origin, institution-specific policies, and geographic location can affect access to health care devices and the frequency of measurements. Inaccuracies in measurements derived from medical devices can also lead to differences in treatment allocation. Therefore, results from automated scoring systems should be interpreted critically.

A recent study evaluating *arterial catheter* use of 300,000 patients across 168 ICUs in the United States reported that these devices were less likely to be placed in women but more likely in Black patients—even after adjusting for age, comorbidities, and severity of illness.[37] In contrast, another study showed that *pulmonary artery catheters* were less likely to be placed in both Black patients and women when adjusting for similar variables.[38] These findings have several implications, including the differential frequency of observational data available to physicians for decision-making through continuous pressure readings and blood tests.

Inconsistencies in the patient subpopulations affected by selection or measurement bias are not uncommon. In fact, differences in ICU admission criteria across medical sites—whether intra- or internationally—may add to the variation in device availability and allocation.[39–41] For instance, a comparative study found that patients admitted to ICUs in the United States had much lower severity of illness at baseline than those admitted in the United Kingdom, which can be explained by the higher number of critical care beds available in the former.[40] Moreover, other aspects of ICU triage exhibit variability: determining when a patient is ready for discharge is a function of both local hospital guidelines and health care provider judgment.[42,43] Overall, these examples highlight how health care access, device allocation, and measurement frequency can influence which patients contribute to ICU datasets and the corresponding range of outcomes that algorithms trained on such cohorts can capture.

Differences in Health-Seeking Behavior and Clinical Practice Between Rural and Urban Academic Centers

Across the world, differences between rural and urban areas persist not only in the availability of medical technology at care centers but also in the health-seeking behavior of populations. These differences affect the management of both chronic and acute conditions. For example, although the proliferation of mHealth in China could be particularly useful to rural communities,[44] critical measurements such as blood pressure (BP) are poorly accessible in rural areas, owing in part to lower rates of individual sphygmomanometer ownership for frequent self-monitoring of vital signs: in a survey,[45] the urban/rural difference in BP measurement frequency was statistically significant even after controlling age, gender, marital status, education level, income, and self-rated health. In the United States, although health service utilization for primary care was found to be similar in a recent observational study of IQVIA Medicare claims data,[46] the frequency of specialty care check-ups (eg, eye examination, mammogram) was significantly lower among beneficiaries cared for at rural centers. Potential causes include impaired perception of care needs among patients,[47] lower rates of recommended examinations by rural practitioners, and difficulty in accessing centers for evaluation.[48] Further afield, in Mozambique, a recent study has highlighted geographic differences in the readiness of health care facilities to deliver oxygen therapy to patients in need and identified that northern rural areas critically lacked medical resources.[49]

Additional Sources of Bias in Clinical Model Development, Beyond Biases Related to Medical Devices

The development of clinical models that are unbiased or have limited biases relies heavily on the quality of underlying data collection processes. The examples discussed earlier highlight how health care access, device allocation, and measurement frequency can influence which patients contribute to ICU datasets and the corresponding range of outcomes that algorithms trained on such cohorts can capture. Moreover, the performance and applicability of models to a given population depends on its similarity to those from which policies were initially derived, that is, to training sets.

Challenges related to persisting disparities among patients or health care systems and to the documentation of medical facts affect both the completeness of patient profile characterization and the definition of health outcomes. For example, disease incidence rates vary not only with the health of underlying patient populations but also the type, size, and reputation of hospitals, which are known to affect self-selection based on patient preferences as exemplified by rural hospital bypass.[50] Therefore, rates of acute events (eg, septic shock, ARDS, maternal complications at birth) and prevalence of patients with complex disease phenotypes differ from one hospital to another.[51,52] Beyond differences in patient characteristics, issues tied to disparate access to care and uneven availability of EHR systems by geography or provider type also arise. For instance, the open MIMIC-III dataset including patients cared for at Beth Israel Deaconess Medical Center in Boston comprises 56.6% male patients and only 2.4% Asian patients,[53] whereas male and Asian individuals account for 48.9% and 7.5% of the Massachusetts' population, respectively.[54] Unfortunately, patients from underrepresented minorities or without private insurance do not necessarily equally benefit from the increasing availability of EHR systems at primary care practices.[55,56] Racial differences also appear in the documentation of health status in clinical notes: a recent computational analysis identified significant differences in note style and content between Black and White patients, including a greater use of negative emotional tone and social dominance language in the former group.[57] Although methodological developments to quantify the extent of different types of biases from medical data are ongoing, not all differences in clinical practice and markers of societal bias can be extracted from retrospective data only and require investigation through surveys and qualitative studies.[58,59] The main consequence of patient selection biases for algorithm development and validation is the lack of generalizability in the model testing phase and further once deployed to target populations.

However, efforts are being made to increase the diversity and representability of clinical data and provide more services to underserved populations. For example, the NIH All of Us research program started in 2018 aims to collect data more inclusively, while also providing participants with more information about their health status and genetic or environmental risk factors.[60] In parallel, a growing body of literature focuses on the just deployment of clinical machine learning models. An increasing number of model audits[61] also signal a willingness to address equity and fairness concerns[62] associated with the practical use of prescriptive and predictive algorithms in medicine,[63-65] including in intensive and critical care.[66] Moreover, regulatory interest is growing, with governments aiming to protect patients from harm due to clinical decision-making based on algorithmic outputs.[67,68] Notably, the COVID-19 pandemic accelerated the appeal for remote monitoring through wearables in clinical trials,[69] for chronic disease management,[70,71] after discharge from the hospital or ICU,[72,73] and in everyday life.[74] In resource-limited settings, low-cost wearable equipment could even be a solution to the challenge of monitoring critically ill patients.[75] However, the pandemic has also shed light on potential biases in algorithms of AI systems developed for respiratory diseases and in health care more broadly.[7] mHealth and critical care provide relevant examples. Despite 20% of US adults using a wearable device,[76] their utilization rates are lower among low-income and minority populations, underscoring the need to avert racial and ethnic disparities related to the use of wearable device data in health research.[77] In critical care, a recent case study raised fairness concerns for Black and publicly insured ICU patients; the investigators advocated for the widespread use of comprehensive frameworks to assess the performance of benchmark pipelines built on open datasets such as MIMIC-III.[78] In doing so, multiple evaluation metrics should be considered: a retrospective analysis of ICU severity scores identified systematic differences in calibration across racial and ethnic subgroups despite discrimination being similar.[79] In addition to medical device biases and the lack of patient diversity in study cohorts used for model training, issues that affect the development of clinical ML algorithms also arise from outcome definition challenges. For example, clinical protocols can influence the frequency of laboratory test and arterial blood gas orders,[80,81] thus yielding a differential likelihood of observing physiologic abnormalities. The presence or absence of outcome labels also affects the overall and subpopulation-specific performance of models. Incentives related to billing can result in the under-[82] or overreporting[83-85] of certain diseases, with implications for the personalization of care in acute settings. Social processes also play an important role: in part because dementia and Parkinson disease are associated with significant stigma,[86,87] these illnesses are often undercoded in EHR data.[88,89] Coding patterns matter because treatments provided during a hospitalization or ICU stay will vary with underlying cognitive function[90] or neurologic profile.[91] Even in scenarios where annotations are more systematic, such as in radiology reports, inconsistencies in outcome labels may appear and subsequently affect diagnostics or prognostics, as with chest radiographs.[92] Importantly, the quality of labels affects downstream tasks, such as the auditing of clinical ML models. Indeed, empirical evidence has shown that dysfunctional data annotation processes can distort the results of algorithmic audits.[93]

Critical Corrections

Measurements obtained from the flawed medical devices described earlier are frequently used in AI-based predictive models, which may generate biased outputs and lead to inadequate, delayed, or unfair clinical care. In this section, the authors outline a framework relying on the following 4 principles deemed necessary to safeguard against and reduce the biases highlighted previously: (1) monitoring medical device performance continuously, (2) investigating differences in measurement bias across patient subpopulations along with other sources of disparities, (3) avoiding post-hoc adjustments of clinical model outputs, and (4) encouraging adaptive regulation of medical devices, as biases and their impacts on clinical care are being identified by practitioners and researchers.

CONTINUOUSLY MONITORING MEDICAL DEVICE PERFORMANCE TO MITIGATE POTENTIAL HARM IN CLINICAL PRACTICE

No single research group can be expected to identify all the drivers of health outcomes using retrospective observational data, particularly when facing the limitation of discontinuous and episodic study designs. Instead, the continuous monitoring of medical device performance should be a collaborative process, spanning hospitals, countries, and regulatory agencies internationally. Restricting the investigation of the sources of health disparities to select time periods and locations may provide a skewed perception of patient care. Indeed, both sampling and measurement biases depend on the patterns of access to health care and the availability of well-calibrated medical devices, which vary across medical sites and countries. Moreover, health inequity is a dynamic process: despite certain disparities being long-lasting, new patient populations may become marginalized in the future; further, shocks such as the COVID-19 pandemic may amplify existing disparities. This reality suggests a shift from the retrospective assessment of bias using passively collected EHR data to the continuous (1) evaluation of the performance of medical devices deployed in the ICU, (2) quantification of differences in treatment allocation and long-term patient outcomes associated with device miscalibration, and (3) modification of go-to-market policy requirements by regulatory agencies such as the Food and Drug Administration (FDA) and European Medicines Agency (EMA) accordingly.

Without these steps, medical risk scores and AI-based clinical models for diagnosis or prognosis will neither be fair nor serve those most burdened by disease. Moreover, although seeking model generalizability might be a desirable outcome, careful consideration for underlying differences in health care access, device availability, and sampling frequency among medical sites and countries should take priority. Indeed, unless a deep understanding of interactions between such factors and measurement bias is achieved, clinical guidelines or predictive models cannot be expected to generalize well across patient populations.

ASSESSING THE PERFORMANCE OF MEDICAL DEVICES ACROSS PATIENT SUBPOPULATIONS AND IMPROVING THE REPRESENTATION OF MINORITY SUBGROUPS

Missing data may prevent researchers and practitioners from assessing the performance of medical devices among different patient subpopulations. For instance, in certain countries, the choice of not recording race or ethnicity in a patient's EHR has been deliberate to limit bias based on their sociodemographic factors. However, not recording such personal attributes brings other challenges, for example, providing guarantees or minimum levels of confidence in model predictions for each subgroup. For instance, the underrepresentation of a given racial or ethnic subgroup in a health care system could hurt the performance and generalizability of models built on such data if deployed elsewhere, for example, on a target population that shares little in common with the training cohort. Yet, if the documentation of patient profiles lacks granularity, the root causes of failures in model deployment may be challenging to diagnose. Even in scenarios when sensitive attributes such as race-ethnicity or sex are available in the EHR but removed at training, sociodemographic biases may still manifest because AI-based models can learn features that approximate them. A recent modeling study in medical imaging—for which root-cause analysis was possible thanks to the availability of protected attributes—has shown that AI algorithms could successfully predict a patient's race from chest radiograph images, computed tomography scans, and mammographies.[94]

MOVING AWAY FROM POST-HOC CORRECTIONS

When building predictive models for critical care, methods such as synthetic minority oversampling technique can only partially compensate for imbalanced clinical datasets suffering from the underrepresentation of certain patient profiles.[95] Similarly, statistical techniques to adjust existing scoring systems a-posteriori can only be a temporary solution, as they do not solve the underlying issues of sampling bias or inaccuracies of measurements obtained from miscalibrated medical devices. Considering pulse oximetry as an example, static correction factors for SpO2 measurements relying solely on race-ethnicity would be an imperfect approximation for the role played by skin tone on light absorption. Indeed, they would not account for interactions among device type, skin pigmentation, and clinical factors, such as presenting with jaundice, liver infection, ARDS, or COVID-19,[96] which can all alter traditional associations captured in existing calculation adjustments.

INCREASING POLICY REQUIREMENTS FOR MEDICAL DEVICE DEPLOYMENT IN CLINICAL PRACTICE

Biases may emerge in one or many steps along the AI algorithm development pipeline, from formulating the clinical problem to collecting the data, building the model, and validating and implementing it.[97] Given that the medical devices discussed earlier would be used by every patient admitted to critical care in the United States, the scale for improvement in the quality and fairness of their measurements is significant. In addition, most AI-based algorithms in critical care incorporate one or more commonly measured vital signs, such as oxygen saturation, body temperature, and blood pressure, when not also including laboratory test results and ECG or EEG signals. Taken together, these 2 considerations should prompt increased and adaptive requirements for testing medical devices on diverse populations before their implementation in the clinic as well as improved postmarket surveillance by regulatory agencies such as the FDA and EMA, alongside data mining of disparities through the retrospective analysis of EHR. To unlock such changes, more significant incentives may be needed—beyond policy requirements—for medical device manufacturers to further invest in technical innovations that reduce measurement bias. Since 2010, the FDA has approved 523 new medical devices for commercialization. As novel medical technologies have arisen to assist clinical teams and facilitate diagnosis by physicians, the FDA has adapted existing regulations. In September 2022, the agency has released new guidance stating that some artificial intelligence tools should be regulated as medical devices as part of the agency's oversight of clinical decision support software.[98]

Indicating how well the medical devices perform across different populations before their release on the market could represent an important factor in mitigating bias; this could imply more rigorous selection criteria during the calibration phase to equilibrate the diversity across different populations.

In summary, leveraging artificial intelligence to allow greater personalization of care, for example, through recommendation systems, will require researchers to provide guarantees about the accuracy of model outputs for all patient subgroups, especially those defined with respect to personal attributes. Ideally, individual-level predictions should be derived from models based on data that are sufficiently representative of the patient's profile. However, researchers should invest in parallel in improved model generalizability and techniques for reliable interpolation-extrapolation of output values beyond the case of patient profiles represented in the training datasets.

FOSTERING COLLABORATIONS AMONG INSTITUTIONS AND HEALTH SYSTEMS

In rural Montana, United States, clinicians reported lacking time to conduct critical assessments of their patient's health status, mainly because of a shortage of providers. Despite the growing use of EHR and IT applications to search for and document patient information, fragmented communication reduces the ability of rural health systems to function as seamlessly as those at academic centers.[99] A promising solution to bridge availability of resources and expertise is through long-term partnerships between urban academic centers and rural practices. They typically rely on a combination of telemedicine and care-based learning. Notable examples include Project ECHO, which connects specialists at the University of New Mexico Health Sciences Center with primary care clinicians in underserved areas to deliver complex specialty care in remote parts of the state.[100] Sharing medical supplies and knowledge is not specific to the United States and other high-income countries; this collaborative approach is also used by rural health care providers in LMICs such as Ghana to remediate challenges with quality care delivery.[101]

AMPLIFYING ORGANIZATIONAL AND EDUCATIONAL INVESTMENTS: THE NEED FOR CONTINUED TRAINING AND QUALITY ASSURANCE

A qualitative assessment among rural practitioners in Wisconsin, United States, revealed a strong interest from clinicians in using emerging medical technology and instrumentation but limited time to explore how they function.[102] To be on par with urban academic centers, rural health care institutions should invest in the development of mobile tools, provide recommendations about their use in clinical practice, and facilitate continued education and hands-on training.

Indeed, along with simplified operations, repetitive use is needed for practitioners to become adepts of new medical technologies.[103] Such interventions will be key to prompt organization-level adoption of best practices and ensure a more frequent and comprehensive monitoring of patient health, irrespective of urbanicity levels. A recent study across the 1400 US Health Resources and Services Administration–funded health centers serving vulnerable populations and spanning both urban and rural areas suggests that improvements in quality of care will depend on supporting programs aimed at increasing the availability of providers, training, and provision of technical resources.[104] Across geographies and care settings, medical centers should thus strengthen organizational and educational efforts, rather than solely improving the availability of medical technology.

Alongside the enhanced distribution of medical devices to ensure frequent monitoring of vital signs and laboratory tests, assessments of geographic differences in the setup and use of information technology applications should be conducted more regularly, for example, through surveys,[105] to respond to the needs of nonacademic medical centers and resource-limited regions in a tailored manner. Indeed, a study performed in Georgia over 15 years ago suggested both within-rural differences and variation by medical area (ie, emergency room services, surgical/operating room, laboratory, and radiology). Going forward, provided funding mechanisms are adequately revised,[103] telehealth could allow the quick delivery of care in emergency settings, such as a stroke.[106] A recent study reported a significant increase in telestroke services over the 2008 to 2015 period in the United States.[107] The continued use and optimization of these services could help address persisting urban/rural disparities in stroke-related outcomes. Furthermore, better monitoring as part of preventive medicine and chronic disease management could improve patient' quality of life, while reducing hospital and ICU admissions.

SUMMARY

The management of critically ill patients relies extensively on the data outputs of sophisticated medical technology. However, it is increasingly evident that measurements from devices commonly used in the ICU may not be equally accurate in all patient populations. In addition, physicians and researchers must acknowledge that clinical data do not perfectly reflect physiology but rather physiology exposed to select methods of measurement. Therefore, pulse oximeter readings, estimated temperature values, blood pressure measurements, ECG and EEG signals, as well as other vital signs and laboratory results assessed continuously or periodically should all be interpreted with caution by clinical teams, who best know the medical history and current context of each patient to make appropriate treatment decisions.

Going forward, mitigating sources of bias present in clinical data demands special consideration for greater representation of patients at trial design or model training, continuous monitoring of device performance in clinical practice, and adaptive regulation of medical technology, as inaccuracies are being reported by practitioners and researchers. Together, these principles will help ensure the broader applicability of AI-based algorithms derived from critical care data.

CLINICS CARE POINTS

- Pulse oximeter readings, estimated temperature values, blood pressure measurements, ECG and EEG signals, as well as other vital signs and laboratory results assessed continuously or periodically should all be interpreted with caution by clinical teams given the potential for measurement biases and differences in medical device performance among patient subgroups.

- Interactions between clinicians and data scientists should be facilitated to foster a better understanding of the multiplicity of biases that can affect data collected in the intensive care unit, including measurement biases, insufficient diversity of patient cohorts, and heterogeneity in patient monitoring frequency, healthcare settings, and patient access to healthcare services.

- The quality and representativity of data utilized to develop clinical prediction algorithms should be evaluated closely to limit the risk for artificial intelligence-based models to yield biased outputs, which could in turn lead to inadequate, delayed, or unfair clinical care.

- To mitigate the risk for medical devices or algorithms to perpetuate health disparities, their performances should also be carefully evaluated across diverse patient populations, with an emphasis on increasing the representation of minority subgroups.

ACKNOWLEDGMENTS

L.A. Celi is funded by the National Institute of Health through the NIBIB, United States R01 grant EB017205.

DISCLOSURE

A.I. Wong has equity and management roles at Ataia Medical. A.I. Wong is funded by the Duke Clinical/Translational Science Institute. The rest have nothing to disclose.

REFERENCES

1. Schrödinger E. An undulatory theory of the mechanics of atoms and molecules. Phys Rev 1926;28:1049–70.
2. Schlosshauer M. Decoherence, the measurement problem, and interpretations of quantum mechanics. Rev Mod Phys 2005;76:1267–305.
3. Zurek WH. Quantum darwinism. Nat Phys 2009;5:181–8.
4. Heisenberg W. Physics and philosophy: the revolution in modern science. New York: Harper; 1958.
5. Obermeyer Z, Powers B, Vogeli C, et al. Dissecting racial bias in an algorithm used to manage the health of populations. Science 2019;366:447–53.
6. Wong A, Otles E, Donnelly JP, et al. External validation of a widely implemented proprietary sepsis prediction model in hospitalized patients. JAMA Intern Med 2021;181:1065–70.
7. Delgado J, de Manuel A, Parra I, et al. Bias in algorithms of AI systems developed for COVID-19: a scoping review. J Bioeth Inq 2022;19:407–19.
8. O'Driscoll BR, Howard LS, Earis J, et al. BTS guideline for oxygen use in adults in healthcare and emergency settings. Thorax 2017;72. ii1–ii90.
9. Severinghaus JW, Honda Y. History of blood gas analysis. VII. Pulse oximetry. J Clin Monit 1987;3:135–8.
10. Chan ED, Chan MM, Chan MM. Pulse oximetry: understanding its basic principles facilitates appreciation of its limitations. Respir Med 2013;107:789–99.
11. Neff TA, oximetry Routine. A fifth vital sign? Chest 1988;94:227.
12. Barker SJ, Tremper KK. Pulse oximetry: applications and limitations. Int Anesthesiol Clin 1987;25:155–75.
13. Jubran A. Pulse oximetry. Crit Care 2015;19:272.
14. Wong AI, Charpignon M, Kim H, et al. Analysis of discrepancies between pulse oximetry and arterial oxygen saturation measurements by Race/Ethnicity and association with organ dysfunction and mortality [Internet]. JAMA Netw Open 2021. https://doi.org/10.1001/jamanetworkopen.2021.31674. Available at.
15. Tobin MJ, Jubran A. Inaccuracy of pulse oximetry in darker-skinned patients is unchanged across 32 years [Internet]. Eur Respir J 2022. https://doi.org/10.1183/13993003.00520-2022. 59.
16. Valbuena VSM, Seelye S, Sjoding MW, et al. Racial bias and reproducibility in pulse oximetry among medical and surgical inpatients in general care in the Veterans Health Administration 2013-19: multicenter, retrospective cohort study. BMJ 2022;378:e069775.
17. Gottlieb ER, Ziegler J, Morley K, et al. Assessment of racial and ethnic differences in oxygen supplementation among patients in the intensive care unit [internet]. JAMA Intern Med 2022 [cited 2022 Jul 11] Available at: https://jamanetwork.com/journals/jamainternalmedicine/article-abstract/2794196.

18. Henry NR, Hanson AC, Schulte PJ, et al. Disparities in hypoxemia detection by pulse oximetry across self-identified racial groups and associations with clinical outcomes* [internet]. Crit Care Med 2022;50:204–11.
19. Magesh S, John D, Li WT, et al. Disparities in COVID-19 outcomes by race, ethnicity, and socioeconomic status: a systematic-review and meta-analysis. JAMA Netw Open 2021;4:e2134147.
20. O'Grady NP, Barie PS, Bartlett JG, et al. Guidelines for evaluation of new fever in critically ill adult patients: 2008 update from the American College of Critical Care Medicine and the Infectious Diseases Society of America. Crit Care Med 2008;36:1330–49.
21. Piaggio D, Castaldo R, Cinelli M, et al. A framework for designing medical devices resilient to low-resource settings. Glob Health 2021;17:64.
22. Nantume A, Shah S, Cauvel T, et al. Developing medical technologies for low-resource settings: lessons from a wireless wearable vital signs monitor-neoGuard. Front Digit Health 2021;3:730951.
23. McLaren ZM, Sharp A, Hessburg JP, et al. Cost effectiveness of medical devices to diagnose pre-eclampsia in low-resource settings. Dev Eng 2017;2: 99–106.
24. Bhavani SV, Wiley Z, Verhoef PA, et al. Racial differences in detection of fever using temporal vs oral temperature measurements in hospitalized patients. JAMA 2022;328:885–6.
25. Charlton M, Stanley SA, Whitman Z, et al. The effect of constitutive pigmentation on the measured emissivity of human skin. PLoS One 2020;15:e0241843.
26. Baker FC, Siboza F, Fuller A. Temperature regulation in women: effects of the menstrual cycle. Temperature (Austin) 2020;7:226–62.
27. Brooks EM, Morgan AL, Pierzga JM, et al. Chronic hormone replacement therapy alters thermoregulatory and vasomotor function in postmenopausal women. J Appl Physiol 1997;83:477–84.
28. Berger A. Oscillatory blood pressure monitoring devices. BMJ 2001;323:919.
29. Fonseca-Reyes S, de Alba-García JG, Parra-Carrillo JZ, et al. Effect of standard cuff on blood pressure readings in patients with obese arms. How frequent are arms of a "large circumference". Blood Press Monit 2003;8:101.
30. Yüksel S, Altun-Uğraş G, Altınok N, et al. The effect of cuff size on blood pressure measurement in obese surgical patients: a prospective crossover clinical trial. Florence Nightingale J Nurs 2020;28:205–12.
31. Mishra B, Sinha N, Ur Rehman H. Quantifying variation in blood pressure measurement through different arm cuffs and estimating its impact on diagnosis of hypertension at community level. J Health Res Rev 2017;4:71.
32. Ringrose J, Millay J, Babwick SA, et al. Effect of overcuffing on the accuracy of oscillometric blood pressure measurements. J Am Soc Hypertens 2015;9: 563–8.
33. Cambiaso-Daniel J, Rontoyanni VG, Foncerrada G, et al. Correlation between invasive and noninvasive blood pressure measurements in severely burned children. Burns 2018;44:1787–91.
34. Rodrigues JCL, McIntyre B, Dastidar AG, et al. The effect of obesity on electrocardiographic detection of hypertensive left ventricular hypertrophy: recalibration against cardiac magnetic resonance. J Hum Hypertens 2016;30:197–203.
35. Etienne A, Laroia T, Weigle H, et al. Novel electrodes for reliable EEG recordings on coarse and curly hair [internet]. bioRxiv 2020. 2020.02.26.965202[cited 2022 Nov 3] Available at: https://www.biorxiv.org/content/10.1101/2020.02.26.965202v1.

36. Zimmerman JE, Seneff MG, Sun X, et al. Evaluating laboratory usage in the intensive care unit: patient and institutional characteristics that influence frequency of blood sampling. Crit Care Med 1997;25:737–48.
37. Gershengorn HB, Garland A, Kramer A, et al. Variation of arterial and central venous catheter use in United States intensive care units. Anesthesiology 2014;120:650–64.
38. Gershengorn HB, Wunsch H. Understanding changes in established practice: pulmonary artery catheter use in critically ill patients. Crit Care Med 2013;41: 2667–76.
39. Tambone V, Boudreau D, Ciccozzi M, et al. Ethical criteria for the admission and management of patients in the ICU under conditions of limited medical resources: a shared international proposal in view of the COVID-19 pandemic. Front Public Health 2020;8:284.
40. Wunsch H, Angus DC, Harrison DA, et al. Comparison of medical admissions to intensive care units in the United States and United Kingdom. Am J Respir Crit Care Med 2011;183:1666–73.
41. Lapsley I, Melia K. Clinical actions and financial constraints: the limits to rationing intensive care. Sociol Health Illn 2001;23:729–46.
42. Sauer CM, Dam TA, Celi LA, et al. Systematic review and comparison of publicly available ICU data sets-A decision guide for clinicians and data scientists. Crit Care Med 2022;50:e581–8.
43. Thoral PJ, Fornasa M, de Bruin DP, et al. Explainable machine learning on AmsterdamUMCdb for ICU discharge decision support: uniting intensivists and data scientists. Crit Care Explor 2021;3:e0529.
44. Ni Z, Wu B, Samples C, et al. Mobile technology for health care in rural China. Int J Nurs Sci 2014;1(3):323–4. https://doi.org/10.1016/j.ijnss.2014.07.003. ISSN 2352-0132.
45. Wang Q, Xu L, Sun L, et al. Rural-urban difference in blood pressure measurement frequency among elderly with hypertension: a cross-sectional study in Shandong, China. J Health Popul Nutr 2018;37(1):25. https://doi.org/10.1186/s41043-018-0155-z.
46. Fraze TK, Lewis VA, Wood A, et al. Configuration and delivery of primary care in rural and urban settings. J Gen Intern Med 2022;37(12):3045–53. https://doi.org/10.1007/s11606-022-07472-x.
47. Gimm G, Ipsen C. Examining rural-urban disparities in perceived need for health care services among adults with disabilities. Front Rehabil Sci 2022;3: 875978. https://doi.org/10.3389/fresc.2022.875978.
48. Cyr ME, Etchin AG, Guthrie BJ, et al. Access to specialty healthcare in urban versus rural US populations: a systematic literature review. BMC Health Serv Res 2019;19(1):974. https://doi.org/10.1186/s12913-019-4815-5.
49. Denhard L, Kaviany P, Chicumbe S, et al. How prepared is Mozambique to treat COVID-19 patients? A new approach for estimating oxygen service availability, oxygen treatment capacity, and population access to oxygen-ready treatment facilities. Int J Equity Health 2021;20(1):90. https://doi.org/10.1186/s12939-021-01403-8.
50. Mohr NM, Harland KK, Shane DM, et al. Rural patients with severe sepsis or septic shock who bypass rural hospitals have increased mortality: an instrumental variables approach. Crit Care Med 2017;45(1):85–93. https://doi.org/10.1097/CCM.0000000000002026.
51. Ike JD, Kempker JA, Kramer MR, et al. The association between acute respiratory distress syndrome hospital case volume and mortality in a U.S. Cohort,

2002-2011. Crit Care Med 2018;46(5):764–73. https://doi.org/10.1097/CCM. 0000000000003015.

52. Creanga AA, Bateman BT, Mhyre JM, et al. Performance of racial and ethnic minority-serving hospitals on delivery-related indicators. Am J Obstet Gynecol 2014;211(6). https://doi.org/10.1016/j.ajog.2014.06.006.

53. Dai Z, Liu S, Wu J, et al. Analysis of adult disease characteristics and mortality on MIMIC-III. PLoS One 2020;15(4):e0232176. https://doi.org/10.1371/journal. pone.0232176.

54. Quick facts about Massachusetts. Population estimates as of july 1, 2021, and july 1, 2022. United states census bureau. Available at: https://www.census.gov/ quickfacts/MA.

55. Hing E, Burt CW. Are there patient disparities when electronic health records are adopted? J Health Care Poor Underserved 2009;20(2):473–88. https://doi.org/ 10.1353/hpu.0.0143.

56. Mack D, Zhang S, Douglas M, et al. Disparities in primary care HER adoption rates. J Health Care Poor Underserved 2016;27(1):327–38. https://doi.org/10. 1353/hpu.2016.0016.

57. Penn JA, Newman-Griffis D. Half the picture: word frequencies reveal racial differences in clinical documentation, but not their causes. AMIA Annu Symp Proc 2022;2386–95.

58. Kunitomo K, Harada T, Watari T. Cognitive biases encountered by physicians in the emergency room. BMC Emerg Med 2022;22(1):148. https://doi.org/10.1186/ s12873-022-00708-3.

59. Coen M, Sader J, Junod-Perron N, et al. Clinical reasoning in dire times. Analysis of cognitive biases in clinical cases during the COVID-19 pandemic. Intern Emerg Med 2022;17(4):979–88. https://doi.org/10.1007/s11739-021-02884-9.

60. The all of us research program. Available at: https://allofus.nih.gov/.

61. Boer A, de Beer L, van Praat F. Algorithm Assurance: Auditing Applications of Artificial Intelligence. In: Berghout E, Fijneman R, Hendriks L, de Boer M, Butijn BJ, editors. Advanced Digital Auditing. Progress in IS. Cham: Springer; 2023. https://doi.org/10.1007/978-3-031-11089-4_7.

62. Chen IY, Pierson E, Rose S, et al. Ethical machine learning in healthcare. Annu Rev Biomed Data Sci 2021;4:123–44. https://doi.org/10.1146/annurev-biodatasci-092820-114757.

63. Oala L, Murchison AG, Balachandran P, et al. Machine learning for health: algorithm auditing & quality control. J Med Syst 2021;45(12):105. https://doi.org/10. 1007/s10916-021-01783-y.

64. Liu X, Glocker B, McCradden MM, et al. The medical algorithmic audit [published correction appears in Lancet Digit Health. Lancet Digit Health 2022; 4(5):e384–97. https://doi.org/10.1016/S2589-7500(22)00003-6.

65. Ovalle A, Dev S, Zhao J, et al.: Auditing Algorithmic Fairness in Machine Learning for Health with Severity-Based LOGAN. arXiv preprint arXiv:2211.08742. 2022 Nov 16.

66. van de Sande D, van Bommel J, Fung Fen Chung E, et al. Algorithmic fairness audits in intensive care medicine: artificial intelligence for all? Crit Care 2022;26: 315. https://doi.org/10.1186/s13054-022-04197-5.

67. Goodman KE, Morgan DJ, Hoffmann DE. Clinical Algorithms, Antidiscrimination Laws, and Medical Device Regulation. JAMA 2023;329(4):285–6.

68. Shachar C, Gerke S. Prevention of Bias and Discrimination in Clinical Practice Algorithms. JAMA 2023;329(4):283–4.

69. Turner JR. New FDA guidance on general clinical trial conduct in the era of COVID-19. Ther Innov Regul Sci 2020;54(4):723–4. https://doi.org/10.1007/s43441-020-00160-0.
70. Kamei T, Kanamori T, Yamamoto Y, et al. The use of wearable devices in chronic disease management to enhance adherence and improve telehealth outcomes: a systematic review and meta-analysis. J Telemed Telecare 2022;28(5):342–59. https://doi.org/10.1177/1357633X20937573.
71. Mattison G, Canfell O, Forrester D, et al. The influence of wearables on health care outcomes in chronic disease: systematic review. J Med Internet Res 2022;24(7):e36690. https://doi.org/10.2196/36690.
72. Kroll RR, McKenzie ED, Boyd JG, et al. Use of wearable devices for post-discharge monitoring of ICU patients: a feasibility study. J Intensive Care 2017;5:64. https://doi.org/10.1186/s40560-017-0261-9.
73. Greysen SR, Waddell KJ, Patel MS. Exploring wearables to focus on the "sweet spot" of physical activity and sleep after hospitalization: secondary analysis. JMIR Mhealth Uhealth 2022;10(4):e30089. https://doi.org/10.2196/30089.
74. Eddahchouri Y, Peelen RV, Koeneman M, et al. Effect of continuous wireless vital sign monitoring on unplanned ICU admissions and rapid response team calls: a before-and-after study. Br J Anaesth 2022;128(5):857–63. https://doi.org/10.1016/j.bja.2022.01.036.
75. Van HMT, Hao NV, Phan Nguyen Quoc K, et al. On behalf of the Vietnam ICU Translational Applications Laboratory (VITAL) Investigators.: vital sign monitoring using wearable devices in a Vietnamese intensive care unit. BMJ Innov 2021;7:s7–11.
76. Zinzuwadia A, Singh JP. Wearable devices-addressing bias and inequity. Lancet Digit Health 2022;4(12):e856–7. https://doi.org/10.1016/S2589-7500(22)00194-7. Epub 2022 Nov 2. PMID: 36335031.
77. Colvonen PJ, DeYoung PN, Bosompra NA, et al. Limiting racial disparities and bias for wearable devices in health science research. Sleep 2020;43(10):zsaa159. https://doi.org/10.1093/sleep/zsaa159.
78. Röösli E, Bozkurt S, Hernandez-Boussard T. Peeking into a black box, the fairness and generalizability of a MIMIC-III benchmarking model. Sci Data 2022;9(1):24. https://doi.org/10.1038/s41597-021-01110-7.
79. Sarkar R, Martin C, Mattie H, et al. Performance of intensive care unit severity scoring systems across different ethnicities in the USA: a retrospective observational study. Lancet Digit Health 2021;3(4):e241–9. https://doi.org/10.1016/S2589-7500(21)00022-4.
80. Agniel D, Kohane IS, Weber GM. Biases in electronic health record data due to processes within the healthcare system: retrospective observational study [published correction appears in BMJ. BMJ 2018;363:k4416. https://doi.org/10.1136/bmj.k1479, 2018;361:k1479.
81. Wong AI, Charpignon M, Kim H, et al. Analysis of Discrepancies Between Pulse Oximetry and Arterial Oxygen Saturation Measurements by Race and Ethnicity and Association With Organ Dysfunction and Mortality [published correction appears in JAMA Netw Open. 2022 Feb 1;5(2):e221210]. JAMA Netw Open 2021;4(11):e2131674. https://doi.org/10.1001/jamanetworkopen.2021.31674.
82. Kesselheim AS, Brennan TA. Overbilling vs. downcoding–the battle between physicians and insurers. N Engl J Med 2005;352(9):855–7. https://doi.org/10.1056/NEJMp058011.
83. Bower JK, Patel S, Rudy JE, et al. Addressing bias in electronic health record-based surveillance of cardiovascular disease risk: finding the signal through the

noise. Curr Epidemiol Rep 2017;4(4):346–52. https://doi.org/10.1007/s40471-017-0130-z.

84. Geruso M, Layton T. Upcoding: evidence from Medicare on squishy risk adjustment. J Polit Econ 2020;12(3):984–1026. https://doi.org/10.1086/704756.

85. Rose S. A machine learning framework for plan payment risk adjustment. Health Serv Res 2016;51(6):2358–74. https://doi.org/10.1111/1475-6773.12464.

86. Rosin ER, Blasco D, Pilozzi AR, et al. A narrative review of alzheimer's disease stigma. J Alzheimers Dis 2020;78(2):515–28.

87. Maffoni M, Giardini A, Pierobon A, et al. Stigma experienced by Parkinson's disease patients: a descriptive review of qualitative studies. Parkinsons Dis 2017; 2017:7203259. https://doi.org/10.1155/2017/7203259.

88. Ford E, Rooney P, Oliver S, et al. Identifying undetected dementia in UK primary care patients: a retrospective case-control study comparing machine-learning and standard epidemiological approaches. BMC Med Inform Decis Mak 2019;19(1):248. https://doi.org/10.1186/s12911-019-0991-9.

89. Okubadejo NU, Bower JH, Rocca WA, et al. Parkinson's disease in Africa: a systematic review of epidemiologic and genetic studies. Mov Disord 2006;21(12): 2150–6. https://doi.org/10.1002/mds.21153.

90. Alcorn S, Foo I. Perioperative management of patients with dementia. BJA Education 2017;17(3):94–8. https://doi.org/10.1093/bjaed/mkw038.

91. Freeman WD, Tan KM, Glass GA, et al. ICU management of patients with Parkinson's disease or Parkinsonism. Curr Anaesth Crit Care 2007;18(5–6):227–36. https://doi.org/10.1016/j.cacc.2007.09.007.

92. Oakden-Rayner L, Dunnmon J, Carneiro G, et al. Hidden stratification causes clinically meaningful failures in machine learning for medical imaging. Proc ACM Conf Health Inference Learn 2020;151–9. https://doi.org/10.1145/3368555.3384468, 2020;2020.

93. Mishra A, Gorana Y. Who decides if AI is fair? The labels problem in algorithmic auditing. Data-Centric AI Workshop at the 2021 edition of the NeurIPS conference in Sydney, Australia. https://arxiv.org/pdf/2111.08723.pdf.

94. Gichoya JW, Banerjee I, Bhimireddy AR, et al. AI recognition of patient race in medical imaging: a modelling study. Lancet Digit Health 2022;4:e406–14.

95. Chawla NV, Bowyer KW, Hall LO, et al. SMOTE: synthetic minority over-sampling technique. jair 2002;16:321–57.

96. Nguyen LS, Helias M, Raia L, et al. Impact of COVID-19 on the association between pulse oximetry and arterial oxygenation in patients with acute respiratory distress syndrome. Sci Rep 2022;12:1462.

97. van de Sande D, Van Genderen ME, Smit JM, et al. Developing, implementing and governing artificial intelligence in medicine: a step-by-step approach to prevent an artificial intelligence winter [Internet]. BMJ Health Care Inform 2022;29. https://doi.org/10.1136/bmjhci-2021-100495. Available at:.

98. Available at: https://healthitanalytics.com/news/fda-releases-guidance-on-ai-driven-clinical-decision-support-tools. Last consulted on January 21, 2023.

99. Coombs NC, Campbell DG, Caringi J. A qualitative study of rural healthcare providers' views of social, cultural, and programmatic barriers to healthcare access. BMC Health Serv Res 2022;22:438. https://doi.org/10.1186/s12913-022-07829-2.

100. Arora S, Kalishman S, Dion D, et al. Partnering urban academic medical centers and rural primary care clinicians to provide complex chronic disease care. Health Aff (Millwood) 2011 Jun;30(6):1176–84.

101. Bawontuo V, Adomah-Afari A, Amoah WW, et al. Rural healthcare providers coping with clinical care delivery challenges: lessons from three health centres in Ghana. BMC Fam Pract 2021;22:32. https://doi.org/10.1186/s12875-021-01379-y.

102. Weichelt B, Bendixsen C, Patrick T. A model for assessing necessary conditions for rural health care's mobile health readiness: qualitative assessment of clinician-perceived barriers. JMIR Mhealth Uhealth 2019;7(11):e11915. https://doi.org/10.2196/11915. PMID: 31702564; PMCID: PMC6874803.

103. Zachrison KS, Richard JV, Mehrotra A. Paying for telemedicine in smaller rural hospitals: extending the technology to those who benefit most. JAMA Health Forum 2021;2(8):e211570.

104. Pourat N, Chen X, Lu C, et al. Assessing clinical quality performance and staffing capacity differences between urban and rural Health Resources and Services Administration-funded health centers in the United States: a cross sectional study. PLoS One 2020 Dec 8;15(12):e0242844.

105. Culler SD, Atherly A, Walczak S, et al. Urban-rural differences in the availability of hospital information technology applications: a survey of Georgia hospitals. J Rural Health 2006;22(3):242–7.

106. Available at: https://www.cdc.gov/chronicdisease/resources/publications/factsheets/telehealth-in-rural-communities.htm. Last consulted on January 21, 2023.

107. Zhang D, Wang G, Zhu W, et al. Expansion of telestroke services improves quality of care provided in super rural areas. Health Aff (Millwood) 2018;37(12):2005–13.

UNITED STATES POSTAL SERVICE ®

Statement of Ownership, Management, and Circulation
(All Periodicals Publications Except Requester Publications)

1. Publication Title	2. Publication Number	3. Filing Date
CRITICAL CARE CLINICS	000 – 708	9/18/2023

4. Issue Frequency	5. Number of Issues Published Annually	6. Annual Subscription Price
JAN, APR, JUL, OCT	4	$274

7. Complete Mailing Address of Known Office of Publication (Not printer) (Street, city, county, state, and ZIP+4®)

ELSEVIER INC.
230 Park Avenue, Suite 800
New York, NY 10169

Contact Person
Malathi Samayan

Telephone (Include area code)
91-44-4299-4507

8. Complete Mailing Address of Headquarters or General Business Office of Publisher (Not printer)

ELSEVIER INC.
230 Park Avenue, Suite 800
New York, NY 10169

9. Full Names and Complete Mailing Addresses of Publisher, Editor, and Managing Editor (Do not leave blank)

Publisher (Name and complete mailing address)

Dolores Meloni, ELSEVIER INC.
1600 JOHN F KENNEDY BLVD. SUITE 1600
PHILADELPHIA, PA 19103-2899

Editor (Name and complete mailing address)

Joanna Collett, ELSEVIER INC.
1600 JOHN F KENNEDY BLVD. SUITE 1600
PHILADELPHIA, PA 19103-2899

Managing Editor (Name and complete mailing address)

PATRICK MANLEY, ELSEVIER INC.
1600 JOHN F KENNEDY BLVD. SUITE 1600
PHILADELPHIA, PA 19103-2899

10. Owner (Do not leave blank. If the publication is owned by a corporation, give the name and address of the corporation immediately followed by the names and addresses of all stockholders owning or holding 1 percent or more of the total amount of stock. If not owned by a corporation, give the names and addresses of the individual owners. If owned by a partnership or other unincorporated firm, give its name and address as well as those of each individual owner. If the publication is published by a nonprofit organization, give its name and address.)

Full Name	Complete Mailing Address
WHOLLY OWNED SUBSIDIARY OF REED/ELSEVIER, US HOLDINGS	1600 JOHN F KENNEDY BLVD. SUITE 1600 PHILADELPHIA, PA 19103-2899

11. Known Bondholders, Mortgagees, and Other Security Holders Owning or Holding 1 Percent or More of Total Amount of Bonds, Mortgages, or Other Securities. If none, check box ► ☐ None

Full Name	Complete Mailing Address
N/A	

12. Tax Status (For completion by nonprofit organizations authorized to mail at nonprofit rates) (Check one)
The purpose, function, and nonprofit status of this organization and the exempt status for federal income tax purposes:
☒ Has Not Changed During Preceding 12 Months
☐ Has Changed During Preceding 12 Months (Publisher must submit explanation of change with this statement)

PS Form **3526**, July 2014 [Page 1 of 4 (see instructions page 4)] PSN 7530-01-000-9931 PRIVACY NOTICE: See our privacy policy on www.usps.com

---

13. Publication Title	14. Issue Date for Circulation Data Below
CRITICAL CARE CLINICS	JULY 2023

15. Extent and Nature of Circulation		Average No. Copies Each Issue During Preceding 12 Months	No. Copies of Single Issue Published Nearest to Filing Date
a. Total Number of Copies (Net press run)		221	142
b. Paid Circulation (By Mail and Outside the Mail)	(1) Mailed Outside-County Paid Subscriptions Stated on PS Form 3541 (Include paid distribution above nominal rate, advertiser's proof copies, and exchange copies)	142	111
	(2) Mailed In-County Paid Subscriptions Stated on PS Form 3541 (Include paid distribution above nominal rate, advertiser's proof copies, and exchange copies)	0	0
	(3) Paid Distribution Outside the Mails Including Sales Through Dealers and Carriers, Street Vendors, Counter Sales, and Other Paid Distribution Outside USPS®	63	54
	(4) Paid Distribution by Other Classes of Mail Through the USPS (e.g., First-Class Mail®)	8	0
c. Total Paid Distribution (Sum of 15b (1), (2), (3), and (4))	►	213	165
d. Free or Nominal Rate Distribution (By Mail and Outside the Mail)	(1) Free or Nominal Rate Outside-County Copies Included on PS Form 3541	7	6
	(2) Free or Nominal Rate In-County Copies Included on PS Form 3541	0	0
	(3) Free or Nominal Rate Copies Mailed at Other Classes Through the USPS (e.g., First-Class Mail)	0	0
	(4) Free or Nominal Rate Distribution Outside the Mail (Carriers or other means)	1	1
e. Total Free or Nominal Rate Distribution (Sum of 15d (1), (2), (3) and (4))	►	8	7
f. Total Distribution (Sum of 15c and 15e)	►	221	172
g. Copies not Distributed (See Instructions to Publishers #4 (page #3))	►	0	0
h. Total (Sum of 15f and g)	►	221	172
i. Percent Paid (15c divided by 15f times 100)	►	96.38%	95.93%

* If you are claiming electronic copies, go to line 16 on page 3. If you are not claiming electronic copies, skip to line 17 on page 3.

PS Form **3526**, July 2014 (Page 2 of 4)

16. Electronic Copy Circulation		Average No. Copies Each Issue During Preceding 12 Months	No. Copies of Single Issue Published Nearest to Filing Date
a. Paid Electronic Copies	►		
b. Total Paid Print Copies (Line 15c) + Paid Electronic Copies (Line 16a)	►		
c. Total Print Distribution (Line 15f) + Paid Electronic Copies (Line 16a)	►		
d. Percent Paid (Both Print & Electronic Copies) (16b divided by 16c × 100)	►		

☒ I certify that 50% of all my distributed copies (electronic and print) are paid above a nominal price.

17. Publication of Statement of Ownership

☒ If the publication is a general publication, publication of this statement is required. Will be printed ☐ Publication not required.

in the OCTOBER 2023 issue of this publication.

18. Signature and Title of Editor, Publisher, Business Manager, or Owner

Malathi Samayan - Distribution Controller *Malathi Samayan* Date 9/18/2023

I certify that all information furnished on this form is true and complete. I understand that anyone who furnishes false or misleading information on this form or who omits material or information requested on the form may be subject to criminal sanctions (including fines and imprisonment) and/or civil sanctions (including civil penalties).

PS Form **3526**, July 2014 (Page 3 of 4) PRIVACY NOTICE: See our privacy policy on www.usps.com

Moving?

Make sure your subscription moves with you!

To notify us of your new address, find your **Clinics Account Number** (located on your mailing label above your name), and contact customer service at:

Email: journalscustomerservice-usa@elsevier.com

800-654-2452 (subscribers in the U.S. & Canada)
314-447-8871 (subscribers outside of the U.S. & Canada)

Fax number: 314-447-8029

Elsevier Health Sciences Division
Subscription Customer Service
3251 Riverport Lane
Maryland Heights, MO 63043

*To ensure uninterrupted delivery of your subscription, please notify us at least 4 weeks in advance of move.

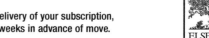

9780443181931